CLEFT PALATE

To Dr. Eugene T. McDonald, creative clinician and skillful scholar, whose innovative and outstanding contributions to the study and treatment of the speech and language disorders of individuals with cleft palate provides the foundation for contemporary approaches to this disorder.

Cover portrait of Eugene T. McDonald by
John Wilson of Austin, Texas.

FOR CLINICIANS BY CLINICIANS
Harris Winitz, Series Editor

This book, *Cleft Palate: Interdisciplinary Issues and Treatment,* is the seventh volume in the For Clinicians by Clinicians series of texts on the diagnosis and clinical management of speech, language, and voice disorders. Each text provides a contemporary perspective on one major disorder or clinical area and is designed for use in clinical methodology courses and continuing education programs. Authors have been selected who represent a broad spectrum of clinical interests and theoretical positions and who hold the common belief that their viewpoints, experiences, and successes should be shared in order to provide a forum for clinicians by clinicians.

Volumes already published in this series are *Treating Language Disorders, Treating Articulation Disorders, Case Studies in Aphasia Rehabilitation, Treating Cerebral Palsy, Alaryngeal Speech Rehabilitation,* and *Treating Disordered Speech Motor Control.*

CLEFT PALATE: INTERDISCIPLINARY ISSUES AND TREATMENT

For Clinicians by Clinicians

Edited by
Karlind T. Moller and
Clark D. Starr

pro·ed
8700 Shoal Creek Boulevard
Austin, Texas 78757

Printed in the United States of America

Library of Congress Cataloging-in-Publication Data

Cleft palate : interdisciplinary issues and treatment / edited by
  Karlind T. Moller and Clark D. Starr.
     p.   cm. — (For clinicians by clinicians)
  Includes bibliographical references and index.
  ISBN 0-89079-567-3
  1. Cleft palate. 2. Cleft lip. 3. Cleft palate children—
Rehabilitation. I. Moller, Karlind T. II. Starr, Clark D.
III. Series.
  [DNLM: 1. Cleft Lip. 2. Cleft Palate. WV 440 C6238]
RD525.C54 1992
617.5′225—dc20
DNLM/DLC
for Library of Congress   92-12022
                                                      CIP

pro·ed
8700 Shoal Creek Boulevard
Austin, Texas 78757

2 3 4 5 6 7 8 9 10   97 96 95 94 93

Contents

Contributors vii

Preface. ix

CHAPTER 1
Interdisciplinary Team Approach: Issues and Procedures 1
   Karlind T. Moller

CHAPTER 2
Development and Genetic Aspects of Cleft Lip and Palate 25
   Robert J. Gorlin

CHAPTER 3
Surgical Issues and Procedures 49
   Alan R. Shons

CHAPTER 4
Oral and Maxillofacial Surgery and the
Management of Cleft Lip and Palate. 79
   Mohamed El Deeb, Daniel E. Waite, and John Curran

CHAPTER 5
Orthodontic Diagnosis and Treatment Procedures 121
   Richard R. Bevis

CHAPTER 6
Prosthodontic Management of Maxillofacial and
Palatal Defects 145
   Herbert A. Leeper, Jr., Paul S. Sills, and David H. Charles

CHAPTER 7
Otologic and Audiologic Concerns and Treatment 189
   Rolf F. Ulvestad and Jane E. Carlstrom

CHAPTER 8
Early Phonological Development and the Child
with Cleft Palate 219
   Patricia A. Broen and Karlind T. Moller

CHAPTER 9
Evaluation of Velopharyngeal Function 251
    Jerald B. Moon

CHAPTER 10
Articulation Assessment Procedures and Treatment Decisions   307
    Judith E. Trost-Cardamone and John E. Bernthal

CHAPTER 11
Behavioral Approaches to Treating Velopharyngeal
Closure and Nasality 337
    Clark D. Starr

CHAPTER 12
Psychological Characteristics Associated with Cleft Palate 357
    Lynn C. Richman and Michele J. Eliason

Author Index 381

Subject Index 391

Contributors

John E. Bernthal, PhD
Department of Special Education
  and Communication Disorders
University of Nebraska–Lincoln
Barkley Memorial Center
Lincoln, NE 68583

Richard R. Bevis, DDS, PhD
Division of Orthodontics
Department of Diagnostic and
  Surgical Sciences
School of Dentistry
University of Minnesota
Minneapolis, MN 55455

Patricia A. Broen, PhD
Department of Communications
  Disorders
University of Minnesota
Minneapolis, MN 55455

Jane E. Carlstrom, MA
Department of Communication
  Disorders
University of Minnesota
Minneapolis, MN 55455

David H. Charles, DDS
Division of Removable
  Prosthodontics
Faculty of Dentistry
University of Western Ontario
and Oral Facial Rehabilitation Unit
University Hospital
London, Ontario, Canada N6G 1H1

John Curran, DDS, FDSRCS
Department of Oral and
  Maxillofacial Surgery
University of Manitoba
Winnipeg, Manitoba, Canada
  R3C 0C8

Mohamed El Deeb, BDS, MS
Division of Oral and Maxillofacial
  Surgery
Department of Diagnostic and
  Surgical Sciences
School of Dentistry
University of Minnesota
Minneapolis, MN 55455

Michele J. Eliason, PhD
College of Nursing
University of Iowa
Iowa City, IA 52242

Robert J. Gorlin, DDS, MS
Division of Oral Pathology and
  Genetics
Department of Oral Sciences
School of Dentistry
University of Minnesota
Minneapolis, MN 55455

Herbert A. Leeper, Jr., PhD
Department of Communicative
  Disorders
Faculty of Applied Health Sciences
University of Western Ontario
and Oral Facial Rehabilitation Unit
University Hospital
London, Ontario, Canada N6G 1H1

Karlind T. Moller, PhD
Cleft Palate Maxillofacial and
  Craniofacial Clinics
Division of Pediatric Dentistry
Department of Preventive Sciences
School of Dentistry
University of Minnesota
Minneapolis, MN 55455

Jerald B. Moon, PhD
Department of Speech Pathology
  and Audiology
University of Iowa
Iowa City, IA 52242

Lynn C. Richman, PhD
Department of Pediatrics
University Hospital
University of Iowa
Iowa City, IA 52242

Alan R. Shons, MD, PhD
Division of Plastic and
  Reconstructive Surgery
Case Western Reserve University
Cleveland, OH 44106

Paul S. Sills, DDS
Division of Removable
  Prosthodontics
Faculty of Dentistry
University of Western Ontario
and Oral Facial Rehabilitation Unit
University Hospital
London, Ontario, Canada N6G 1H1

Clark D. Starr, PhD
Department of Communication
  Disorders
University of Minnesota
Minneapolis, MN 55455

Judith E. Trost-Cardamone, PhD
Department of Communicative
  Disorders
California State University–
  Northridge
Northridge, CA 91330

Rolf F. Ulvestad, MD
Cleft Palate Maxillofacial Clinic
School of Dentistry
University of Minnesota
Minneapolis, MN 55455

Daniel E. Waite, DDS, MS
Department of Oral and
  Maxillofacial Surgery
Baylor College of Dentistry
Dallas, TX 75246

Preface

Some years ago, Harris Winitz approached us to consider developing a text for clinicians, by clinicians, in the area of cleft lip and palate. Collectively, we have had a strong clinical interest in persons with cleft palate for almost 70 years. *Sustaining* interest for this long has not been difficult. In many ways, cleft lip and palate is one of the most rewarding disorders with which to be involved. Clearly, it is an area where we, as speech and language pathologists, have much to offer and, in many instances, what we say has a significant impact on what happens to our patients—they may or may not have surgery based on our evaluation of what they can or cannot do with their present speech mechanisms. We have come to appreciate the true value of working with other medical and dental specialists focusing on a common goal. That goal is a successful outcome—acceptable appearance, dental–facial form and function, communicative ability, and psychosocial skills.

Clinical outcome is something all of us will be hearing much more about as we approach the 21st century. We firmly believe that successful and, indeed, optimal outcome for persons with cleft lip and palate is highly dependent upon the interdisciplinary approach. That is what this book is all about.

Although the primary readership of this book is anticipated to be speech–language pathologists and audiologists, we believe that medical, dental, and other specialists involved in cleft palate management will benefit because of the interdisciplinary nature of the disorder. Additionally, speech–language pathologists should be well informed and knowledgeable, not only about their own discipline as it applies to cleft lip and palate management, but about other professionals who work with them in interdisciplinary diagnosis and treatment planning. For an interdisciplinary team to be successful, there needs to be a mutual respect among team members and for their specialty areas, with a good understanding of what each can and cannot do. The following chapters are written by professionals trained in their specialties so that the readers can appreciate the nature of their training and the issues and procedures involved in cleft palate management. Indeed, we requested the authors of several chapters to specify the training required for their specialties. Although this is a clinical text, we are persuaded that what we do well clinically is grounded in research. Therefore, this book is intended to be a strong research reference to explore in depth what we currently know, what investigative procedures and results have led to our knowledge base, and what we still need to accomplish. Although much of the content of this text could be variously applied to other craniofacial disorders, the clear focus is cleft lip and palate. It is assumed that readers of this text have some knowledge of the anatomy and physiology of the speech and hearing mechanism.

It is not possible to thank all of the people who have influenced and contributed to this venture. We certainly thank Harris Winitz, who first approached us too many years ago. Then it was our responsibility to contact persons in the various disciplines to share their expertise and perspective on cleft lip and palate management. We believe that we have obtained highly skilled clinicians with the appreciation for research methodology, and we thank them for their contributions. In an edited text with multiple authorship, it is difficult to blend all of the pieces (chapters) masterfully; however, the common thread in the fabric is the patient with cleft lip and palate. To those patients and their families, we thank you for all you have taught us. And this book is certainly dedicated to people like Eugene T. McDonald, who not only saw the wisdom of interdisciplinary care, but who, by their example, helped many to see.

Importantly, for the sharing of our time and for understanding that we were doing something worthwhile, we sincerely thank our own families. Their encouragement and gentle, but sometimes firm prodding got the job done.

CHAPTER 1

Interdisciplinary Team Approach: Issues and Procedures

Karlind T. Moller

Moller clearly advocates for interdisciplinary care for persons with cleft lip and cleft palate because this disorder affects appearance, dental function, and speech and hearing. He reviews how and why teams were first formed, as well as contemporary structure and function. Issues relating to the value and quality of team function and their future importance are also discussed.

1. *Moller states that knowledge of the cleft at birth allows for several assumptions regarding management. What are these assumptions and why is it important for parents/caregivers to know about them early?*
2. *Define an interdisciplinary team. Distinguish between multidisciplinary and interdisciplinary teams.*
3. *What factors were influential in the early formation of interdisciplinary teams, and what was the caveat about specialization at that time?*
4. *What does Moller mean by the "desirable" team as opposed to the "core" team?*
5. *Moller lists several functions of organized teams. Discuss one and defend its importance as it relates to other team functions.*
6. *For the interdisciplinary team approach to continue to be successful, will teams need to be "different" in the future?*

The following excerpt from the preamble of the constitution of the American Cleft Palate–Craniofacial Association (1990) points out the range of concerns and the potential impact on the quality of life for persons with cleft palate:

> we wish to encourage by every appropriate method and device the improvement of scientific clinical services to persons suffering from cleft palate and associated deformities in order that they may achieve a more adequate physical, emotional, social, educational, and vocational adjustment. (p. xiii)

The constitution also includes a mission statement: "to foster communication and cooperation among professionals from all disciplines interested in craniofacial anomalies" (p. xiii). These statements clearly suggest that the concerns and problems in persons with cleft lip and palate are multidimensional, and that treatment requires multidisciplinary attention.

It is not uncommon for a person with a cleft palate, in the growing years, to be evaluated and/or treated by as many as 10 medical, dental, and other specialists. Periodic evaluations and treatment by these specialists will take many years and require family resources of time, energy, and finances. That is the difficult news; the good news is that cleft lip and palate is a very treatable condition. With the cooperative efforts of the patient and family and several medical, dental, speech, hearing, and psychosocial specialists, acceptable appearance, communication, social skills, and oral function are very realistic. However, successful treatment does not merely happen. This chapter focuses on the approach I believe has the best chance of ensuring success—the interdisciplinary approach. First, however, I consider some aspects of the nature of clefting and the assumptions, biases, and definitions pertaining to interdisciplinary care.

NATURE OF CLEFTING AND ASSUMPTIONS ABOUT TREATMENT

Cleft lip and palate is one of the most frequent congenital anomalies. The incidence of clefting of some kind in the caucasian population is approximately 1 in 600 births; it is higher in the oriental groups and lower in the black groups.

Not all clefts are alike. Clefts can involve only the lip and alveolar ridge (primary palate), only the hard and soft palate (secondary palate), or both the primary and secondary palates. Clefts involving the primary palate, the secondary palate, or both vary in severity. Clefts of the lip may not extend to the floor of the nostril, may not involve all of the primary palate or secondary palate, and may occur on one or both sides.

Some clefts, such as submucous cleft palate, are difficult to detect. Considering the heterogeneous nature of clefting, treatment needs to be planned in accordance with the specific problems and needs of each patient. More specific information on the developmental aspects and types of clefts is included in Chapter 2. Because cleft lip and palate can be seen, felt, and heard (Lis, Pruzansky, Koepp-Baker, & Kobes, 1956), it is a somewhat unique disorder. It is, or should be for the most part, identifiable at birth. If a cleft lip and palate is detected at birth, several assumptions can be made relative to management. There will be concerns—not necessarily problems—with appearance, dental and jaw relationships, speech and hearing, and the potential these have to affect psychosocial adjustment.

Care of cleft lip and palate will be long term. Treatment will begin immediately after birth and may extend into late adolescence before completion of the final treatment. The medical disciplines such as pediatrics, reconstructive surgery, and otolaryngology (ear, nose, and throat) are most typically involved from a very early age; however, information and counseling services from genetics, psychology, social work, speech, audiology, preventive dentistry, and others, are also appropriate and encouraged. As the child grows and matures physically and behaviorally, treatment priorities may shift among specialists, but each discipline contributes throughout the growing years.

Appropriate treatment for any child with cleft lip or palate must be closely aligned with physical and behavioral growth and development. State-of-the-art knowledge dictates times when certain treatment is most appropriate and times when it is not. For example, speech development and proficiency (behavior aspects), as well as facial growth and development (physical aspects), directly influence the timing of certain physical management procedures.

The patient and the family/caretakers need to be well informed and actively involved in the treatment program. The patient and the family must make the ultimate decision whether to proceed with treatment. Patients and families who have not been well informed, are misinformed, or do not understand the rationale for certain treatments tend to be less actively involved in and less compliant with treatment recommendations. The effect is compromised outcome.

The foregoing may lead the reader to believe that optimal cleft palate management is rather painstaking, arduous, and perhaps does not occur very often. Quite the contrary! However, professionals and parents/caregivers need to recognize and accept these assumptions and have a good understanding of the disorder. When the treatment is well planned and coordinated, with each phase of treatment correlated with growth and development, persons with cleft lip and palate are likely to achieve their physical, educational, social, and vocational potentials.

THE INTERDISCIPLINARY APPROACH—BIASES AND DEFINITIONS

Clinicians need to accept that cleft lip and palate is a multifaceted, complex disorder requiring several specialty areas for optimal treatment, and that an approach, or system, is necessary to achieve the best possible outcome. Various specialists involved with cleft palate habilitation have stated that no one person has the expertise to address the range of concerns for persons with cleft palate. The contributors to this book share the strong bias with many other specialists that the interdisciplinary team approach is the best, most effective, and most efficient way to achieve optimal outcome, appearance, dental form and function, and communication and social skills.

Various authors have both espoused the benefits and recognized the potential problems of the interdisciplinary approach in cleft lip and palate management (Bleiberg & Leubling, 1971; Cooper, 1953; Koepp-Baker, 1963, 1979; Krogman, 1979; McWilliams, Morris, & Shelton, 1990; Morris, 1980; Nackashi & Dixon-Wood, 1989; Ross & Johnston, 1978; Spriestersbach & Sherman, 1968; Wells, 1971). All concluded that the cooperative and integrative efforts of several specialists, over many years, is the best way to achieve the optimal result. Dynamics of team activities and characteristics that contribute to positive and negative team function are discussed later in this chapter.

Many adjectives have been used in conjunction with teams: interdisciplinary, multidisciplinary, intradisciplinary, interprofessional, intraprofessional, transprofessional, and transdisciplinary. Although specialists can argue about terminology differences and preferences, the professions involved in cleft palate management are clearly between (inter-) and not within (intra-) disciplinary boundaries. Just as clear is the fact that several disciplines are required. Therefore, multidisciplinary team or interdisciplinary team would appear the most appropriate terminology. Nevertheless, the involvement of several specialists does not necessarily ensure optimal team function. Koepp-Baker (1979) distinguished between multidisciplinary teams and interdisciplinary teams:

> we have come to regard the word multidisciplinary as reflecting the quality of immaturity. The proper adjective describing the mature and effective team, as we conceive it, is interdisciplinary. It better suggests the attributes of the interpersonal and interprofessional intervention that distinguishes this form of human enterprise. (p. 61)

Because the treatments required for the patient are highly interrelated, that element of person-to-person interaction is necessary if the team concept is to be worthwhile and productive and to yield optimal outcome.

Therefore, we consider interdisciplinary to be the most appropriate term, and it will be used in this text.

Writers addressing interdisciplinary care in general (Ducanis & Golin, 1979; Valletutti & Christoplos, 1977) also stress that a team is not merely a collection of people and input, but is a system to make collaboration effective in best meeting the needs of the patient. Team care is the antithesis of fragmented care. The team needs to operate as one unit with the specified goal of providing the best care for the patient. Indeed, the effective team cannot deviate from being totally patient centered. Ducanis and Golin (1979) provided the following definition of any interdisciplinary team: "a functioning unit composed of individuals with varied and specialized training, who coordinate activities to provide services to a client or group of clients" (p. 3).

Herbert Cooper (1979), an orthodontist and early proponent of interdisciplinary care for persons with cleft lip and palate, commented on the importance of team effort with patient focus:

> individualism and initiative are to be respected, but a team can succeed only with smooth cooperation by men and women who, while feeling free and independent, are willing to do what is expected of them without friction. They must be motivated to act in the greatest interest of the patient, and in my opinion, the only way to make this philosophy work is to follow the three "C's"—communication, cooperation, and coordination of effort. (p. 9)

Morris (1980) defined the interdisciplinary team by the function performed: "to bring to bear, on the problem-solving process, for the patient, the expertise of relevant science, basic and clinical in an effective and efficient and practical manner" (p. 106).

Many words can describe what an effective team is supposed to do: communicate, discuss, collaborate, integrate, synthesize, recommend, coordinate, prioritize, cooperate, follow up, and surely many more. All of these tasks are a part of interdisciplinary function; however, not all teams do equally well with all activities. Better functioning and more mature and effective teams may perform more of these tasks successfully. Assembling a certain number of people into a team for some purpose initially may allow for discussion and some level of communication, but certainly does not ensure coordination, cooperation, or integration. Valletutti and Christoplos (1977), in discussing interdisciplinary approaches to human services, pointed out that communication is prerequisite to cooperation. They stated,

> Sharing interdisciplinary information is an initial step toward providing a mechanism through which the collective wisdom of individual team members may be marshalled for the purpose of arriving at the most logical,

productive, efficient means to remediate the difficulties that clients experience. (p. 1)

Interdisciplinary management for persons with cleft palate requires a cooperative effort to effectively identify the concerns; recommend, prioritize, and coordinate the treatment plan; and follow up on treatment objectives. Clearly, the range of concerns that exist for a patient with cleft lip and palate are best addressed by the interdisciplinary approach.

DEVELOPMENT AND HISTORY OF TEAMS

The advent of health care teams as we know them today dates back to the 1920s. Around that time, there was considerable interest in medical specialization and much discussion of the potential dangers of specialization if findings were not satisfactorily coordinated (Barker, 1922).

According to Ducanis and Golin (1979), establishment of teams was influenced by three major factors: (a) importance of treating the "whole" client, (b) needs of the organization, and (c) external mandates. Participants in the White House Conference of 1930 espoused the philosophy that treatment of patients must include the whole person and not an isolated part. At the same time, with the increasing trend toward medical and dental specialization, specialty consultations and interdisciplinary coordination of effort became necessary within organizations rather than fragmented care. The interdisciplinary team offered a way of organizing personnel to enhance communication and exchange of information concerning clients or patients. In more recent years, external mandates by third-party payers, governmental agencies, and others, have demanded professional accountability and improvement in the quality of care. Currently, the team concept is applied to many health disorders, as well as educational, vocational, and social programs.

Health care teams have long been a part of rehabilitation services. Whitehouse (1951), a rehabilitative specialist, emphasized the importance of treating the whole person and the importance of teamwork: "Fundamentally, no treatment is medical, social, psychological, vocational—all treatment is total" (p. 45). The team concept for diagnosis and treatment of patients with cleft lip and palate, which became visible in the 1930s, was likely influenced by similar factors. The first functioning cleft palate team was reported to be in the shared office of James Maby, a maxillofacial surgeon, and Albert MacDougal, an orthodontist (R. Kersten, personal communication, 1970).

Cooper, the orthodontist mentioned previously, was a leader in advocating the team concept for patients with cleft lip and palate. In 1938, he established the first cleft palate clinic devoted to interdisciplinary diagnosis and treatment in Lancaster, Pennsylvania. Cooper, who lobbied for federal support for these patients for several years, pointed out (1953, 1979) that although the National Society for Crippled Children and Adults was established in 1919, this society did not consider patients with cleft lip and palate to be eligible for their services. Eligibility was primarily for patients with orthopedic problems. Cooper spoke convincingly for considering patients with cleft palate as "facially crippled." As a result of Cooper's work, most states today provide services and financial assistance for cleft lip and palate from what was formerly called Crippled Children's Services and administered federally through the Maternal and Child Health Program.

The interdisciplinary approach for persons with cleft palate became more prevalent yearly, and in 1943, the Academy of Cleft Palate Prosthesis was established. This academy was the beginning of what is now the American Cleft Palate–Craniofacial Association. A significant factor in the emergence and subsequent growth of interdisciplinary cleft palate teams may have been the increasing interest and recognition of the effect of surgical procedures on facial and dental growth and development. This interconnectedness of surgical repair, physical growth and development, and speech function made cleft lip and palate a natural for the team approach. Wells (1971) discussed the success of the interdisciplinary approach and rightly pointed out the abundance of interdisciplinary activity related to cleft palate in publications, conferences, and professional organizations over the years. The interested reader is referred to a history of the first 36 years of the interdisciplinary American Cleft Palate Association (Wells, 1979).

In summary, it appears that the interdisciplinary team concept is alive and very well. Over 200 teams are listed in the 1990 American Cleft Palate–Craniofacial Association Directory. Requirements for being listed as a team include having a minimum of a plastic surgeon, dentist, and speech pathologist on the team; holding regular team meetings; and membership in the association of at least one team member.

STRUCTURE AND FUNCTION OF INTERDISCIPLINARY TEAMS

Structure

The structure of teams and the manner in which they organize themselves vary considerably. Decisions regarding who serves, who leads, and what format the operation and procedures should take depend in large part on the team's primary function and the physical setting in which it operates. The optimal setting for team activities and meetings appears to be based on the diagnostic and treatment needs of the patient population served. For persons with cleft lip and palate and other cranio-facial anomalies, that setting would be a medical or dental facility. In certain geographic areas, however, this is not possible, and teams need to meet in less optimal facilities.

Morris (1980) listed several factors that determine any health team's structure: an identifiable common objective, a workable administrative system, a basis for regular team activities, and an atmosphere of respect among members and for the system. Cooper (1979) emphasized that the varying structures of teams depend on goals and function. He stated,

> there is the "vertical" team in which the decisions and the instructions originate at the top, with one person; the other members merely carry out their assigned duties. This works well on the football field where the goal is a straight white line. In a clinic addressing itself to the complex shifting ramifications of cleft lip and palate, however, it is our experience that a more even distribution of input, a wider sharing of ideas and opinions, among team members, achieves a better result. (p. 9)

Although a team may assume a variety of organizational configu-rations, the focus on cleft lip and palate and other craniofacial anoma-lies requires information and opinions from several specialty areas and a sharing and discussion of that information to contribute to the optimal treatment for the patient. Ultimately, the contribution of the team approach to patient management must be greater or better than the sum of its parts.

Team composition. Recognition as a team by the American Cleft Palate–Craniofacial Association requires that at least a reconstructive surgeon, dentist, and speech pathologist meet on a regular basis. Although there is reasonable justification for these professionals to con-stitute a "core" team, including representatives of several other dis-ciplines would create a "desirable" team. What is desirable in terms of size and representation depends upon the constellation of concerns of the particular clinical disorder or population. With cleft lip and palate, there is usually a medical component, which may consist of reconstruc-tive surgery, otolaryngology, pediatrics, nursing, and radiology; a dental component, comprising orthodontics, pediatric or family dentistry, pros-thodontics, oral surgery, and dental hygiene; a speech and hearing com-ponent, consisting of speech and language pathology and audiology; a psychosocial component, consisting of psychology and social work; and a genetic component. This composition has remained quite stable over time. Although not all specialists in each component may be represented at all visits or with every patient, each component is usually represented or readily available for most teams. Team representation would be simi-lar for patients with disorders involving craniofacial structures, but with the addition of at least neurosurgery and ophthalmology.

All teams need a leader or an identifiable person to direct and coordinate the team activities, chair the interdisciplinary conference, seek information, facilitate and summarize discussion of the interdisciplinary team conference, and communicate findings to parents, patients, and the professional community. Although some teams change the leader as treatment focus changes with the patient's growth and development, there is value in having the same person assume the various leadership functions for an extended time period. In this way, the consumers of the team product (patient, parent, and care provider) experience the stability and assurance of communicating with one person. Surgeons are frequently the team leaders; however, teams can be led effectively by persons in any of the involved disciplines. Valetutti and Christoplos (1977) argued that no single profession should assume constant hegemony over any team, and that change in leadership should correlate with the patient's changing needs and with the team setting. However, they also noted that leadership function involves execution of the team's decision and reception of the team's advice. Furthermore, it is frequently this person who communicates and interprets the team's findings and recommendations to the patient and/or family. They stated,

> Unless a special rapport exists, successful implementation may be severely threatened. It is no small task to identify and establish the modus operandi for selecting the effective leader(s) to structure organizational pattern, to develop operating rules of the team, and to provide the most effective communication with the client. (p. 11)

Team operation and procedures. The interdisciplinary team approach for persons with cleft lip and palate and other craniofacial anomalies involves referring and identifying patients, scheduling appointments, documenting results of evaluations, and distributing interdisciplinary reports. In addition, for any scheduled appointment, team activity requires interdisciplinary examinations, interdisciplinary conferencing to determine appropriate treatment recommendations, and a sharing of that information with the patient and family. These activities are necessary for any team. Specific procedures utilized in performing these activities, however, vary from team to team and from clinic to clinic. Again, the variability often depends on specific team functions and physical setting. For example, in a setting such as a large university medical–dental complex, sophisticated radiographic equipment for dental and surgical evaluations, oral and speech physiology, and instrumental evaluation of speech are often available. Therefore, team operation and procedures involve time spent to obtain and review this information in interdisciplinary patient examinations and conferencing. In a setting where little, if any, of this equipment is available, patient examinations are more cursory and based on observable clinical findings. In this situation, referral to another physical facility is frequently required for needed diagnostic radiographs and instrumental assessments.

The manner in which patients are examined by teams may differ. Some patients are examined by all team members at the same time in one room. Subsequently, an interdisciplinary conference is held to determine the appropriate treatment plan. The patient and family may or may not be present at this meeting. If they are not present, usually the team leader, coordinator, social worker, or someone else shares the findings and recommendations with the patient and family. Other patients are examined individually by the team members and, although some interdisciplinary consultation and discussion may occur at that time, full discussion of observations occurs after all the individual examinations. Unfortunately, in some clinics, not all team members participate in the interdisciplinary conference. Following the individual examination, some specialist's findings and recommendations are recorded or written for the patient's report, but the specialist does not (or cannot) attend the interdisciplinary conference. The "heart" of the interdisciplinary approach, however, is the members of the team sharing, discussing and interpreting the findings, determining the needs, inquiring about observations, examining and determining the priorities of treatment, and deciding on a treatment plan. This works best for the patient when all members are present and actively participating in a meeting. As Koepp-Baker (1979) aptly stated,

> The way to obtain the most fruitful outcomes for such a patient is to keep in mind the steadying, illuminating and responsible inquiry: What is the best thing to do for the patient and what is the best way to do it, at this particular stage of his or her growth and development? (p. 55)

Function

As noted above, the structure of a given team is dependent on its function. The primary functions of interdisciplinary teams are (a) to provide consultation regarding treatment and/or (b) to prescribe and carry out the treatment. In the first situation, the members examine and evaluate patients and, through interdisciplinary discussion, recommend treatment or a treatment plan. Final decisions are at the discretion of the family and the direct treatment provider. In the second situation, the interdisciplinary team members are the providers; that is, the team is the treatment team in addition to the diagnosis and evaluation team. This is an important distinction and, of course, related directly to how clinics and teams obtain their patients. The professional referring a patient to a team needs to understand the function of a particular clinic or team: to consult regarding treatment of the professional's patient (Situation 1) or to evaluate *and* treat the patient (Situation 2).

Valletutti and Christoplos (1977) discussed the implications of these primary team functions and noted that responsibility of the direct provider, not the team, is crucial in Situation 1, whereas accountability for the treatment outcome rests with the team in Situation 2. Thus, the team functions are similar, but for different purposes. The most important function of any team is to provide the best possible service to the patient. To fulfill that purpose, the team organized with a focus on cleft lip and palate has several related functions, which include the following:

1. Diagnosis and evaluation
2. Discussion of findings
3. Treatment planning
4. Communication with patient/family
5. Communication with care providers
6. Facilitation and coordination
7. Follow-up on treatment

Diagnosis and evaluation.   Optimal team function and service requires correct diagnosis and complete evaluation of the patient's status at his or her stage of growth and development. This information-gathering function must be carried out by all team members before they can contribute to the interdisciplinary discussion. Information gathering, or data collection as described by Ducanis and Golin (1979), involves thorough review of available information about the patient based on observation and examination according to each discipline's clinical protocol and perspective, identification of the patient's problems and concerns, and judgment of the patient's treatment needs from a growth and development standpoint. Quantitative and qualitative results of certain physical, physiological, or psychosocial assessments may be available for the patient or performed at the time of the examination. Again, the techniques and methods available for these assessments depend on the team's physical facility. In some instances, the diagnosis and evaluation phase may consist only of clinical observation and examination of the patient.

Discussion of findings.   Following the information gathering, the team discusses the findings in an interdisciplinary conference. Although some interdisciplinary discussion occurs when two or more members are examining the patient, the opportunity for full team discussion of each specialist's observations, examination results, problems and concerns, and treatment needs is important. What occurs in the interdisciplinary discussion of findings can be described by various appropriate words: sharing, collaborating, learning, convincing, checking, compromising, and so forth. However, it is critical in this phase for the discussion to be, as Koepp-Baker (1979) stated, a "free and open communication." The outcome of discussion should result in an *integration* of the information gathered in order to most efficiently and effectively establish treatment plans. Integration involves interpretation and reporting of the findings so that it is understandable to all team members.

Treatment planning. Once the team has sufficiently discussed the findings and integrated the information, the team establishes the treatment plan for the patient. Ducanis and Golin (1979) discussed that treatment planning involves evaluation of the options. For persons with cleft lip and palate and other craniofacial disorders, evaluation of options must include determining the best or most ideal recommendation for treatment; however, alternatives need to be considered. Indeed, the optimal outcomes are not dependent only on one mode of treatment and the timing of that treatment. An example would be in the treatment of excessive hypernasality due to an inadequate velopharyngeal closure mechanism. Based on all diagnostic information available, the patient may be an excellent candidate for a surgical procedure such as a pharyngeal flap, but also an excellent candidate for construction of a speech prosthesis. Each treatment has advantages and disadvantages that the patient and the family need to fully understand before making a decision.

The treatment planning function for patients with cleft lip and palate involves *prioritizing* treatment plans. Prioritization of treatment, both short term and long term, can be accomplished effectively with full interdisciplinary participation. For example, surgical repair of the alveolar cleft, orthodontic treatment, speech articulation treatment, and restorative dental care may be strongly indicated for a 9-year-old patient. The key to the treatment plan is the priority or desired order of those treatments. Initiating speech treatment may depend on timing and extensiveness of orthodontic treatment. Orthodontic crossbite correction (upper arch expansion) may be desirable before the alveolar cleft can be repaired; however, it may be that orthodontics cannot be initiated until the dental restorative work has been completed and the oral hygiene has been improved. Therefore, the most appropriate treatment plan may require (a) establishing immediate dental care and home program of oral hygiene, (b) initiating a phase of orthodontic treatment to correct the crossbite, (c) proceeding with repair of the alveolar cleft when orthodontic treatment is completed, and (d) deferring active speech treatment for articulation until bone grafting has been completed. With good facilitation, cooperation, and coordination, it may be possible that speech treatment could be initiated in approximately 9 months.

The treatment-planning function directly implies decision making. With all pertinent information gathered, discussed, and integrated, the guiding question for the clinical decision making regarding the treatment plan is, What is the optimal treatment for this patient at this time and for the future? The patient is at the "heart" and center of all that occurs.

Communication with patient/family. The team's optimal treatment plan may be less successful if it is not effectively communicated to the patient and family. Although the team has reached a decision, the patient and family must ultimately *agree* with the plan and, furthermore, *proceed* with the plan. Therefore, an important team function is to communicate the findings, recommendations, and decisions in an understandable manner. It is reasonable to assume that the degree to which patients and families pursue team recommendations is related to communication between teams and patients/families. Studies have been sparse on compliance with team recommendations by patients with cleft lip and palate and their families. Paynter, Jordan, and Finch (1985) investigated the rate of compliance with interdisciplinary team recommendations. They examined responses of patients/families to a questionnaire that requested information about patient characteristics, compliance with team recommendations made at the most recent visit, opinions about the team's performance, financial issues, nature and severity of the problems, and so forth. Paynter et al. found that 95% complied with at least one team recommendation, but that 88% did not comply with all recommendations. Obviously, there was considerable variability. No factors were found to be significantly related to compliance. In this study and others carried out on patient/family compliance (Topic, 1987; Westra, 1982), patient/family understanding of the treatment recommendations was not assessed. However, it seems intuitively reasonable that increased understanding of treatment recommendations and the rationale for specific treatment on the part of the patient/family results in increased compliance.

Communication with care providers. Similarly, the interdisciplinary team needs to communicate its findings, recommendations, treatment plan, and so forth, to persons involved in the patient's welfare and persons providing direct care. As previously discussed, the consultative team may not comprise any of the patient's providers. In this case, because final decisions to carry out treatments must rest with the family and direct care provider, communication is an important and necessary team function. Usually, a team distributes a clinic report and/or letter to the appropriate providers, agencies, and payers.

Facilitation and coordination. Team functions of facilitation and coordination may occur during the interdisciplinary conference or after the conference. These functions relate directly to the often-cited advantages of the team approach—efficiency and effectiveness. For example, a patient requires surgical revision of the nose (perhaps at 16 to 18 years of age), removal of the wisdom teeth, and exploratory middle ear surgery. All these procedures can be done at the same time, thus avoiding multiple hospitalizations, outpatient visits, and administrations of anesthesia. This facilitation and coordination of treatment is most likely to occur with the interdisciplinary team approach.

Follow-up on treatment. It should be obvious that interdisciplinary team care for persons with cleft lip and palate is not a one-time event. Treatment is long term and correlated with physical and behavioral growth and development. Follow-up, or follow-through (Koepp-Baker, 1979), is an integral function of the team. Through this activity, the team can measure patient progress toward optimal outcome. Patient records consisting of speech recordings, audiometric data, photographs/radiographs, speech physiological data, psychosocial and growth and development information, and so forth, can be evaluated and compared. Through the team function of follow-up, treatment can proceed in the right direction—one step at a time—most effectively and efficiently.

Although not listed as a specific team function, research and education is another important function of interdisciplinary teams. Interdisciplinary teams in academic institutions and/or medical–dental environments can serve as a rich resource for training future members of health teams and providers of care for persons with cleft lip and palate and other craniofacial disorders. Furthermore, data obtained through patient observation and examination over many years can be fertile ground for research activities. Systematic, detailed, and standardized documentation by all specialties can contribute to better understanding of the effect of certain treatments that ultimately lead to improved care.

INTERDISCIPLINARY TEAM ISSUES

To this point, I have considered some assumptions and biases about interdisciplinary management, reviewed historical development of teams, and discussed team structure and function. It should be of no surprise that some teams flourish better than others and, by a variety of criteria, are more successful. Although interdisciplinary teams with satisfactory structure and defined goals and functions *can* provide the best and most effective and efficient management, not all teams succeed. Several issues can be explored regarding interdisciplinary team management for persons with cleft lip and palate and other craniofacial disorders; however, discussion here is limited to issues related to *team value, team quality,* and *team future.*

Team Value

Reasonable questions and issues have been raised over many years about the advantages and, in fact, need for interdisciplinary teams. As mentioned previously, Barker (1922) cautioned about the dangers of increasing specialization without adequate coordination and integration. In 1962, Curtin asked several questions about cleft palate teams: Does a team of specialists threaten the time-honored and personal doctor–patient relationship? Do teams tend to submerge and inhibit individual initiative? Is the team approach an efficient method of providing health services? He, too, strongly supported the interdisciplinary approach: "We can no longer thrive in the backwoods of individual specialities but need to join with allied disciplines in an effort to increase our understanding of all dimensions of the patient's needs and to improve standards of care" (p. 292).

Current support of the value of interdisciplinary cleft palate and craniofacial care is not hard to find. The specialization versus holistic controversy seems nicely resolved with effective interdisciplinary management. Although a good deal of manpower, time, and energy are involved in interdisciplinary activity, Valletutti and Christoplos (1977) pointed out that teams provide a check against hasty decisions made by individuals who do not face peer accountability. At the same time, however, teams sometimes stifle creativity and unorthodox approaches to solving problems. This is not always true: Creativity *can* and, in fact, *should* flourish on teams while checks and balances are maintained. In a very real sense, teams can offer the best of both worlds—the best treatment may be new and innovative, but also appropriate and practical.

Although there appears to be overwhelming support for interdisciplinary activity—not only in cleft palate and craniofacial disorders, but in a variety of medical–dental, social, educational, and vocational areas—there is no scientific evidence for concluding it is the best. According to Whitehouse (1965), "Team work as a method has been so logically appealing and so seemingly an obvious solution to the 'whole man' commitment as well as to the issue of specialization, that the practice has developed without examination of the premises" (p. 16). Valletutti and Christoplos (1977) noted that there are no guidelines for patients to determine whether a team effort is more beneficial than an individual effort. There are no "hard data" regarding comparative effects of team versus individual effort. In the absence of clear support, decisions are left to chance or to the inclinations and sophistication of the patient and to persons and agencies referring patients.

Ducanis and Golin (1979) summarized some of the limited research concerning evaluation and research of team effectiveness. Other than the previously mentioned studies of patient compliance, no recent controlled or comparative studies have investigated effectiveness of cleft palate or craniofacial teams. Ducanis and Golin raised some interesting evaluation issues in investigating team effectiveness, including what to evaluate and how to measure "effectiveness" or "success." Research issues about team systems might involve relationships among team variables such as structural aspects, function, and outcome.

Questions such as "Does therapy work?" or "Is treatment approach A more effective than treatment approach B?" are not easy to answer in the scientific sense. Siegel (1987) commented that these questions are not appropriate for research. He wrote that research on clinical outcome is confounded by so many variables that cannot be controlled that any conclusions are rendered meaningless. Siegel stated that science is a "very powerful tool for answering the questions it was designed to answer, but there are realms where science is not the most effective approach to elucidating and solving problems" (p. 311). Perhaps, as he suggested, the issue is not whether therapy or a therapy approach works, but whether the benefits exceed the costs, and these are questions of values. Kent (1990) argued that it is indeed appropriate to ask whether one treatment approach is more effective than another and that answers are possible only through therapeutic outcome research. He stated that outcome research is needed to determine how treatment can be more efficient and effective. Kent clearly felt that clinical service issues should not be dissociated from research.

More on patient outcome appears later in this chapter; however, the primary test or measure of team value and success in cleft lip and palate and other craniofacial disorders seems to be patient outcome. Regardless, the success of the team approach needs to be evaluated in terms of all factors that eventually contribute to outcome—clinical service, research, and education.

Team Quality

What are the characteristics of the excellent team? Why are some teams more "successful," "smooth running," and "healthy" than others? Although these are very subjective descriptions, nobody would argue with the notion that some teams seem to function more efficiently and effectively than others. Certainly, some aspects of organizational structure and function are important, but team dynamics and personal interaction also contribute significantly to team quality and health. Valletutti and Christoplos (1977) stated that efficiency is meaningless without effectiveness.

Koepp-Baker (1979) postulated that outcomes of group interaction to make effective decisions and solve problems are contingent on meeting two conditions: the *quality* of the decision based on the objective information available and the *acceptability* of the decision based on human feelings, attitudes, and biases. Clearly, the interdisciplinary approach in determining treatment in craniofacial disorders involves *people* making clinical decisions. We are not yet near the situation where appropriate bits of subjective information can be fed into a computer that ultimately prints out the most appropriate treatment. There are simply too many important pieces of information, some of which are not quantifiable and some of which are people-generated judgments based on quantitative as well as qualitative information.

Whitehouse (1965) described team work as a dynamic system. He pointed out that the successful team

> is effective not primarily because of the quality of its individual components but to the extent to which each component is complementary to, contributes to, and mutually enhances each other so that the main purposes and goals may be achieved. (p. 17)

He likens the effective team to a computer: Correct data input is valuable, self-correcting feedback occurs, and effective control of relationships of components (team members) occurs so that the entire system operates according to the established purposes.

Personal characteristics of team members. Interdisciplinary teams consist of people with varying backgrounds, training, and experience. A myriad of personal characteristics—both good and poor—contribute to team quality. The following represent, in my judgment, some of the more important ones:

1. *Interest in the patient and the disorder*—A strong interest in contributing to the welfare of patients with cleft lip and palate and other craniofacial disorders is essential. Team members must view team participation as contribution to the whole patient, not to isolated parts.
2. *Willingness to share openly*—Team recommendations and decisions are based on complete information and input from all specialists involved. There needs to be frequent and open communication of findings and judgments.
3. *Mutual respect*—Each team member must respect each other member as a person and respect each discipline. There needs to be a good understanding of what each discipline can and cannot do.
4. *Equal partnership*—There should be a feeling or perception that all members contribute equally to the team function. All members need to be confident in themselves as professionals and feel that their profession contributes to the whole. Equal partnership and team function is critical because it "encourages freedom to grow, gives

opportunity for open presentation of opinions, tends to educate each member of the group, develops mature responsibility, and strengthens pride in professional integrity" (Whitehouse, 1951, p. 52).

5. *Motivation to learn*—A characteristic of persons associated with high-quality teams is the desire to learn from each other about the disorder and to remain knowledgeable about new findings in their respective disciplines. Team members should not be satisfied with current techniques for evaluation and management, but should continually update their knowledge and understanding. Certainly, contributing new information through research enhances team quality and health.

Successful teams communicate results to appropriate persons effectively and efficiently. Immediate feedback to the patient and family, direct care providers, appropriate agencies, and third-party payers is important to good team function. When there is open communication, the interdisciplinary approach can be very successful.

Interdisciplinary problems and cautionary notes.   Effective team function does not merely happen with the formation of a team. Over the years, writers have commented on certain problems of interdisciplinary approach. Whitehouse (1951) pointed out that just because a group of persons admits interest in a problem does not guarantee cooperation and efficiency. He discussed several factors that inhibit what team work attempts to accomplish: (a) Professionals are not necessarily cooperative persons, (b) some professionals are unwilling to admit that others can accomplish a goal more effectively and efficiently, and (c) the team's goals may be too high and not practically obtainable.

Team evaluation and treatment planning for persons with cleft lip and palate may confuse the patient/family because a variety of opinions and treatment possibilities are inherent in the process. Indeed, determining various options is one of the functions of the interdisciplinary approach. Spriestersbach (1973) concluded that inadequate communication between the family and the team is a potential major problem. He noted that patients/families do not always understand all the information, do not always know what they want to know, are afraid to ask "silly" questions, and are confused by the "conflicting" advice from experts on the team. The antidote for this situation is more effective communication by the team leader or coordinator to summarize and explain to the patient/family the team discussion, differences, conclusions, and decisions. Thus, the team enterprise is not merely a listing of things that each specialist considers appropriate from his or her area of expertise, but a unified and cohesive plan developed by all the specialists.

Another frequently cited complaint is that teams seem impersonal to patients/families. Again, teams need to take precautions to prevent this feeling from occurring. At least one team member—someone with whom the family feels comfortable—needs to be identified as the effective communicator with the patient/family. Typically, that person is the leader or coordinator, but any member of the team can serve this function. In fact, this contact person may change as the patient's needs change with growth and development. The patient/family must perceive the team's recommendations as a well-integrated whole, not as unrelated parts. Again, no treatment is medical, social, psychological, or vocational—all treatment is total (Whitehouse, 1951). Similarly, no treatment is related solely to oral surgery, orthodontics, speech, or otology. Campbell and Gooch (1988) suggested that interdisciplinary course instruction "should look seamless to the students" (p. 8). Similarly, interdisciplinary treatment should look seamless to the patient. Patients need to view the team as one large provider. They should avoid seeing distinct professional boundaries.

Although team operation and procedure can be cumbersome and may appear to lack efficiency, teams enable the patient to see, and have the opportunity to consult with, several professionals at one visit. An added bonus is that those professionals can communicate with each other to make appropriate interdisciplinary decisions. Interdisciplinary activity is more time-consuming than one individual making a decision; however, if that one professional attempted to obtain information from all appropriate specialists, the time and energy would be greater than with established interdisciplinary procedures.

Another potential problem with interdisciplinary team activity is lack of patient focus. At times, teams can get caught up with their own activities and concerns with professional overlap of treatment, which can result in defensive behavior. The focus then becomes more directed at the team members themselves rather than the patient.

Koepp-Baker (1979) noted that team procedures can become routine and pedestrian behavior, resulting in a feeling of weariness or dissatisfaction on the part of some members. He suggested that research and continued education are corrective measures for ennui. Each interdisciplinary conference can and should be an educational experience; the desire to inform and be informed must be prevalent on teams.

Team Future

What is the future of interdisciplinary teams? Will the importance and impact of team management for persons with cleft lip and palate and other craniofacial disorders increase? The factors discussed early in this chapter contributing to the development and formation of interdisciplinary teams continue to exist—the concept of the whole person, the needs of the organization (specialization), and external mandates (Ducanis & Golin, 1979). Indeed, it is likely that increased numbers of specialists will be providing care for each patient with a particular disorder. Furthermore, there is increasing demand for professionals to deliver the highest standards of care, as efficiently and economically as possible. This demand comes from several sources: consumers of services (patient/ families), referral sources (private practitioners, professional groups, agencies), and third-party payers.

The concept of establishing regional centers for cleft palate and craniofacial evaluation and treatment based on criteria determined by others likely will be debated in the 1990s and into the next century. Brown and Cohen (1990) discussed a 10-year experience in New Jersey. Three centers were selected to provide interdisciplinary diagnostic services and treatment to persons with cleft lip and palate and/or associated craniofacial anomalies and/or velopharyngeal problems, "thus bringing to an end the isolated, independent approach of earlier years with its lack of beneficial cost-effectiveness and quality control" (p. 2). The specific guidelines and criteria that had to be met were established by the state before the centers were selected. Brown and Cohen reported that regionalization and creation of state standards with this contractual system of providing service have significantly reduced the cost of the care. They also believed that quality of care is improved when specialized care is provided in a limited number of centers. Although cost-effective, quality service is a laudable goal, an important issue is who sets the standards. Shprintzen (1990), referring to the New Jersey government sanction formula, questioned whether it is ethical for the state to determine the standards and raised issues of patient and provider rights.

Morris, Jakobi, and Harrington (1978) reported the results of two conferences conducted to identify standards of care for cleft lip and palate management. They cited several reasons why standards are needed: significant advances in treatment over time, the need for treatment goals and results to be evaluated and assessed, the fact that many practitioners are legally qualified to provide services but have little experience or knowledge about the disorder, and the variability of the disorder and its effects on patients and families.

Treatment providers must keep abreast of rapid advancement of knowledge. Clearly, the interdisciplinary approach is likely to foster state-of-the-art thinking and provide quality care. Although many states do not have written standards of care for cleft lip and palate and craniofacial management, several are now involved in this process. Interdisciplinary evaluation and treatment planning should be an integral part of those standards.

Some individual team members may feel that participation on teams for some length of time yields interdisciplinary expertise so that the team approach is no longer valuable. Curtin (1962) stated, "the mission of our team is in fact to do away with the team. Our purpose is to make every practitioner more completely self-sufficient" (p. 291). I disagree, and I suspect at this time that Curtin would also disagree, that team work should become obsolete. Again, no one person has the expertise necessary to provide the optimal interdisciplinary care for persons with cleft lip and palate. The need for interdisciplinary care is unlikely to diminish with time.

Effective and efficient interdisciplinary function must continue to be the primary goal of treatment teams. In the future, the value of the interdisciplinary team approach needs to be systematically investigated by carrying out studies designed to evaluate team effectiveness and determine relationships among variables that have the greatest impact on team function. Better and more standard ways to assess the various outcome parameters are needed, since outcome is the criterion by which any therapeutic process is measured.

According to Paul Ellwood (1990), president and chairman of the Board of Interstudy, a nonprofit research group dealing with health care issues, little is known about outcome, and it is important to determine precisely what outcome is desirable. For example, in heart bypass surgery, is the outcome an issue of life versus death or pain versus no pain? What is the outcome in the treatment of persons with cleft lip and palate— acceptable appearance, dental function, and communication skills? Career success? And how are these to be measured? Ellwood challenges practitioners with a concept called "outcomes management"—the effect of treatment on patients' well-being. This concept is based on continuous clinical trials with no one person, group, or category excluded. Outcomes management must be based on sound epidemiological principles, not merely casual observations, to determine the impact of treatment on quality of life. Perhaps practitioners need to focus on how outcome can be assessed in a standard fashion. Can a protocol be developed on how to describe patients and specify desirable outcomes? Ellwood concluded, perhaps correctly, that practitioners need to be assured that what they are doing in health care produces a beneficial effect. Interestingly, he compliments interdisciplinary management for persons with cleft lip and palate as an example of doing the appropriate thing for many years.

Ducanis and Golin (1979) stated that training, focusing on competence in team work, is important. There should be increased emphasis on education of professionals in the interdisciplinary process at the undergraduate, graduate, and professional continuing education levels. Furthermore, workshops, symposia, and conferences are helpful for persons currently serving on interdisciplinary teams.

The following chapters of this text are written by persons trained in specific professions and committed to the interdisciplinary approach. This book is intended to give the reader knowledge about the disciplines, required training, clinical issues, and management of cleft lip and palate, as well as to provide a strong reference base for further study. This chapter closes with a statement made by L. F. Barker in 1922 to his New York State medical colleagues. The message is relevant today, and will be for a long time to come.

> The conception of a diagnostic survey of a patient as a whole (with full consideration of all the somatic, psychic, and social elements concerned), though relatively new, is rapidly growing in appreciation in the minds as well as in those of the producers of medical services. All are coming to recognize the dangers of an ever-increasing medical specialization that does not provide for proper coordination of the activities of the specialists and the suitable integration of the results of their work; only through such coordination and integration can unified diagnostic conclusions be safely arrived at, conclusions on which a comprehensive therapeutic regimen dare be based and executed. (p. 777)

REFERENCES

American Cleft Palate–Craniofacial Association. (1990). *Membership–Team Directory.*

Barker, L. F. (1922, March 18). The specialist and the general practitioner in relation to team-work in medical practice. *Journal of the American Medical Association, 78* (11), 773–779.

Bleiberg, A. H., & Leubling, H. E. (1971). *Parent's guide to cleft palate habilitation: The team approach.* New York: Exposition Press.

Brown, A. S., & Cohen, M. A. (1990). The New Jersey experience. *Cleft Palate Journal, 27*(1), 1–2.

Campbell, W. E., & Gooch, V. (1988). Philosophical biology or biological philosophy? In V. Turdik (Ed.), *Focus on teaching and learning* (Vol. 3, No. 3). Office of Educational Development Program, University of Minnesota, Minneapolis.

Cooper, H. K. (1953). Integration of services in the treatment of cleft lip and palate. *Journal of the American Dental Association, 47,* 27–32.

Cooper, H. K. (1979). Historical perspectives and philosophy of treatment. In H. K. Cooper, R. L. Harding, W. M. Krogman, M. Mazaheri, & R. T. Millard (Eds.), *Cleft palate and cleft lip: A team approach to clinical management and rehabilitation of the patient.* Philadelphia: W. B. Saunders.

Curtin, J. W. (1962). A surgeon's evaluation of the cleft palate team. *Plastic and Reconstructive Surgery, 29,* 289–292.

Ducanis, A. J., & Golin, A. K. (1979). *The interdisciplinary health care team.* Germantown, MD: Aspen Systems.

Ellwood, P. (1990). *Patient outcome research: Trends in the 90's.* Invited presentation to the American Cleft Palate–Craniofacial Association, St. Louis.

Kent, R. D. (1990). Fragmentation of clinical service and clinical science in communicative disorders. *National Student Speech Language Hearing Association Journal, 17,* 4–16.

Koepp-Baker, H. (1963). Cleft palate: Multidisciplinary management. In H. L. Morris (Ed.), *Cleft palate criteria for physical management.* Iowa City: University of Iowa Press.

Koepp-Baker, H. (1979). The craniofacial team. In K. R. Bzoch (Ed.), *Communicative disorders related to cleft lip and palate.* Boston: Little, Brown.

Krogman, W. (1979). The cleft palate team in action. In H. K. Cooper, R. L. Harding, W. M. Krogman, M. Mazaheri, & R. T. Millard (Eds.), *Cleft palate and cleft lip: A team approach to clinical management and rehabilitation of the patient.* Philadelphia: W. B. Saunders.

Lis, E. F., Pruzansky, S., Koepp-Baker, H., & Kobes, H. (1956). Cleft lip and cleft palate: Perspectives in management. *Pediatric Clinics of North America, 3*(4), 995–1028.

McWilliams, B. J., Morris, H. L., & Shelton, R. L. (1990). *Cleft palate speech.* Philadelphia: B. C. Decker.

Morris, H. L. (1980). The structure and function of interdisciplinary health teams. In C. F. Salinas & R. J. Jorgenson (Eds.), *Dentistry in the interdisciplinary treatment of genetic diseases* (Birth Defects: Original Article Series, Vol. 16, No. 5). New York: Alan R. Lis.

Morris, H. L., Jakobi, P., & Harrington, D. (1978). Objectives and criteria for management of cleft lip and palate and the delivery of management services. *Cleft Palate Journal, 15,* 1–5.

Nackashi, J. A., & Dixon-Wood, V. L. (1989). The craniofacial team: Medical supervision and coordination. In K. R. Bzoch (Ed.), *Communicative disorders related to cleft lip and palate.* Austin, TX: PRO-ED.

Paynter, E., Jordan, W., & Finch, D. (1985). *Patient compliance with cleft palate team regimens.* Paper presented at the Texas Speech–Language–Hearing Association, Corpus Christi, TX.

Ross, R. B., & Johnston, M. C. (1978). *Cleft lip and palate.* Baltimore: Williams and Wilkins.

Shprintzen, R. J. (1990). Editorial—Who sets the standards. *Cleft Palate Journal, 27*(2), 92–93.

Siegel, G. M. (1987). The limits of science in communication disorders. *Journal of Speech and Hearing Disorders, 52,* 306–312.

Spriestersbach, D. C. (1973). *Psychosocial aspects of the cleft palate problem* (Vol. 1). Iowa City: University of Iowa Press.

Spriestersbach, D. C., & Sherman, D. (1968). *Cleft palate and communication.* New York: Academic Press.

Topic, M. (1987). *A study of compliance of patient/families seen in a cleft palate clinic.* Unpublished master's thesis, University of Minnesota, Minneapolis.

Valletutti, P. J., & Christoplos, F. (1977). *Interdisciplinary approaches to human services.* Baltimore: University Park Press.

Wells, C. (1971). *Cleft palate and its associated speech disorders.* New York: McGraw-Hill.

Wells, C. (1979). The American Cleft Palate Association: Its first 36 years. *Cleft Palate Journal, 16,* 86–123.

Westra, S. E. (1982). *Velopharyngeal insufficiency: Treatment recommendations, treatment implementations, and effects on speech in a selected cleft palate population.* Unpublished master's thesis, University of Minnesota, Minneapolis.

Whitehouse, F. A. (1951). Teamwork—A democracy of professions. *Exceptional Children, 18,* 45–52.

Whitehouse, F. A. (1965). Teamwork as a dynamic system. *Cleft Palate Journal, 2*(1), 16–27.

CHAPTER 2

Development and Genetic Aspects of Cleft Lip and Palate

Robert J. Gorlin

Gorlin points out the clinical variability of cleft formation and the types of clefts. He discusses how clefts develop embryologically from approximately the 5th through the 10th week and some possible mechanisms of cleft formation. Multifactorial inheritance is discussed and presumed to be the cause for most examples of clefting. The genetics of clefting and the importance of genetic counseling to families with cleft members are presented.

1. *What are the two basic types (entities, diagnoses) of clefting? How does incidence vary in males versus females and among racial groups?*

2. *Explain what Gorlin means by the forming and merging of facial prominences from the 5th through the 10th weeks of embryological development. What can we conclude embryologically about a child born with a cleft uvula?*

3. *Why do we know so little about specific mechanisms of cleft production?*

4. *Define multifactorial inheritance. What is the recurrence risk in first-degree relatives for multifactorial traits? Can you think of other multifactorial traits? What autosomal-dominant conditions frequently involve clefting?*

5. *What does Gorlin mean by nondirective genetic counseling?*

Clinically, there is great variability in the degree of cleft formation. Relatively minor degrees of involvement include bifid uvula, linear lip indentations, so-called intrauterine-healed clefts, and submucous palatal clefts. Clefts may involve only a portion of the upper lip or may extend to the nostril and may be combined with defects of the hard and/or soft palates. Isolated palatal clefts may be limited to the uvula, or they may be more extensive, cleaving the soft palate or both soft and hard palates to just behind the incisor teeth.

TYPES OF CLEFT FORMATIONS

Cleft Lip and Cleft Palate

A combination of cleft lip and cleft palate (CLP) is more common than cleft lip (CL) only or cleft palate (CP) only. The breakdown according to types seems to differ somewhat among several large surveys depending, in part, upon whether the data are gathered at birth or at the time of surgery. Data obtained from birth records are notoriously unreliable. Roughly, however, CLP comprises about 50% of cases, and CL only and CP only each represent about 25% of cases, irrespective of race. However, CL only and CP only are far less common in the Native American than is CLP. Fogh-Andersen (1942), by sorting clefts into three groups— isolated cleft lip, cleft lip and cleft palate, and isolated cleft palate— was able to show that there are two separate entities: (a) cleft lip with or without cleft palate and (b) isolated cleft palate. Cleft lip with or without cleft palate appears to occur in about 1 per 1,000 white births (range 0.6–1.3 per 1,000). The prevalence is higher in Japanese and Chinese populations (about 1.7 per 1,000 live births) and lower among blacks (approximately 1 per 2,500 births) (Abyholm, 1978; Altemus, 1966; Bear, 1976; Emanuel, Huang, Gutman, Yu, & Lin, 1972; Leck, 1984; Lowry & Trimble, 1977; Vanderas, 1987).

Isolated Cleft Lip

CL only may be unilateral (80% of occurrences) (see Figure 2.1) or bilateral (20%) (see Figure 2.2). When unilateral, the cleft occurs on the left side about 70% of the time, although it is no more extensive than right clefts. About 85% of cases of bilateral cleft lip and 70% of cases of unilateral cleft lip are associated with cleft palate. Cleft lip with or without cleft palate is more common in males. Clefts of the lip do not always extend into the nostril, and in about 10% of the cases, there are bridges of skin (Simonart's bands) across the cleft.

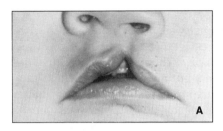

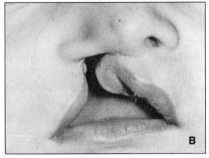

Figure 2.1 Unilateral cleft lip. Unilateral cleft lip may be incomplete (i.e., barely through the vermilion) as in A, or complete (i.e., extending to the nostril) as in B. (From "Lippen-, Kiefer-, Gaumenspalten" by W. Hoppe, 1965, *Archiv fur Kinderheikunde, 171,* Suppl 52:1, pp. 22, 27. Copyright 1965 by Springer-Verlag Publishing Co. Reprinted with permission.

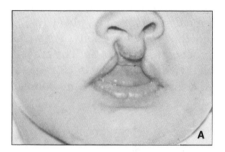

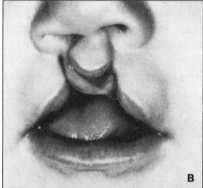

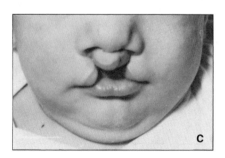

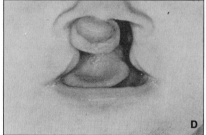

Figure 2.2 Bilateral cleft lip. Note the various degrees of clefting. In D, the primary palate is attached only to the columella. (From "The Management of Bilateral Cleft of the Primary Palate" by T. Skoog, *Plastic and Reconstructive Surgery, 35,* p. 40. Copyright 1965 by Williams and Wilkins Co. Reprinted by courtesy of the Estate of Tord Skoog.)

Isolated Cleft Palate

CP only (Figure 2.3) appears to be an entity separate from cleft lip with or without cleft palate. Numerous investigators have pointed out that siblings of patients with cleft lip with or without cleft palate have an increased frequency of the same anomaly but not of isolated cleft palate, and vice versa. The frequency of CP only among both whites and blacks appears to be between 1 per 2,000 and 1 per 2,500 births (Owens, Jones, & Harris, 1985). It may be a bit more common among Japanese (Natsume & Kawai, 1986). CP only occurs somewhat more often in females, comprising about 60% of the cases. However, studies of the extent of cleft palate clearly indicate that although there is a 2:1 (female:male) predilection for complete clefts of the hard and soft palate, the ratio approaches 1:1 for clefts of the soft palate only.

Cleft Uvula

Cleft or bifid uvula varies in degrees of completeness, with incomplete clefts being much more common. The incidence of cleft uvula (1 in 80 white individuals) is much higher than that for cleft palate. As with clefts of the soft palate, cleft uvula approaches a 1:1 sex ratio. The prevalence in parents and siblings of persons with clefts (probands) ranges from approximately 7% to 15% (Chosack & Eidelman, 1978; Lindemann,

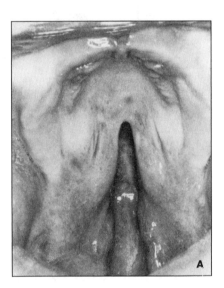
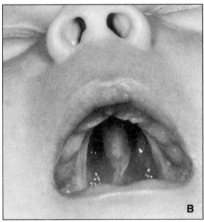

Figure 2.3   Cleft palate. Like cleft lip, cleft palate may be of variable extent. In this patient, note that cleft involves all of the soft palate and about one-half of the hard palate.

Riis, & Sewerin, 1977). The frequency of cleft uvula among Native American groups is quite high, ranging from 1 per 9 to 1 per 14 individuals, depending upon the tribal group. It is much less frequent in blacks: Estimates have ranged from 1 per 350 to 1 per 400 (Cervenka & Shapiro, 1970; Jaffe & DeBlanc, 1972; Schaumann, Peagler, & Gorlin, 1970).

Microforms

Minimal expressions (microforms) of cleft lip and/or cleft palate include cleft uvula, submucous palatal cleft, hairline indentation of the lip, and palatal defects demonstrated by laminographic examination (Heckler, Oesterle, & Jabaley, 1979). *Minimal cleft lip* has varied from intra-uterine-healed clefts of the lip (see Figures 2.4 and 2.5) to clefts extending through the vermilion (red portion of the lip). More extensive examination of these patients reveals occasional nasal deformity, alveolar deformity, and anomalous tooth development on the affected side (Lehman & Artz, 1976). Velopharyngeal inadequacy for speech may also occur in the absence of an overt cleft palate. This may be associated with bifid or absent uvula, short soft palate, or submucous cleft of the palate.

Submucous Palatal Cleft

Submucous cleft palate (SMCP) refers to imperfect muscle union across the soft palate underlying the mucous membrane. The palate is short and velopharyngeal closure is inadequate for acceptable speech in some, but certainly not all, cases. Clinicians frequently describe the classic

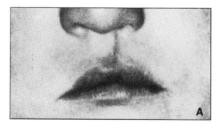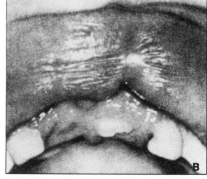

Figure 2.4   Intrauterine-healed unilateral cleft lip. Note the defect in the orbicularis oris. (From "Zur Histologie und Klinik der Lateralen Oberlippen-Furcher" by G. Leutert and H. Heiner, 1962, *Archiv Klinische Chirurgiae, 299,* p. 791. Copyright 1962 by Springer-Verlag Publishing Company. Reprinted with permission.)

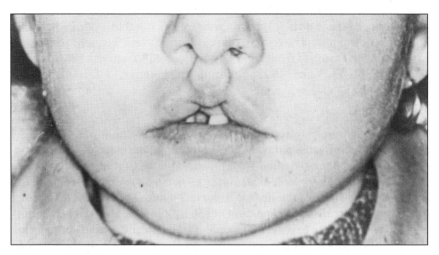

Figure 2.5 Intrauterine-healed bilateral cleft lip. (From "Zur Histologie und Klinik der Lateralen Oberlippen-Furcher" by G. Leutert and H. Heiner, 1962, *Archiv Klinische Chirurgiae, 299,* p. 792. Copyright 1962 by Springer-Verlag Publishing Company. Reprinted with permission.)

triad of symptoms for SMCP: bony notch in the posterior border of the hard palate, cleft uvula, and thin, bluish appearance of the midline of the soft palate. There is usually a median deficiency or notch in the bone at the posterior edge of the hard palate (Figure 2.6). This can be detected by palpation or by means of a light probe placed within the nose. Among those with SMCP, approximately 30% have cleft uvula and over 60% have a short palate, with poor mobility demonstrated in 20% of all cases (Poswillo, 1979). SMCP is relatively uncommon, being seen in 1 in 1,200 children, and there appears to be no sex predilection.

EMBRYOLOGY OF THE PRIMARY AND SECONDARY PALATES

The nature of this text does not permit me to "begin at the beginning." Many excellent treatises can guide the reader from the formation of the fertilized egg through development to the three-germ cell layer embryo. In this section, I discuss the period of embryonic development when the facial prominences form and merge, that is, roughly the 5th to 10th weeks after conception. However, reference is made to earlier events that play a critical role (Johnston, Hassell, & Brown, 1975; Johnston & Sulik, 1979).

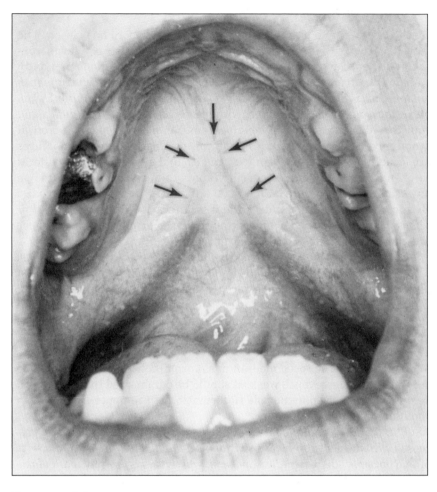

Figure 2.6 Submucous cleft palate. Arrows indicate the extent of the bony defect. (From *Syndromes of the Head and Neck,* 3rd ed., by R. J. Gorlin, M. M. Cohen, Jr., and L. S. Levin, 1990, New York: Oxford University Press. Reprinted with permission. Courtesy of H. W. Smith, New Haven, CT.)

The Neural Crest

Neural crest cells play an integral part in facial morphology. At about the time when the neural folds fuse to form the neural tube, ectodermal cells adjacent to the neural plate migrate into the underlying regions. Those in the head and face form essentially all the skeletal and connective tissues of the face: bone, cartilage, fibrous connective tissue, and all dental tissues except enamel.

Formation of the Primary Palate

By the end of the fourth week, the anterior neuropore has closed. The face, if one can call it that at this period of time, consists of a large frontal prominence overlying the first or mandibular arch. If one manually elevates the frontal prominence, one can see into the *primary mouth or stomodeum*. The primary mouth is separated from the foregut by the *buccopharyngeal membrane,* which undergoes selective cell death and ruptures about this time in development. On both sides of the frontal prominence, the *nasal placodes* are forming. These bilateral structures are located just above the primitive mouth and are represented by local thickening of the surface ectoderm. Rapid proliferation of tissue known as *nasal swellings* occurs both lateral and medial to the nasal placodes. By means of selective cell death and proliferation of tissues, *nasal or olfactory pits* are formed, which extend into the primitive mouth. These are the primitive nostrils. (See Figure 2.7.)

Extremely active growth occurs during the fifth and sixth weeks. The maxillary swellings, which represent the upper portion of the first pharyngeal arch, enlarge considerably and, by pushing the nasal swellings or prominences medially, cause them to approach one another in the midline. When the two prominences meet, merging takes place between the median nasal prominences and the maxillary swellings. Thus, the upper lip is formed laterally by the maxillary prominences and medially by the fused median nasal prominences (Figure 2.8). This occurs around the seventh week. It should be emphasized that the lateral nasal prominences play no role in formation of the upper lip, but form the alae or wings of the nose.

The *primary palate* consists of the two merged medial nasal processes, which form the *intermaxillary segment.* This, in turn, consists of two portions: (a) a *labial component,* which forms the philtrum of the upper lip (i.e., the indented area flanked by roughly parallel ridges that run from the columella of the nose to the middle of the upper lip) and (b) the triangular *palatal component* of bone (premaxilla) that includes the four maxillary incisor teeth. The primary palate extends posteriorly to the incisive foramen or, clinically, to the incisive papilla.

Formation of the Secondary Palate

The so-called secondary palate makes up at least 90% of the hard and soft palates, or all except the anterior portion that houses the incisor teeth. Its development appears to be somewhat more complicated than originally thought. The palatal shelves originate as swellings or shelflike burgeonings of the medial surfaces of the maxillary prominences. They appear in the sixth week and grow downward, lateral to, and somewhat beneath the tongue. Elevation of the palatal processes to a hori-

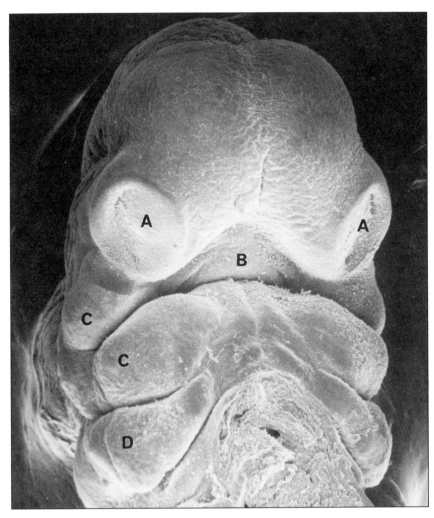

Figure 2.7 Scanning electron micrograph of 32-day-old embryo showing bilateral olfactory pits (A), buccopharyngeal membrane (B), mandibular arch (C), and hyoid arch (D). (From J. Jirasek and B. Shapiro, Minneapolis, MN. Courtesy of Burton Shapiro, Minneapolis, MN.)

zontal plane is more "rigorous" anteriorly, that is, in the part nearer the primary palate. Elevation begins during the seventh week.

What promotes the elevation has been called "intrinsic shelf force," which has a complex biochemical and physiochemical basis. The tongue appears to play little role in shelf elevation. This has been demonstrated in mouse embryos, where removal of the tongue prior to shelf elevation

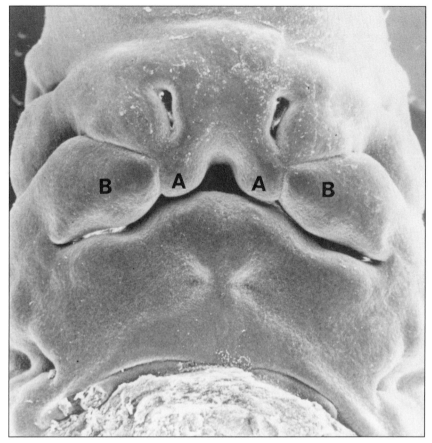

Figure 2.8 Scanning electron micrograph of 44-day-old embryo. Note that the upper lip
will be formed from fusion of the median nasal prominence (A) and the
maxillary part (B) of the mandibular arch bilaterally. (From K. Sulik, Chapel
Hill, NC.)

has been followed by partial elevation of the shelves to the horizontal
plane.

In mammals, elevation of the shelves is associated with widening
and forward growth of the mandible (Figure 2.9A). This seems to be
dependent upon growth of Meckel's cartilage, the evanescent stiffener
of the first pharyngeal arch. Once the shelves are elevated to the horizontal plane, there is programmed cell death of the overlying epithelium.
This has been demonstrated by noting the absence of certain cellular
enzymes (cytochrome oxidase) by histochemical study and by observing
increased activity of other enzymes (e.g., cyclic adenosine monophos-

phate). When the shelf edges touch, the epithelium has thinned and is undergoing advanced stages of degeneration (Figure 2.9B). This allows a flow of ectomesenchyme from each side to close the gap. Complete fusion takes place by the 10th week. In some infants, there is cystic degeneration of the epithelial remnants, which produces evanescent midline palatal microcysts.   *F goes away*

MECHANISMS OF CLEFT PRODUCTION

By definition, cleft lip involves the failure of closure of the primary palate, whereas cleft palate involves the failure of closure of the secondary palate. Our knowledge regarding mechanisms involved in regulation of embryonic growth is, at best, sparse. The blueprints for the rate at which facial prominences grow or burgeon, and in what direction they grow, is in part determined by the genetic template. The template is the deoxyribonucleic acid (DNA) code located in the nucleus of each cell. However, hereditary factors do not act alone. Growth patterns can be affected by environmental factors as well. For example, several mouse models exist for cleft lip and cleft palate. There are both susceptible and nonsusceptible strains. Furthermore, various teratogenic substances (corticosteroids, vitamin A, phenytoin, various folic acid antagonists, etc.) produce clefting in rodents. However, there is little evidence that any of these agents plays a role in cleft palate production in humans.

Cleft lip and/or cleft palate or, for purposes of general discussion, any malformation evident at birth results from some failure in a normal embryologic event. For example, various genetic and/or environmental

5 wks

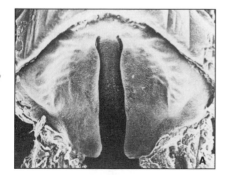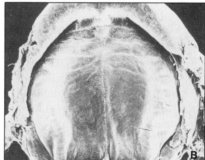

8 wk 3 days

Figure 2.9 Scanning electron micrograph of a palate. In the 35-day-old embryo (A), fusion of primary palate only has occurred. At 59 days (B), there is complete fusion of secondary palate. (From L. Russell, Chapel Hill, NC.)

factors may inhibit the flow of neural crest cells or may affect their volume or mass so that contact between prominences is impossible or inadequate. The epithelium covering the ectomesenchyme may not undergo programmed cell death so that fusion cannot take place. Exact timing and exact positioning play critical roles. For example, Johnston and Sulik (1979) showed that if the bilaterally formed nasal placodes contact one another, the result is severe to complete suppression of development of median nasal prominences.

Perhaps altered positioning of the nasal placodes or abnormal direction of growth of the facial prominences is responsible for cleft of the primary palate (cleft lip). This has been supported not only by animal models, but by the clinical observation that parents of children with cleft lip exhibit some degree of reduction in overall midface size.

Many mechanisms may lead to cleft of the secondary palate (cleft palate); however, some suggested mechanisms are doubtful causes. For example, it is extremely unlikely that a markedly large tongue could interfere with palatal closure. There is no known association with congenital hypothyroidism or macroglossia–omphalocele syndrome, although it may be argued that tongue enlargement in those disorders occurs late in gestation. Failure of growth of the mandible (microretrognathia) may inhibit elevation of the shelves since the Robin sequence and mandibulofacial dysostosis are associated with cleft palate.

Clefts of both primary and secondary palates occur in association in about half the cases. Researchers have sought a common mechanism of production. One suggestion is that the tongue tip becomes wedged in the labial cleft produced by failure of fusion of the median nasal and maxillary prominences. This, it has been argued, would not allow the tongue to drop and, consequently, would interfere with midline contact and resultant closure. This explanation appears too simplistic, however. Reduction in size of both the labial maxillary prominence *and* the palatine process of the maxillary prominence seems to be a far more reasonable explanation (see Gorlin, Cohen, & Levin, 1990, for discussion).

Clefts of the secondary palate most likely result from either hypoplasia (underdevelopment) of the shelves or delay in timing of shelf elevation. Experiments carried out on susceptible strains of mice have suggested that both mechanisms are operative, but at different times of gestation. For example, large doses of vitamin A given early in gestation inhibit palatal shelf growth, whereas cortisone, given later in gestation, inhibits palatal shelf elevation.

MULTIFACTORIAL INHERITANCE

Because most examples of cleft lip and/or cleft palate appear to have multifactorial inheritance, a short discussion of this type of hereditary transmission appears relevant. Multifactorial inheritance is far less familiar to most people than is single-gene inheritance. The latter is presented in some form in pre–high school years and emphasized in high school biology courses. Study of multifactorial inheritance is usually reserved for college courses in genetics or human genetics. This is surprising in view of the major role that this form of inheritance plays in our lives. Such diverse traits as height, hair color, and intelligence depend on the additive properties of many genes and environmental factors, as do schizophrenia, club foot, dislocated hips, most types of congenital heart disease, and most cases of cleft lip and/or cleft palate. Multifactorial disorders tend to cluster in families and follow different rules from those of single-gene inheritance.

A multifactorial disorder, by definition, is influenced by a combination of genetic and environmental factors. However, researchers do not know for such disorders how many genes are involved, whether each gene has an equal influence (unlikely), or, in most cases, what environmental factors are operating. Multifactorial traits, such as stature, are unimodal. They generally follow a normal curve if we ignore the blips in the tails due to gigantism at one end and such conditions as achondroplasia or other rare disorders of growth retardation at the other. Development, in general, follows a continuous distribution. Failure in a developmental process due to whatever cause will interrupt the continuous distribution. If the failure in development after a certain point results in malformation, there are two classes, normal and abnormal, separated by a threshold. This is termed *quasi-continuous variation.*

Recurrence risks for multifactorial disorders are calculated from surveys of various populations. Analyses are then carried out on the frequencies of the disorder in assorted relatives: parents, children, uncles, aunts, nieces, nephews, grandparents, grandchildren, cousins, and so forth. From this data, empirical risk figures are calculated. An estimate that approximates the empirical risk in first-degree relatives may be easily calculated. This figure, known as the Edwards or Falconer approximation, equals the square root of the frequency of the specific disorder in the population. Thus, if a disorder has a population frequency of 1 in 2,500, the recurrence risk in first-degree relatives will be 1 in 50 or 2%. From this, it necessarily follows that the lower the population frequency, the greater the relative increased risk for affected siblings. For example, a disorder with a population frequency of 1 in 10,000 would have a recurrence risk of 1 in 100 (a 100-fold increase), whereas a disorder with a frequency of 1 in 900 would have a recurrence risk of 1 in 30 (a 30-fold increase).

Multifactorial disorders often occur more frequently in one sex. It follows that an affected individual of the less susceptible sex who needs greater genetic and/or environmental factors to manifest the disorder, endows his or her offspring with a greater risk.

Multifactorial inheritance also differs from single-gene inheritance in that the recurrence risk increases as additional family members are affected. For single-gene traits, the risks stay the same regardless of the number of relatives affected. Risks for cleft lip and/or cleft palate are dealt with in great detail in the following sections. Another observation regarding multifactorial inheritance is that the more severe the malformation, the higher the risk of recurrence. The risk to subsequent siblings is also higher if there is parental consanguinity or marriage among relatives.

Twin studies are often employed for investigation of multifactorial traits to show the relative strengths of genetic and environmental factors. Concordance for a trait is compared in both monozygotic (MZ) and dizygotic (DZ) twins. Concordance among MZ twins should be complete for single-gene disorders, but is rarely complete for multifactorial disorders. (The reader should remember that DZ twins are no different from siblings born during different gestations.) Thus, if the concordance rate is more than twice as great in MZ twins as in DZ twins, simple dominant inheritance can be excluded, whereas if concordance is more than four times as great, simple recessive inheritance can be excluded. A comparison between MZ and DZ twins will be made in the case of cleft lip and/or cleft palate below.

GENETICS OF FACIAL CLEFTING

Following the belief in the single-gene inheritance of clefting expressed during the early decades of this century, it became evident that recurrence risks did not correspond to any simple pattern of inheritance. This was bolstered by twin studies, which indicate the relative roles played in cleft production by genetic and nongenetic influences. Table 2.1 reveals that among twins with cleft lip with or without cleft palate, concordance is far greater in monozygotic (36.2%) than in dizygotic twins (4.7%). In twins with CP only concordance is not quite as large between the two groups (monozygotic, 22.2%; dizygotic, 4.6%) (Blake & Wreakes, 1972; Gorlin et al., 1990; Schweckendiek, 1973; Shields, Bixler, & Fogh-Andersen, 1979). These data suggest a stronger genetic basis for cleft lip with or without cleft palate than for CP only. Microforms such as velopharyngeal incompetence and submucous palatal cleft could alter the data markedly. Although many investigators believe that cleft lip with or without cleft palate follows the rules of multifactorial threshold inheritance, others express skepticism that CP only obeys the rules and have suggested that environmental factors play a major role. They have further suggested that cleft palate represents a heterogeneity.

TABLE 2.1

Concordance in Facial Clefts in Twin Studies (1922–1988)

	Monozygotic Twins		Dizygotic Twins	
	Cleft Lip ± Palate	Cleft Palate	Cleft Lip ± Palate	Cleft Palate
N studied	84	27	191	44
Concordance (n) *(ie both twins have condition?)*	34 *←would be much higher if grown only?*	6	9	2
Percentage concordance	36.2	22.2	4.7	4.6

Note. Adapted from *Syndromes of the Head and Neck* (3rd ed., p. 697) by R. J. Gorlin, M. M. Cohen, Jr., and L. S. Levin, 1990, New York: Oxford University Press.

Both cleft lip with or without cleft palate and CP only consist of three groups: sporadic (75% to 80%), familial (10% to 15%), and syndromal (1% to 5%).

Clefting is heterogeneous, the variation and liability probably being determined by a number of major genes, minor genes, environmental insults, and a developmental threshold (Fraser, 1974; Reich, 1979). As indicated, cleft palate does not fit the multifactorial model very well. It is probably more heterogeneous than cleft lip with or without cleft palate (Ching & Chung, 1974; Chung, Bixler, Watanabe, Koguchi, & Fogh-Andersen, 1986; Melnick, Bixler, & Shields, 1980; Shields, Bixler, & Fogh-Andersen, 1981). Because one cannot, at this time, distinguish clearly among the multifactorial (polygenic) model, a major gene with reduced penetrance, and a mixture of sporadic cases, it seems foolish to argue for one or the other until more convincing evidence has been presented. Little error is made using empirical risk data or, in fact, mathematical model data described below. The parents and relatives of an affected individual should also be examined carefully for such minor stigmata as bifid uvula, submucous cleft palate, or velopharyngeal incompetence.

RISK

In the random population, the risk for the occurrence of cleft lip and/or cleft palate ranges from 1 in 2,500 for CP only to essentially 1 in 2 for cleft lip with or without cleft palate if in association with paramedian fistulas (pits) of the lower lip. In the vast majority of cases, the cleft is either isolated or associated with a constellation of anomalies that do not form a recognizable syndrome. Although there may well be over 250 recognized cleft syndromes, they constitute a small number (2% to 4%) of the total cases. However, efforts *must* be made to recognize a cleft syndrome, since the pattern of inheritance may be a simple one and the genetic risk for future affected children may then be made more precise. More specific reference is made to these syndromes in the next section, Associated Anomalies.

In the event of failure to recognize such a pattern, we must resort to empirical risk figures based on pooled data. These have been calculated by several investigators (Bonaiti et al., 1982; Bonaiti-Pellie & Smith, 1974; Tolarová, 1972, 1987a, 1987b; Tolarová & Morton, 1975; Woolf, 1971). The reader is also referred to a mathematical model devised by Spence, Westlake, Lange, and Gold (1976) that yields results remarkably close to the empirical risk. In the use of tables, it should be borne in mind that the data apply only to risks for similar anomalies; for example, a parent with CP only has no greater risk than anyone else of having a child with cleft lip with or without cleft palate, and vice versa.

As the reader can see from Tables 2.2 and 2.3, in the case of uncomplicated clefts, the risk to a first-degree relative of an affected individual (proband) is on the order of 2% to 4%. This is very close to the Falconer estimation of the square root of 1 in 900 (i.e., 1 in 30 or 3.3%). The risks increase as more individuals are affected. For example, if a parent and child have clefts, the risk for a future affected sibling increases to about 9%. These and other situations are presented in detail in Tables 2.2 and 2.3.

The severity of a facial cleft affects the recurrence risk. For example, if a parent has isolated unilateral cleft lip, the recurrence risk is about 2.5%. If there is unilateral cleft lip and cleft palate, the risk increases to 4%, whereas if there is bilateral cleft lip with cleft palate, the risk is over 5.5% (Gorlin et al., 1990).

ASSOCIATED ANOMALIES

Cleft lip and/or cleft palate most often occur as isolated anomalies. In these cases, several thorough patient examinations conducted over several years have revealed no other primary abnormalities. This state-

TABLE 2.2

Facial Clefts—Empirical Recurrence Risks (%)

| Parents | Siblings | | Cleft Lip ± Palate | Cleft Palate |
	Affected	Normal		
Normal parents	1	0	4.0	3.5
	1	1	4.0	3.0
	2	0	14.0	13.0
One parent affected	0	0	4.0	3.5
	1	0	12.0	10.0
	1	1	10.0	9.0
	2	0	25.0	24.0
Both parents affected	0	0	35.0	25.0
	1	0	45.0	35.0
	1	1	40.0	35.0
	2	0	50.0	45.0

Note. Derived from "Empirical Recurrence Risk Figures for Genetic Counseling of Clefts" by M. Tolarová, 1972, *Acta Chirurgiae Plasticae* (Praha) *14*, p. 235. Copyright 1972 by Czechoslovak Medical Press. Adapted with permission.

TABLE 2.3
Comparative Empirical Risks (%) for Cleft Lip ± Cleft Palate and for Cleft Palate

Relative	Cleft Lip ± Palate Proband		Cleft Palate Proband	
	Male	Female	Male	Female
Brother	6.7	6.8	1.8	2.8
Sister	2.8	4.4	3.7	1.7
Father	3.0	3.1	1.2	1.2
Mother	1.6	3.1	4.8	5.5
Son	6.7	2.4	11.5	6.0
Daughter	4.0	8.7	5.6	17.2

Note. Adapted from *The Etiology of Cleft Lip and Cleft Palate* (pp. 239 and 243) by M. Melnick, D. Bixler, and E. D. Shields (Eds.), 1980, *Progress in Clinical and Biological Research* (vol. 46), New York: Alan R. Liss. Copyright 1980 by Alan R. Liss. Adapted with permission.

ment would exclude, for example, middle ear infections, which frequently occur *secondary* to cleft palate.

Data secured at birth differ from data obtained at surgery, because those patients with more serious defects often succumb prior to surgery. When data are broken down according to subtype, there is general agreement that other congenital anomalies are far more often associated with CP only (20% to 50%) than with either CL only (7% to 13%) or CLP (2% to 11%). Emanuel et al. (1972) found that the frequency with which one or more malformations accompanied clefts of all types was almost 28%.

More malformations have been found in infants with bilateral cleft lip with or without cleft palate than in those with unilateral cleft lip. Associated anomalies are more frequently noted in patients without a family with clefts than in patients with affected relatives. Congenital velopharyngeal incompetence has been found to be frequently associated with cervical anomalies. The more malformations a child has, the lighter the birth weight.

As noted earlier, some of these associated findings form recognizable cleft syndromes. Perhaps as much as 5% of facial clefting is syndromal, and approximately 50% of cleft syndromes have single-gene inheritance (Shprintzen, Siegel-Sadowitz, Amato, & Goldberg, 1985). In 1971, Gorlin, Cervenka, and Pruzansky listed 72 such syndromes. This was increased to 133 such disorders by Cohen in 1978 and to over 204 cleft conditions by Lynch and Kimberling in 1981. The latter authors listed 47 autosomal-dominant, 55 autosomal-recessive, 6 X-linked, 32 chromosomal, and 64 disorders of unknown nature that are associated with facial clefting. A current estimate of the number of cleft syndromes is in excess of 250, with new ones described each year.

GENETIC COUNSELING

Genetic counseling is sometimes sought by parents of a child with a craniofacial anomaly, such as cleft lip and/or palate, who want to know why it happened and whether it will happen to subsequent children. A counselee may be the individual with the disorder, or perhaps a close family member, or even someone who plans to marry into the family. The counselee may represent a social agency involved in adoption. Not uncommonly, a couple will seek genetic counseling prenatally or even during pregnancy. Some couples become concerned when they learn that they are distantly related to affected individuals.

The definition of genetic counseling has changed with time and is still in flux. One role of the genetic counselor is to help provide answers to these individuals' questions. However, genetic counseling is much broader than merely communicating facts and probabilities regarding certain specific disorders. It also should help the person to cope with fear, anger, and guilt. The counselor also helps the counselee to understand the diagnosis or lack of diagnosis, the nature of the disorder, and the probable course of the condition if diagnosis has been established. Counseling should also involve a discussion of management of the condition. The counselor should discuss various options or courses of action available to the counselee based on the risks in each case and the ethical and religious views of each family. An inordinate number of concerns are of greater immediate importance in the counseling role than the presentation of a recurrence risk. These concerns often require the counselor to play a role in psychological support, trying to eliminate guilt if it exists or, if that fails, at least to distribute the guilt as much as possible, so that it becomes more easily vitiated.

The background of genetic counselors until recently has been quite variable. Some have had intensive training in human genetics. Others have developed an interest in counseling for only a single disorder or for a limited number of conditions. With the relatively recent establishment of the American Board of Medical Genetics, it is reasonable to assume that all major health science centers will have certified genetic counselors and that requirements concerning training programs and qualifications will become more exacting.

Counselors' approaches to patients vary. In general, most genetic counseling is nondirective; that is, the genetic counselor attempts to stay removed from ultimate decision making, being careful not to transmit personal bias to the patient. Directive counselors, however, feel that some patients need to be led. They argue that the patient is asking for help and that it is the counselor's role to direct the patient in a positive manner toward reaching that goal. Many patients either consciously or unconsciously place the counselor in the position of making the decision for them by asking, "What would you do if you were I?" Most counselors respond by saying that they cannot be placed in such a position because they cannot know all the factors involved and that there are emotional aspects to the case that are not transferable. Most counselors try to be uninvolved and to avoid exhibiting preference for any single option. They believe that their function has come to an end when the risk of recurrence has been estimated. Nevertheless, subtle movements or facial expressions (body language) often convey the counselor's bias to the counselee.

To counsel, one first needs the correct diagnosis. The counselor may or may not be the diagnostician. To blindly accept an unconfirmed diagnosis and to base one's discussion of the case on possibly spurious evidence is an untenable situation. Because of the desire to have a disorder labeled (which pleases both patient and diagnostician), individuals will be understandably discomfited if the original diagnosis is replaced with "disorder unknown." Even if the prognosis of the erroneously named disorder were grim, its replacement by an unknown prognosis produces fear. This fear and the attendant resentment, even though not articulated, may often inhibit the process of counseling. The counselor's use of specialists, whether local, national, or international, to establish a diagnosis should be encouraged. The specialist should be supplied with a thorough history, laboratory findings, and excellent-quality color transparencies and radiographs (if relevant). Computer-assisted diagnostic services are available, but the answers obtained are only as good as the information supplied. A good clinician can often prevent countless dollars from being expended on myriad useless laboratory tests.

Once the diagnosis has been established, the counselor enters an informative role. A family pedigree should *always* be constructed, even in the "simplest" situations. It may not be possible to complete the pedigree in a single session; bits and pieces of information may be gathered over weeks or even months. Contacts may have to be made with various health professionals or agencies. Relatives who might provide useful information may be less than cooperative, resenting intrusion into matters they consider personal. In the process of data gathering, the skilled counselor may encounter information that could be detrimental were it to fall into the hands of unethical persons. Questions arise as to whether all information acquired regarding a patient or family should be made available to the person who seeks counsel, and whether other relatives are entitled to this information.

One cannot emphasize strongly enough the importance of keeping accurate records. They should be kept up to date and in good order, and should be easily accessible. Counseling sessions that are highly charged with emotion may be tape-recorded and a transcript sent to the counselee. It is important that the counselee's nodding in agreement seldom be considered to reflect understanding or, in fact, total hearing. The psychological trauma of the birth of an abnormal infant often works against communication. A reasonable test is to ask the counselee to repeat in his or her own words what the counselor has said. The revealed lack of understanding or fabricated misinformation is often shocking to the neophyte. In any event, a follow-up letter that summarizes the findings (both positive and negative), the diagnosis (if one has been determined), and the counseling information given (or nature of disorder) should be as explicit as possible. It is a good idea to have counselees sign a statement that they have received counseling and have understood the material presented (if they have, of course). A copy of this *signed and witnessed* statement should be kept in the patient's file.

Sometimes, especially in the case of an isolated malformed infant, a counselor cannot give the odds of recurrence because the underlying condition has not been identified. In those cases, should a counselor "bracket" the odds? For example, in the case of a mentally retarded male infant, a study of banded chromosomes reveals a normal karyotype. Does the statement, "The chance for recurrence is somewhere between 0 and 25 percent" completely cover the situation? Although 25% would be the recurrence risk of a disorder with autosomal or X-linked recessive inheritance and 0% (or near that) would represent a new dominant mutation, the estimate would *not* cover the much higher chance of recurrence if a mother were still subject to the same unknown teratogen. Nor would it cover unaffected parents who have two or more children with a known dominant disorder due to segmental mutation in a testis or ovary. Although these are extremely rare examples, they are *real* examples. Obviously one has to compromise lest one scare parents of a malformed child from having future children.

Another aspect of counseling involves dealing with caveats reported by the "sensationalist" media. Most caveats are based on isolated case reports, rarely on prospective studies; however, retrospective data are always suspect. The associated feeling of guilt in having parented a malformed child may be transferred to something done or not done or to some agent consumed or not consumed during pregnancy. The media may inappropriately expound on such a report. It is important to remember that *because an agent is teratogenic in a mouse does not mean that it is teratogenic in a rat, no less in man.*

Finally, a few words about the role of the genetic counselor and the law. A marked increase has occurred in litigation regarding genetic malpractice. These cases have been largely concerned with "wrongful birth" and/or "wrongful life." These cases have involved the failure of the health professional to meet a certain standard of care because of omission or commission that injures or harms a patient. The genetic counselor may fail to advise the counselee (a) that the risk for recurrence is greater than normal or (b) to what degree the risk is enhanced. This failure could lead to a claim of *wrongful birth* (the parent's claim) or *wrongful life* (the child's claim).

REFERENCES

Abyholm, F. E. (1978). Cleft lip and palate in Norway. *Scandinavian Journal of Plastic and Reconstructive Surgery, 12,* 29–34.

Altemus, L. A. (1966). The incidence of cleft lip and cleft palate among North American Negroes. *Cleft Palate Journal, 3,* 357–361.

Bear, J. C. (1976). A genetic study of facial clefting in Northern England. *Clinical Genetics, 9,* 277–284.

Blake, G. B., & Wreakes, G. (1972). Clefts of the lip and palate in twins. *British Journal of Plastic Surgery, 25,* 155–164.

Bonaiti, C., Briard, M. L., Feingold, J., Pavy, B., Psaume, J., Migne-Tufferand, G., & Kaplan, J. (1982). An epidemiological and genetic study of facial clefting in France: I. Epidemiology and frequency in relatives. *Journal of Medical Genetics, 19,* 8–15.

Bonaiti-Pellie, C., & Smith, C. (1974). Risk tables for genetic counselling in some common congenital malformations. *Journal of Medical Genetics, 11,* 374–377.

Cervenka, J., & Shapiro, B. (1970). Cleft uvula in Chippewa Indians: Prevalence and genetics. *Human Biology, 42,* 47–52.

Ching, G. H., & Chung, C. S. (1974). A genetic study of cleft lip and palate in Hawaii: I. Interracial crosses. *American Journal of Human Genetics, 26,* 162–176.

Chosack, A., & Eidelman, E. (1978). Cleft uvula: Prevalence and genetics. *Cleft Palate Journal, 15,* 63–67.

Chung, C. S., Bixler, D., Watanabe, T., Koguchi, H., & Fogh-Andersen, P. (1986). Segregation analysis of cleft lip with or without cleft palate: A comparison of Danish and Japanese data. *American Journal of Human Genetics, 39,* 603–611.

Cohen, M. M., Jr. (1978). Syndromes with cleft lip and palate. *Cleft Palate Journal, 15,* 306–328.

Emanuel, I., Huang, S-W., Gutman, L. T., Yu, F-C., & Lin, C. C. (1972). The incidence of congenital malformations in a Chinese population: The Taipei collaborative study. *Teratology, 5,* 159–170.

Fogh-Andersen, P. (1942). *Inheritance of harelip and cleft palate*. Copenhagen: A. Busck.

Fraser, F. C. (1974). Updating the genetics of cleft lip and palate. *Birth Defects, 10*(8), 107–111.

Gorlin, R. J., Cervenka, J., & Pruzansky, S. (1971). Facial clefting and its syndromes. *Birth Defects, 7*(7), 3–49.

Gorlin, R. J., Cohen, M. M., Jr., & Levin, L. S. (1990). *Syndromes of the head and neck* (3rd ed.). New York: Oxford University Press.

Heckler, F. R., Oesterle, L. G., & Jabaley, M. E. (1979). The minimal cleft revisited: Clinical and anatomic correlations. *Cleft Palate Journal, 16*, 240–247.

Hoppe, W. (1965). Lippen-, Kiefer-, Gaumenspalten. *Archiv fur Kinderheilkunde, 171* (Suppl. 52), 1–54.

Jaffe, B. F., & DeBlanc, G. B. (1972). Cleft palate, cleft lip and cleft uvula in Navajo Indians. *Cleft Palate Journal, 7*, 301–305.

Johnston, M. C., Hassell, J. R., & Brown, K. S. (1975). The embryology of cleft lip and palate. *Clinics in Plastic Surgery, 2*, 195–203.

Johnston, M. C., & Sulik, K. K. (1979). Some abnormal patterns of development in the craniofacial region. *Birth Defects, 15*(8), 23–42.

Leck, I. (1984). The geographical distribution of neural tube defects and oral clefts. *British Medical Bulletin, 40*, 390–395.

Lehman, J. A., & Artz, J. S. (1976). The minimal cleft lip. *Plastic and Reconstructive Surgery, 58*, 306–309.

Leutert, G., & Heiner, H. (1962). Zur histologie und klinik der lateralen oberlippen-furcher. *Archiv Klinische Chirurgiae, 299*, 791.

Lindemann, G., Riis, B., & Sewerin, I. (1977). Prevalence of cleft uvula among 2,732 Danes. *Cleft Palate Journal, 14*, 226–229.

Lowry, R. B., & Trimble, B. K. (1977). Incidence rates for cleft lip and palate in British Columbia 1952–1971 for North American Indian, Japanese, Chinese and total populations: Secular trends over twenty years. *Teratology, 16*, 277–283.

Lynch, H. T., & Kimberling, W. J. (1981). Genetic counseling in cleft lip and cleft palate. *Plastic and Reconstructive Surgery, 68*, 800–815.

Melnick, M., Bixler, D., Fogh-Andersen, P., & Conneally, P. M. (1980). Cleft lip ± cleft palate: An overview of the literature and an analysis of Danish cases born between 1941 and 1968. *American Journal of Medical Genetics, 6*, 83–97.

Melnick, M., Bixler, D., & Shields, E. D. (Eds.). (1980). *The etiology of cleft lip and cleft palate. Progress in clinical and biological research*. (vol. 46). New York: Alan R. Liss.

Natsume, N., & Kawai, T. (1986). Incidence of cleft lip and cleft palate in 39,696 Japanese babies born during 1983. *International Journal of Oral Surgery, 15*, 565–568.

Owens, J. R., Jones, J. W., & Harris, F. (1985). Epidemiology of facial clefting. *Archives of Diseases in Childhood, 60*, 521–524.

Poswillo, D. (1979). The pathogenesis of submucous cleft palate. *Scandinavian Journal of Plastic and Reconstructive Surgery, 8*, 34–41.

Reich, T. (1979). The use of multiple thresholds and segregation analysis in analyzing the phenotypic heterogeneity of multifactorial traits. *Annals of Human Genetics, 42,* 371–390.

Schaumann, B. F., Peagler, F. D., & Gorlin, R. J. (1970). Minor craniofacial anomalies among a Negro population. *Oral Surgery, Oral Medicine and Oral Pathology, 29,* 566–575.

Schweckendiek, W. (1973). Further findings concerning the occurrence of clefts in twins. *Journal of Maxillofacial Surgery, 1,* 109–112.

Shields, E. D., Bixler, D., & Fogh-Andersen, P. (1979). Facial clefts in Danish twins. *Cleft Palate Journal, 16,* 1–6.

Shields, E. D., Bixler, D., & Fogh-Andersen, P. (1981). Cleft palate: A genetic and epidemiologic investigation. *Clinical Genetics, 20,* 13–24.

Shprintzen, R. J., Siegel-Sadowitz, V. L., Amato, J., & Goldberg, R. B. (1985). Anomalies associated with cleft lip, cleft palate, or both. *American Journal of Medical Genetics, 20,* 585–595.

Skoog, T. (1965). The management of bilateral cleft of the primary palate. *Plastic and Reconstructive Surgery, 35,* 40.

Spence, M. A., Westlake, J., Lange, K., & Gold, D. P. (1976). Estimation of polygenic recurrence risk for cleft lip and palate. *Human Heredity, 26,* 327–336.

Tolarová, M. (1972). Empirical recurrence risk figures for genetic counseling of clefts. *Acta Chirurgiae Plasticae (Praha), 14,* 234–235.

Tolarová, M. (1987a). Orofacial clefts in Czechoslovakia. Incidence, genetics and prevention of cleft lip and palate over a 19-year period. *Scandinavian Journal of Plastic and Reconstructive Surgery, 21,* 19–25.

Tolarová, M. (1987b). A study of the incidence, sex ratio, laterality and clinical severity in 3,660 probands with facial clefts in Czechoslovakia. *Acta Chirurgiae Plasticae (Praha), 29,* 77–87.

Tolarová, M., & Morton, N. E. (1975). Empirical recurrence risks in facial clefts. *Acta Chirurgiae Plasticae (Praha), 17,* 97–112.

Vanderas, A. P. (1987). Incidence of cleft lip, cleft palate, and cleft lip and palate among races: A review. *Cleft Palate Journal, 24,* 216–225.

Woolf, C. M. (1971). Congenital cleft lip: A genetic study of 496 propositi. *Journal of Medical Genetics, 8,* 65–83.

CHAPTER 3

Surgical Issues and Procedures

Alan R. Shons

Shons points out that the surgeon is only one member of the interdisciplinary team and "outlines" a surgical approach for the patient with a cleft lip and palate. Surgical repair of the cleft lip and palate is presented from historical, timing, and current techniques perspectives.

1. *Why does Shons caution against rapid introduction of new surgical techniques as applied to persons with cleft lip and palate?*
2. *What are the general goals of cleft lip and palate repair?*
3. *How does Shons feel about presurgical orthopedics prior to lip repair? Can you think of disadvantages to presurgical orthopedic appliances in infants?*
4. *Why do you think bilateral cleft lip repair is more than twice the problem of unilateral cleft lip repair?*
5. *Explain the general procedures involved in the surgical construction of a pharyngeal flap as opposed to sphincter pharyngoplasty. What is the primary indication for the use of each?*
6. *Defend Shons's statement "the surgical care of the cleft lip and/or palate patient represents a continuum from birth to adulthood." Does it make any sense to say how many surgeries a child with cleft lip and palate needs to have?*

Plastic and reconstructive surgery is the surgery of defects and deformities of the skin and underlying musculoskeletal framework. The specialty originated with the early developments in facial reconstruction. The work of Tagliacozzi in 16th-century nasal reconstruction is a cornerstone of modern plastic surgery. Today, a significant component of any plastic surgeon's practice is related to aesthetic and reconstructive facial surgery. The educational background of the typical plastic surgeon involved with cleft work today includes 4 years of medical school, 5 years of general surgical residency, followed by 2 or 3 years of plastic surgical residency, and often 1 or 2 years of additional craniofacial fellowship.

Beginning in the Middle Ages, plastic surgeons pioneered the development of techniques for the correction of deformities relating to cleft lip and palate. Cleft lip and palate surgical repair is an example of a surgical problem compounded by the effects of growth and development. The surgery performed may have a profound effect on growth, and growth may have a significant effect on the ultimate result of the surgical procedure. The development of new techniques is fraught with uncertainty because the final result of a surgical procedure on an infant will not be known until growth is complete. What may appear brilliant in the short run may ultimately prove harmful if the effects of growth are not favorable.

Because there is a 20-year time span between application of the technique on a newborn and appreciation of the final result, careful long-term follow-up is essential. Due to the long time span, analyses of the results of surgical procedures are frequently not performed by the individuals responsible for their development. On the one hand, this lends an element of objectivity to long-term studies; on the other hand, investigators may lack interest in someone else's work, and their analyses may be less than complete. In the discussion that follows, the reader should keep in mind that rapid evolution of surgical techniques continues to occur and controversies exist in many areas. Although there is constancy in general principles, the surgical techniques of today will not be the surgical techniques of tomorrow.

In this chapter, I outline a surgical approach to the patient with cleft lip and/or palate. I believe the plastic surgeon is only one member of a comprehensive, interdisciplinary team. As suggested in Chapter 1, the approach to the complex longitudinal problem of a patient with cleft lip and/or palate must be a patient-oriented rather than a specialty-oriented effort. Input from the various members of the specialty team must be assembled by a team director/coordinator, and a coherent plan of treatment set forth. The direction of the team must not be dominated by a single specialist. The team leader may be a member of any specialty, but must have leadership experience and a genuine interest in the proper management of a team effort. The skilled leader improves the quality of team decisions, and the method employed by the capable leader ensures the acceptance of those decisions by the group (Maier, 1963).

The birth of a child with cleft lip and/or palate is a psychological blow to any family. The parents feel initial shock and distress, and often guilt. The parents may express multiple concerns, including "What did we do wrong?" "What could we have done to prevent it?" and "What is the chance that another child will be born with the same problem?" The plastic surgeon is often one of the first members of the specialty team to meet with the parents. During the initial examination of the child and the discussion with the parents, the surgeon must take great care to be supportive and optimistic in assuring the parents of the steps that can be taken to correct the deformity.

The surgical considerations are complex, the current surgical techniques are limited, and the healing process cannot be well controlled. Nevertheless, the surgeon can take a positive approach and outline a general plan of treatment. In early discussions with parents, the surgeon should emphasize the long-term sequential order of events and provide details primarily for the first step which, in many patients, is lip repair. It is unrealistic to think that all questions can be answered initially because much information will be forgotten or not understood by parents who are just beginning to cope with the realities of their child's deformity and its management.

In the initial discussion with the parents, the surgeon needs to present a general timetable of surgical events to provide the parents with an appreciation that surgical treatment must be closely related to the child's growth and development. Lip repair can be accomplished any time from the first few days of life to several months of age. The palate can be repaired from a few months to several years of age. Nasal work is often begun at the time of lip repair, but may not be definitively completed until facial growth is complete in the middle to perhaps late teens. The timing of the various steps is discussed in more detail when the surgical techniques are outlined later in this chapter. Although the surgeon should not emphasize the detailed timing of procedures in the initial discussion with parents, he or she should stress the concept of a continuity of care requiring several steps from the neonatal period to adulthood.

The objective of surgery for the child with cleft lip and/or palate is the achievement of a functionally and aesthetically normal individual. Specifically, lip alignment and muscle function should be normal; surface scars should be minimally visible; the nose must display symmetry with the airways functionally open; alveolar integrity must be present, permitting preservation of teeth within the cleft area and permitting orthodontic correction of tooth malalignment; the palate must be intact to allow normal speech development; and palate repair should not adversely affect maxillary growth.

CLEFT LIP

History

The first recorded cleft lip repair was performed by an unknown Chinese surgeon in approximately 390 AD (Boo-Chai, 1966). A 16th-century French surgeon, Pierre Franco, is considered the father of cleft lip surgery, having published a clear description of an operative repair for cleft lip (Franco, 1561). The next 300 years saw little progress, although numerous surgical advances were made during the Renaissance. The early techniques involved simply paring the cleft edges, allowing healing of the raw surfaces (Pare, 1575). Later, the cleft edges were sharply incised and some type of suture material, frequently combined with pins, was used (Veau, 1938). In the early 19th century, Von Graefe suggested a curving incision to prevent notching of the straight-line closure used previously (Lexer, 1904). Malgaigne (1834) first described cleft lip repair using flaps of local tissue. He designed inferiorly based flaps, medial and lateral to the cleft, that were turned down and closed back to back. This procedure added fullness at the vermillion border and was designed to prevent the whistle deformity or notching of the lip. In 1844, Mirault refined Malgaigne's technique and, by discarding a portion of Malgaigne's medial flap, developed a technique involving a lower lateral flap turned across the cleft. This technique was the forerunner of today's flap closure operations (Mirault, 1844).

Modern techniques of lip repair, like the ancient methods, are commonly associated with individual names. Straight-line operations involving paring the edges of the cleft with closure began with Von Graefe and were refined by Rose (1891) and Thompson (1912). Lower one-third operations include techniques by Owen (1904), in which a flap is rotated from the medial to the cleft side, and by Brown and McDowell (1945), in which a flap is rotated from the lateral to the medial side. Lower one-third triangular flap operations involving a three-limb incision evolved into the widely used Tennison (1952) method. A lower one-third flap operation involving a quadrilateral flap was first suggested by Hagedorn (1884) and refined and popularized by LeMesurier (1962). Upper one-third flap operations in which a modification of the Z-plasty technique is employed is illustrated by the Millard rotation advancement technique (Millard, 1960, 1968). The Millard technique has gained wide acceptance over the last 15 years and is now the method of choice of most craniofacial surgeons around the world. The Skoog repair (1969) combines an upper and lower flap within the upper lip.

Preoperative Care

A child with an isolated incomplete cleft lip may be breast fed; however, children with complete clefts of the lip and palate may present feeding problems. Feeding is usually not a significant problem, and most children can be managed effectively. Holding the child in the semi-upright position during feeding will minimize nasal regurgitation. Because the child with a cleft palate cannot suck normally, special feeding devices and techniques have been developed. The simplest is a nipple with an enlarged crosscut hole, which may be attached to a soft squeezable container or a feeder with a collapsible reservoir. These devices prove satisfactory for most infants. If the child's cleft is unusually wide, modification of nipple feeders may not be adequate, and some type of bulb syringe with a catheter tip may be necessary.

Timing of Cleft Lip Repair

Repair of the lip can be accomplished at any time after birth, even before the child initially leaves the hospital. Lip repair in the first 2 to 3 days of life is frequently done under local anesthesia. The healing process is most favorable in utero, where experimental cleft lip repairs in mice have produced no visible scar (Hallock, 1985). The healing process becomes relatively less favorable with each day following birth.

I believe that 3 to 4 weeks of age is an ideal time for lip repair. At this point, the total status of the patient is known, weight gain is established, and general anesthesia is an acceptable risk. The healing process is still very favorable, and the lip scar should be much less obvious than in a repair performed at 2 to 3 months of age following the old rule of 10s for surgical timing: 10 weeks, 10 lb, and 10 g of hemoglobin. The medial alveolar segment in complete unilateral clefts and the premaxilla in bilateral clefts will mold easily in response to soft tissue pressure of the repaired lip at 3 to 4 weeks of age. Alveolar remodeling is slower and less certain in a child 2 or 3 months old.

Bilateral lip repairs are done completely at 3 to 4 weeks of age. Complete unilateral clefts in which there is reasonable alignment of the alveolus also are repaired at 3 to 4 weeks. For the complete unilateral cleft lip with marked forward displacement of the medial alveolar segment, a lip adhesion is performed at 2 to 3 weeks of age and formal lip repair is completed 2 months later.

Preoperative Maxillary Positioning

Presurgical maxillary orthopedics, using a variety of intraoral and extraoral appliances, can improve alignment of the alveolar segments prior to lip repair (Georgiade & Latham, 1975; Hagerty, Mylin, & Hess, 1969).

The lip adhesion technique of Randall (1965) is an alternative to orthopedics in the wide cleft. I believe, generally, that presurgical orthopedics
is unnecessary if the lip is repaired within the first month. Soft tissue
pressure from a lip adhesion or definitive lip repair provides the most
natural force for the development of satisfactory alveolar dental arch
form. In clefts repaired later, orthopedic repositioning may be necessary to achieve movement of the more firmly fixed alveolar segments.

Unilateral Cleft Lip Repair Techniques

Lip adhesion.   A lip adhesion may be indicated in the wide complete
cleft to achieve molding of the underlying alveolus and to stretch the
tissues surrounding the cleft prior to definitive lip repair. The technique
is not required in complete clefts in which the alveolar segments are
well aligned. The technique of Randall (1965, 1971; Randall & Graham,
1971) is widely used.

The operation is performed under general anesthesia. Lip markings
are placed to be used for the definitive repair (see Figure 3.1A). Flaps
are devised within tissue that would be discarded in the definitive repair.
An anterior rectangular flap on the medial cleft margin is raised, including mucosa and some of the underlying muscle. Similarly, a posterior
rectangular flap is created from mucosa and underlying musculature
on the lateral side (Figure 3.1B). Finally, 5-0 vicryl sutures are used
to approximate the mucosa and muscle layers, and 7-0 chromic sutures
are used on the skin (Figure 3.1C).

The technique provides a reasonably secure soft tissue closure. If
a dehiscence or wound breakdown occurs, the wound is treated conser-
vatively until surface healing is complete, and a definitive repair is then
performed. A more extensive lip adhesion technique has been advocated
by Furnas (1984).

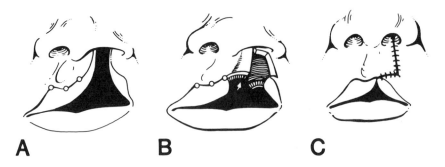

A   **B**   **C**

Figure 3.1 Lip adhesion.

Straight-line repair (Rose–Thompson technique). The straight-line repair technique should be used only for the minimal cleft or prenatal scar (Rose, 1891; Thompson, 1912). The resulting suture line is in good position, being near the line of the philtral ridge. Measurements can be precise, and with the inclusion of a Z-plasty in the mucosal area, a very satisfactory lip can result. The procedure is a poor choice for a wide or a complete cleft in that too much marginal cleft tissue is discarded.

As shown in Figure 3.2A, points 4 and 5 are marked in the nostril floor at the base of the columella. The apexes of the cupid's bow are marked (1 and 3), as is the center of the cupid's bow (2). If the nostril floor is wide on the cleft side, an additional point 6 is placed, and the distance from point 5 to point 6 is the width to be excised. The length of the lip along the philtral crease on the normal side (between points 1 and 4) is then transferred to the cleft side by measuring from 6 to 7 on the vermillion margin. The distance from 4 to 1 must equal that from 6 to 7 and that from 5 to 3. Both elements on the cleft side are usually shorter; thus, a curving incision is indicated to gain length. The back cut of the curve into both medial and lateral segments of the lip must be conservative to preserve the maximum amount of tissue. The wound is repaired in layers, first securely closing the muscle with 5-0 vicryl sutures (Figure 3.2B), and then the skin with 7-0 chromic sutures (Figure 3.2C). A Z-plasty is employed on the mucosal portion of the incision to prevent notching (Figure 3.2D).

Upper one-third flap repair (Millard rotation advancement). Millard's rotation advancement technique can be used for all clefts (Millard, 1960, 1968, 1976a, 1976b). The technique is best suited to the incomplete or narrow cleft. There are technical difficulties in the application of the technique to the wide complete cleft, for which some surgeons prefer the triangular flap Tennison–Randall technique, described below. The incision line in Millard's technique is a curving approximation of the philtral ridge. This produces a more normal appearing cupid's bow and philtrum than the triangular or the rectangular techniques, which create an irregular scar superior to the cupid's bow. Deficiency of the nostril sill is improved. Revisions are easier than with other techniques. I use this technique as the procedure of choice for unilateral cleft lip repair regardless of the cleft configuration.

As shown in Figure 3.3A, the lateral points of the cupid's bow (points 1 and 3) and the midpoint (2) are marked. The rotation incision is outlined, curving upward from point 3 across the base of the columella to point 5, which is medial to the philtral ridge. A back-cut (from 5 to X) may be necessary to allow downward rotation of the medial lip element. The back-cut is normally no more than 2 to 3 mm. The distance from the normal commissure (point 6) to the lateral margin of the cupid's bow

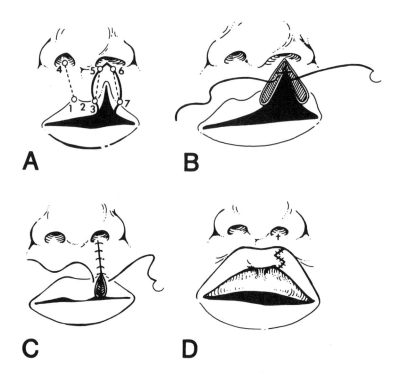

Figure 3.2 Unilateral straight-line repair.

(point 1) is measured and marked on the cleft side from the commissure (point 7) to point 8. The incision along the cleft lateral side then extends superiorly from 8 to 9, the upper extent of adequate skin thickness, and the incision curves laterally to points 10 and 11 around the left alar base. The distance from 3 to 5 to X must equal that from 8 to 9 and the distance from 1 to 2 must equal that from 8 to 10. Incisions are made, and flap C is used to achieve columella lengthening. A relaxing incision in the sublabial sulcus is necessary to mobilize the lateral flap (Figure 3.3B). The lateral portion of flap C joins the alar base flap. A small interdigitating flap at the vermillion border of the lateral segment is created to be transposed medially to break up the scar line and give additional fullness at the vermillion border (Figure 3.3C). The wound is closed in layers, using interrupted 5-0 vicryl sutures on the muscle layer and interrupted 7-0 chromic sutures on the skin edge (Figure 3.3D).

Randall (1971) described a muscle flap technique utilizing the rotation advancement incision. A flap of orbicularis oris muscle is dissected

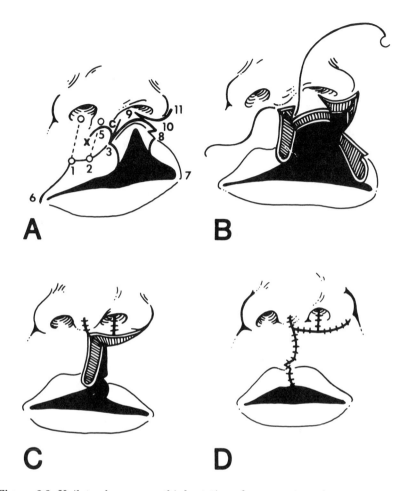

Figure 3.3 Unilateral upper one-third rotation advancement repair.

from the lateral edge of the cleft, detached from its insertion into the area of the alar base, and transposed in a horizontal fashion across the cleft. A tunnel is created on the cleft side, and the muscle is securely sutured. This approach is typical of the emphasis now properly placed on muscle realignment in both unilateral and bilateral cleft repairs. Surgeons must perform an extensive dissection of the muscle to the lateral margins of the upper lip in all cleft repairs to achieve a well-aligned muscle continuity.

Lower one-third flap repair (Tennison–Randall). The triangular flap technique is preferred by some surgeons for repair of the wide complete cleft. The cupid's bow is preserved and well aligned with this method. Requisite fullness is produced in the area of the mucocutaneous border. Very little tissue is discarded. Disadvantages of the technique include a scar in the lower portion of the lip, which is not as favorable as the scar produced by the rotation advancement method. The operation requires careful preoperative marking and measuring. Very little adjustment can be made once initial incisions are made. The technique used was described by Randall as a modification and clarification of the Tennison procedure (Hagedorn, 1884; Randall, 1959).

As shown in Figure 3.4A, the lateral margins of the cupid's bow (points 1 and 3) and the midpoint (2) are marked. Point 5 is marked at the base of the columella on the cleft side, and point 6 is the corresponding position lateral to the cleft at the alar base. A line is drawn from a midpoint of the columella to the midpoint of the cupid's bow. Another line is drawn perpendicular to this midline, intersecting the lateral margin of the cupid's bow on the cleft side. Point 7 is marked halfway between the intersection of the two perpendicular lines and the midpoint of the cupid's bow. Point 8 on the lateral segment is marked at the medial extent of a normal vermillion cutaneous ridge. The distance from 4 to 1 equals that from 5 to 3 *plus* that from 7 to 3. Point 9 is placed so that the distance from 6 to 9 equals the distance from 5 to 3. Point 10 is placed so that the distance from 9 to 10 equals that from 7 to 3. The interposed lateral triangular flap allows downward rotation of the cupid's bow. The technique rotates the orbicularis oris muscle in the lower portion of the lip to a more normal transverse position. By preserving all possible muscle in the superior segment of the lateral lip element and discarding only vermillion, it is possible to create an upper flap that can be detached from the alar base insertion and brought transversely across the repair. This flap adds an important functional component to the repair (Figure 3.4B). The flaps are approximated using interrupted 5-0 vicryl sutures to the muscle layers and interrupted 7-0 chromic sutures to the skin edge (Figure 3.4C).

Combined upper and lower lip flap repair (Skoog). The Skoog (1969) technique discards little or no tissue. The nostril floor is supplemented by a superior lateral flap. The lower lateral triangular flap is designed in a fashion similar to that in the Tennison–Randall repair. An irregular suture line is created, which produces an acceptable scar. The technique as described by Skoog can be combined with a periosteal flap closure of the alveolar defect. Because multiple small flaps are created in this repair, it is technically demanding. The creation of multiple small flaps places an absolute limitation on intraoperative adjustment.

As seen in Figure 3.5A, markings are similar to those in the triangular flap method (Figure 3.4A). The difference is in the creation of

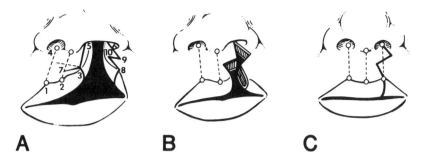

Figure 3.4 Unilateral lower one-third flap repair.

a small superiorly based flap on the lateral lip. Following initial lip incisions, attention is directed to flap closure of the alveolar cleft. Bilateral posteriorly based periosteal flaps are elevated, turned across the defect, and sutured (Figure 3.5B). The lateral lip segment is undermined and elevated off the underlying maxilla. A periosteal flap based superiorly and medially near the alar base is then developed laterally and transposed medially across the defect (Figure 3.5C). Medial lip incisions are made, and the cupid's bow is displaced downward (Figure 3.5D). The superior lateral flap is interposed at the base of the columella. An inferiorly based muscle flap is developed laterally, detaching the orbicularis oris muscle from the insertion near the base of the ala. This is transposed across the defect and sutured using interrupted 5-0 vicryl sutures (Figure 3.5E). The skin is closed with interrupted 7-0 chromic sutures (Figure 3.5F).

Bilateral Repair Techniques

The bilateral cleft lip represents a far more difficult problem than the unilateral cleft lip. A bilateral cleft lip is commonly associated with a complete cleft of the palate, although the deformity may involve only a cleft of the primary palate. The clefting may be asymmetrical and complete or incomplete. In the case of a bilateral complete cleft of the lip and palate, the premaxilla may protrude at an awkward angle and the prolabium may be diminutive and attached to the nose by what appears to be an almost nonexistent columella. The repair should be done in a single stage. Staged bilateral lip repairs create an obligatory asymmetry of scar and produce a short-term distorting force upon the premaxilla.

Cronin (1957) discussed the following principles for the plan of a bilateral cleft lip repair. The prolabium belongs in the upper lip and should be used to form the full vertical length of the midportion of the

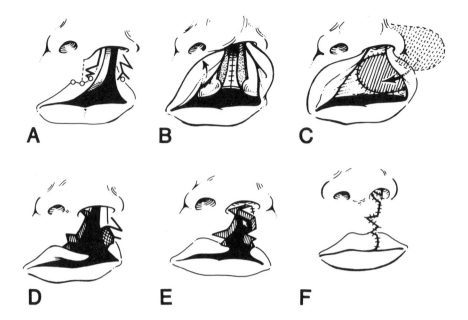

Figure 3.5 Unilateral combined upper and lower lip flap repair.

lip; the vermillion ridge of the prolabium should be preserved; the thin prolabium should be supplemented with mucosa–muscle flaps from the lateral lip elements; prior to lip closure, repositioning of the premaxillary segment should be accomplished; and collapse of the lateral maxillary segments should be prevented by an obturator.

I believe primary bilateral lip repair should be performed at 3 to 4 weeks of age. Orbicularis oris muscle continuity should be established if possible. Provision should be made for subsequent columella lengthening.

Marked protrusion of the premaxilla is common in the complete bilateral cleft. Deformity increases during the first few weeks of life due to unopposed forward pressure on the structure resulting from feeding and tongue movement. The easiest solution is early complete bilateral lip repair. The premaxilla is extremely mobile in the first month and, given the balanced pressure of lip repair, will mold back into position within a few days. Randall (1971) advocated bilateral lip adhesion to achieve setback of the premaxilla. This can achieve proper positioning of the premaxilla; however, lip adhesion in the bilateral cleft lip provides a tenuous soft tissue bridge that may easily dehisce (separate), compromising the integrity of the already inadequate medial soft tissue available for definitive lip repair. Maximum repair strength is obtained in formal lip repair.

If lip repair is delayed beyond 1 month, orthopedic repositioning of the premaxilla may be necessary before definitive lip repair. External elastic traction employing some type of head cap and lip band can be used (Clodius, 1964). All external elastic methods have the disadvantage of requiring constant care and supervision by the parents. Two types of intraoral traction devices have been described by Georgiade (1972; Georgiade & Latham, 1975). He first suggested a through-and-through maxillary wire placed in the pterygoid area with a Dacron strap around the premaxillary segment, attached to the anchoring transverse wire by a spring device. A later technique uses an intraoral expansion device that provides bilateral support, preventing collapse of the lateral maxillary segments, along with a pin device that permits slow repositioning of the premaxillary segment. A surgical setback of the premaxilla is an option that is rarely necessary (Kahn & Winsten, 1960). The surgical setback must be a conservative one that will permit lip closure under reasonable tension, but without compression of the premaxilla back into the confines of the arch as defined by the lateral maxillary segments.

Technical considerations in the repair of the bilateral cleft lip are similar to those described for the unilateral cleft lip.

Straight-line repair (Veau III).   Straight-line repair produces the shortest scars, which are in the area of the philtral ridge; however, the prolabial segment is usually too wide for this technique. Revisions of lips repaired by this technique are relatively easy, and the approach can yield a good result in the bilateral cleft (Brauer, 1971).

As shown in Figure 3.6A, point X is placed at the midline of the prolabial segment. Points 1 and 3 are placed at the lateral aspects of the prolabial segment, 4 to 5 mm from X. Points 4, 5, 6, and 8 are placed near the cleft edge. Points 7 and 9 are placed at the medial extent of normal fullness of the lateral lip segment vermillion. Lines 1 to 4 and 3 to 5 are slightly curved to provide adequate length. This distance should be no less than 9 mm. The vermillion border of the prolabial segment can be preserved, and a mucosal flap based inferiorly is turned down. Vermillion muscle flaps are created from the lateral lip segments and brought to the midline, supplementing soft tissue of the prolabial segment. These flaps should contain only mucosa and underlying muscle. Skin from the lateral lip segment should not be brought beneath the prolabial segment. Orbicularis oris muscle flaps can be developed from the lateral lip segments, detached from their alar base insertions, and sutured to rudimentary muscle of the prolabial segment or the subcutaneous tissue of the prolabial segment (Figure 3.6B). The lateral flaps

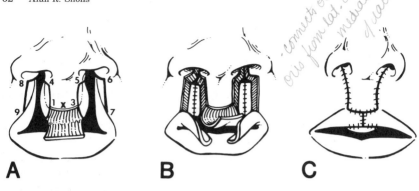

connects orbic. oris from lat. and medial part of each cleft

Figure 3.6 Bilateral straight-line repair.

are sutured in the midline or, if excess length is available, they can be crisscrossed. Muscles are sutured using interrupted 5-0 vicryl sutures, and skin is closed with interrupted 7-0 chromic sutures (Figure 3.6C).

Straight-line muscle repair with forked flaps (Millard). Millard's (1976a) two-stage technique is probably the most widely used technique today for bilateral cleft lip repair. An adequate prolabium is required for this technique. Bilateral forked flaps are developed and stored in the nostril sill for future use in columella lengthening. The alar bases are repositioned medially. Muscle continuity is reestablished through the prolabial segment, and a prolabium of normal dimension is achieved. Reentry into the well-healed lip is avoided at a later stage by creation of the forked flaps and storage of the flaps at the time of the initial operation.

As shown in Figure 3.7A, a new prolabial segment that will provide the philtrum is outlined. The distance between points 2 and 3 should be approximately 6 mm. The vertical height of the philtrum (from 3 to 5) should be 8 to 12 mm. The additional width of the prolabium, 1 to 2 and 3 to 4, is used for the creation of the forked flaps. Point 6 is placed at a position that will achieve adequate upper lip length. The distance from 6 to 7 should be 18 to 22 mm. The distance from 6 to X is one-half the distance from 2 to 3. The mucocutaneous ridge of the prolabium can be preserved if it is of good quality; otherwise, the mucocutaneous ridge is turned down in an inferiorly based mucosal flap. The prolabial skin is raised on a superior base with attached lateral forked flaps. Orbicularis oris musculature is dissected out laterally, detached from its alar base attachment, and brought across the midline. The mucosal flap based upon the premaxilla is turned superiorly to provide the inner portion of the labial gingival sulcus. Vermillion flaps based superiorly on the

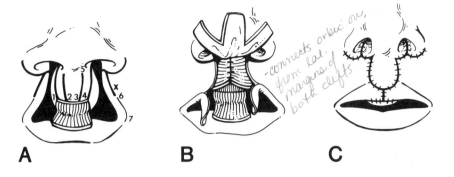

Figure 3.7 Bilateral straight-line muscle repair with forked flaps.

lateral lip elements can be used to provide lateral release of the nostrils (Figure 3.7B). The forked flaps are sutured temporarily into the nostril sill area. Lateral mucosal flaps from the lateral lip elements are approximated in the midline (Figure 3.7C).

The most commonly used lip repair techniques have been outlined above. Although this is not meant to be a handbook of surgical technique, the repairs are illustrated with sufficient detail for the reader to understand and appreciate the complexities of the surgical techniques and the basis for imperfections that may occur.

Alveolar Bone Grafting

Bone grafting of the alveolar cleft in complete unilateral or bilateral clefts has gained wide acceptance (see Chapter 4 for a more detailed discussion). The bone graft can provide stability of the dental arch and support of the alar base. The graft provides periodontal support for teeth at the cleft margins and allows stable eruption and preservation of permanent teeth in the cleft area.

The timing of the bone graft has been a continuing controversy. Bone grafting of the alveolar cleft during the first few months of life was advocated more than 30 years ago (Nordin & Johanson, 1955; Schmid, 1955). Long-term studies unfortunately showed a significant incidence of growth problems, including maxillary retrusion and lateral crossbite, developing in children who had undergone early bone grafting (Jolleys & Robertson, 1972). A group at Northwestern University has reported excellent results with a technique of alveolar cleft grafting using rib before 6 months of age (Bauer, 1989). Using a limited dissection technique, maxillary growth restriction has not been a problem.

The majority of cleft palate teams advocate alveolar cleft grafting during late primary dentition or early mixed dentition at 5 to 8 years of age. At this time, maxillary molars are present, allowing the placement of expansion devices, and the graft can provide stability for the eruption of the permanent dentition (Sadove, Nelson, & Jones, 1989). Cancellous iliac bone grafts are commonly used. Cranial bone is an alternative, and may provide a donor site with lower morbidity than the iliac crest. The characteristics of the cranial bone are not as ideal as the cancellous iliac bone for molding into the alveolar defects.

CLEFT PALATE

History

Whereas a cleft lip may represent a severe deformity of physical appearance, a cleft palate may represent a severe functional problem. In the isolated cleft palate patient, outward appearance is normal, yet the problems of swallowing, nasal regurgitation, velopharyngeal incompetence for speech, and middle ear problems can be very significant.

Throughout the Middle Ages, the problems of palatal clefts were recognized, but only crude remedies were offered. Obturators of various types were constructed by the dentists of the period. Various techniques were tried, including freshening the edges of the cleft and treatment with hot cautery. This apparently led to scarring closure in some cases. The modern approach to cleft palate repair began with Von Graefe (1817), who described a simple closure of a cleft palate. Dieffenbach in 1826 described closure of the hard palate by the use of lateral relaxing incisions. Further refinements of this technique were described by Von Langenbeck (1861). Lateral release incisions with hamular infractures plus elevation of full thickness mucoperiosteal flaps were used. In an attempt to improve speech results following palatal closure, various techniques of palatal retrodisplacement have been devised, leading to the development of the pushback Kilner–Veau–Wardill technique described by Peet (1961). The Furlow double Z-plasty cleft palate repair first presented by Furlow in 1978 has gained increasing recognition for improved speech results in clinics experienced in earlier techniques (Randall, LaRossa, Solomon, & Cohen, 1986). The Furlow repair achieves proper soft palate muscle realignment and added length, while minimizing anterior hard palate dissection.

Abnormalities of mid-facial growth are common in the long-term follow-up of repaired cleft palate patients. It is believed, but not conclusively proven, that surgical manipulation in the anterior palate area interferes with growth of the maxilla. Schweckendiek (1962) proposed early closure of only the soft palate, with obturator closure of the hard palate defect, in an effort to obviate the problems of facial growth retardation. The hard palate would then be closed at around age 13. In a follow-up study of patients treated in this fashion, Bardach, Morris, and Olin (1984) reported that facial growth was satisfactory and similar to growth seen with repairs by other techniques; however, the speech results were inferior. In a similar study of 30 patients assessed at age 7 following the Schweckendiek method, although a very low incidence of lateral crossbite was noted, speech results were inferior to patients in whom the hard and soft palate had been closed in one stage at the usual 8- to 18-month age (Jackson, McLennan, & Scheker, 1983).

Goals of Treatment

The objectives of cleft palate closure are creation of a mechanism capable of producing normal speech, preservation of hearing, and minimal interference with facial growth. The normal velopharyngeal valve is composed of the soft palate and the pharyngeal walls. The valving function of the soft palate is served primarily by the paired levator veli palatini muscles, which arise from the petrous portion of the temporal bone. The levator veli palatini muscles elevate the soft palate and draw it posteriorly while also causing medial movement of the lateral pharyngeal walls. The levator veli palatini muscles insert into the posterior margin of the hard palate in the cleft palate patient. Levator contraction with the abnormal hard palate insertion actually causes an enlargement of the velopharyngeal orifice (Trier, 1985).

As more is understood about the normal and abnormal soft palate muscle function, there is increasing emphasis on restoration of normal soft palate muscle anatomy in cleft palate repairs. No well-designed prospective studies have compared various methods of palate closure on final speech results. In a summary of multiple reports employing several different operative techniques, an overall percentage of normal speech in 3,743 children with repaired cleft palates was 71%. Normal speech ranged from 44% to 94% (Grabb, 1971). Recent reviews of the results of two palate repair techniques, the Von Langenbeck (Trier, 1985) and the Furlow (Randall et al., 1986), reported similar 80% velopharyngeal competence rates. In general, of the children who fail to develop normal speech following palate repair, one-half will have problems of velopharyngeal incompetence, and the remaining one-half will have inadequate speech based upon other neuromuscular abnormalities.

Middle ear problems are common in cleft palate patients (see Chapter 7 for a more detailed discussion). The abnormal muscular anatomy produces inadequate opening of the Eustachian mechanism. Previous studies have reported that 30% to 50% of cleft palate patients will have some hearing loss (Skolnick, 1958). The percentage of actual hearing loss is much lower today due to the vigilance of cleft palate teams in audiometric assessment and middle ear examination; however, the majority of cleft palate patients will require PE (pressure equalizing) tube placement at some point. Middle ear problems and depressed hearing are generally treatable conditions.

Timing of Cleft Palate Repair

Complete closure of the hard and soft palate has been most commonly performed at 12 to 18 months of age. The child at this age is a reasonable anesthetic risk, the structures are sufficiently developed, and it was thought that this time frame antedated the development of meaningful speech. However, it is now known that important elements of speech development occur much earlier. Dorf and Curtin (1982) found a 10% incidence of pharyngeal and glottal articulation in children who underwent palate repair before age 1 and an 86% incidence of the same problems in patients repaired after age 1. No hypernasality was noted in a series of children whose palates were repaired by the Kilner–Veau–Wardill technique at 16 weeks (Desai, 1983).

The current approach to palate repair timing is determined by balancing the speech requirements for early repair with the limitations of the cleft anatomy. The narrow cleft of the secondary palate can probably be closed easily within the first 3 to 9 months. Because closure of the wide complete cleft palate is far more difficult and prone to fistula formation and incomplete healing, it is best to wait until about 12 months before repairing the wide complete cleft palate.

Cleft Palate Repair

A V–Y pushback procedure is the most widely used technique for cleft palate repair. Theoretically, this operation provides additional palatal length. As shown in Figure 3.8A, bilateral mucoperiosteal flaps are outlined, beginning at the anterior edge of the cleft. The edge of the cleft is incised, mucoperiosteal flaps are elevated, and the major palatine vessels are preserved. The hamular process may be infractured to release lateral tension on the flaps (Figure 3.8B). The oral mucosa is elevated off the muscular layer of the soft palate. The nasal mucosa is elevated off the hard palate and the nasal surface of the muscles of the soft palate. The abnormal insertion of the levator into the posterior edge of the hard palate can then be appreciated, and the muscles are separated at the muscle–hard palate interface (Figure 3.8C). The muscles are turned medially and reoriented approximately 90 degrees. The nasal mucosa layer can be lengthened by a Z-plasty (Figure 3.8D). The muscles are securely sutured in the midline (Figure 3.8E). The three-layer closure is accomplished with the final suturing of the oral mucoperiosteal layer using 4-0 chromic sutures (Figure 3.8F).

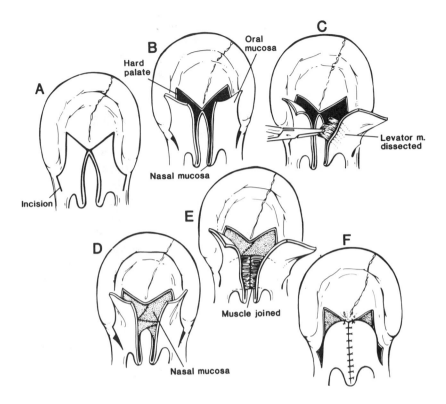

Figure 3.8 V–Y pushback cleft palate repair.

Submucous Cleft Palate

In a submucous cleft palate, there is a separation of the soft palate musculature beneath an intact mucosa. A bifid uvula and a palpable notch in the posterior border of the hard palate may be present. Diagnosis of submucous cleft palate may be difficult, and once the diagnosis is made, there may or may not be reason to repair the defect.

The patient with a submucous cleft palate should be thoroughly evaluated by a speech–language pathologist to determine whether physical improvement of velopharyngeal closure is required. There may be neuromuscular abnormalities in addition to the anatomical problem of the submucous cleft. A trial with a prosthetic speech appliance may be indicated to determine the contribution of the velopharyngeal abnormality to the total speech problem. In those patients in whom surgical improvement of velopharyngeal closure is required, simple muscle repair is often inadequate and a pharyngeal flap may be necessary. Sometimes a submucous cleft palate or congenitally short palate may be masked by large tonsils, adenoids, or nasal obstruction.

THE CLEFT LIP NOSE

The cleft lip nose represents a complex component of the facial deformity in the patient with cleft lip and palate. The asymmetrical deformity of the unilateral cleft lip nose consists of a combination of deforming elements. The nasal septum is bowed to the cleft side with the base angled to the cleft side. The nasal floor and sill are absent. The alar cartilage on the cleft side is buckled, flattened, and tipped inferiorly. The alar base is flared on the cleft side. The deformity is symmetrical in the bilateral cleft lip nose. The problem consists primarily of a short or essentially absent columella and a flared position of the alar bases associated with deficiencies in the nasal sill and floor. The surgical details of correction of the cleft lip nasal deformity are beyond the scope of this discussion; however, a general outline of the surgical plan is presented.

The timing of the various corrective nasal surgical procedures is controversial. Certain abnormalities are corrected at the time of lip repair. There is a trend toward more extensive alar cartilage and nasal tip reconstruction at the time of initial unilateral lip repair. I perform an extensive dissection of the alar cartilage on the affected side to gain a normal position of the cartilage at the time of lip repair. I believe that much of the late nasal deformity results from growth of normal structures (alar cartilage) in an abnormal position. If the position can be corrected early in the growth period, better long-term results are obtained. Further nasal tip work can be performed before school age, and any final reshaping of the nose is accomplished when facial growth is complete in the mid-teen years (see Chapter 7).

In the bilateral cleft lip, the initial repair technique must include provisions for subsequent columella lengthening. Prolabial tissue can be preserved within the prolabium or in forked flaps for later columella lengthening. The nasal floor is reconstructed and the alar base position is corrected at the time of initial lip repair. Bone or cartilage grafts to provide support of the nasal tip are frequently needed later in the cleft lip nose. Final reshaping, often with narrowing of the nasal bone framework, is performed when facial growth is complete.

The patient with the overoperated nasal tip, the result of multiple and inadequately performed early procedures, creates a most distressing problem. Whenever nasal tip surgery is undertaken, the procedure must be carefully planned and performed because a certain amount of irreversible scarring will be created with each procedure. The potential for optimal results decreases with each additional procedure.

SECONDARY SURGICAL PROCEDURES

The surgical care of the patient with cleft lip and palate represents a continuum from birth to adulthood. Several major operative events occur in this continuum, including lip repair, palate repair, and nasal repair. A wide variety of secondary surgical procedures of a lesser nature may be due to problems arising from primary procedures or may be planned as a second step in a sequential correction of the deformity. In each primary step, careful diagnosis of the problem, planning of the operation, and execution of the operation, will reduce the need for secondary procedures. The potential for optimal results is always greatest with the primary procedure, and with each succeeding secondary procedure, the results are compromised. Secondary surgical procedures for velopharyngeal incompetence, columella lengthening, the Abbe flap, and palatal fistula closure are described below to illustrate the types of soft tissue procedures that may be needed.

Velopharyngeal Incompetence

The diagnosis of velopharyngeal incompetence, or the inability to separate the nasal cavity from the oral cavity adequately for acceptable speech, is based primarily on thorough evaluation of the speech characteristics by a speech–language pathologist. Multiview radiographic assessment and nasendoscopy are helpful in defining the anatomical and physiological problem. The action of the soft palate and lateral pharyngeal walls can be observed and the proper surgical procedure chosen. If the problem is abnormal muscle action in a repaired palate in which the levator has not been restored, a secondary repair with muscle reorientation is carried out. If the soft palate is short and diffusely immobile with good lateral pharyngeal movement, a pharyngeal flap procedure is performed (Hogan, 1973). If soft palate movement appears normal and lateral wall immobility is the problem, a sphincter pharyngoplasty is indicated (Jackson et al., 1983; Jackson & Silverton, 1977).

Radiographic and nasendoscopic evaluations are technically difficult in the young child. Most children needing surgical correction of the velopharyngeal mechanism can be diagnosed by speech evaluation 2 or 3 years before they will tolerate instrumental assessment. Early correction of the velopharyngeal mechanism is extremely important to minimize the development of maladaptive articulation mechanisms, which may be difficult to correct at a later date (see Broen & Moller, Chapter 8). Therefore, we appreciate the added information that can be provided by radiographic and endoscopic techniques, but we will not wait for these if the diagnosis of velopharyngeal incompetence can be made early by speech assessment alone.

Surgical repair of the velopharyngeal mechanism is the treatment of choice in most patients. In some patients, the velopharyngeal incompetence is of a minor degree or is inconsistent, and a speech prosthesis such as a palatal lift may be of benefit prior to consideration of surgery. Another speech prosthesis such as a speech bulb may be used as an approach to improving velopharyngeal closure. In conjunction with speech therapy, the lift or bulb can be progressively reduced in size. Some patients are able to compensate for these size reductions with increased movement of the palatal and/or pharyngeal muscles, and eventually the appliance can be removed. However, most patients eventually require surgical correction.

In the complex patient with a variety of neuromuscular abnormalities, a speech prosthesis can be tried to determine the result likely to be achieved with improved velopharyngeal closure. We do not favor the long-term use of a speech prosthesis. If it is judged that velopharyngeal closure is incompetent for speech and that speech treatment or a prosthetic approach will not or cannot result in competent closure, a surgical approach is needed. The interdisciplinary team makes these decisions.

Pharyngeal Flap Operation

I have used a superiorly based lateral port control pharyngeal flap procedure for those patients in whom lateral pharyngeal wall movement is normal but soft palate abnormalities are present. The superiorly based pharyngeal flap has produced uniformly satisfactory results. Although calibration of the lateral ports using the catheter adds precision to the procedure, variabilities of soft tissue tension in the closure can result in hypo- or hypernasality. Rarely, a secondary correction of port size is necessary.

As shown in Figure 3.9A, the soft palate is divided at the midline and a superiorly based posterior pharyngeal wall flap is elevated at the level of the prevertebral fascia. The posterior pharyngeal wall donor is closed in the midline. Bilateral nasal mucosa lining flaps based laterally are developed from the turned-up soft palate flaps. A 14 French catheter is used to calibrate the lateral port area. The border of the elevated flap is sutured to the nasal surface of the soft palate. Following complete suturing of the flap to the nasal mucosa, the laterally based nasal mucosa flaps are turned across the raw surface of the flap and sutured in place to provide lining tissue and prevent late contracture of the flap (Figure 3.9B). The soft palate is then closed in layers using 4-0 chromic sutures (Figure 3.9C).

Sphincter Pharyngoplasty

A sphincter pharyngoplasty is employed in those patients in whom lateral pharyngeal wall movement is the primary problem in achiev-

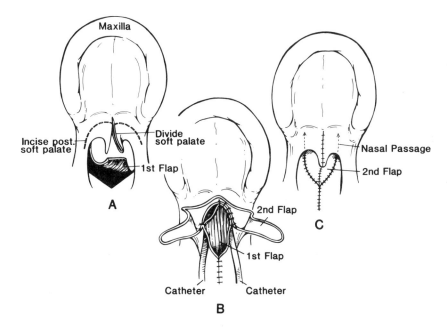

Figure 3.9 Superiorly based pharyngeal flap.

ing competent velopharyngeal closure for speech. The technique has the potential to produce a dynamic sphincter; however, in some cases, the result is only a static narrowing of the velopharyngeal space.

As seen in Figure 3.10, two superiorly based lateral pharyngeal wall flaps are incised. The flaps contain segments of palatopharyngeus musculature. The flap bases are connected by a transverse incision (Figure 3.10A). The flaps are then turned transversely and sutured with a midline closure. The lateral donor areas are closed primarily (Figure 3.10B).

Columella Lengthening

Two procedures are commonly used to lengthen the columella. The V–Y rotation advancement of the nostril sill is used if the columella is only moderately short. This technique has the advantage of not reentering the well-healed lip. It cannot recreate the full-length columella, which is often required. As shown in Figure 3.11, incisions are made along the alar base and extending into the midline of the columella. An alar base wedge may be resected (Figure 3.11A). The alar incisions are made, and a bipedicle flap of nasal floor is developed. The membranous columella is separated from the cartilaginous septum, and the skin is under-

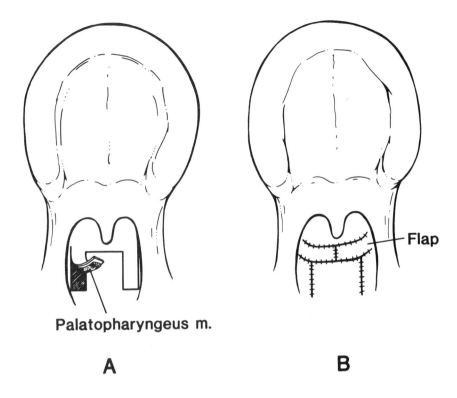

Figure 3.10 Sphincter pharyngoplasty.

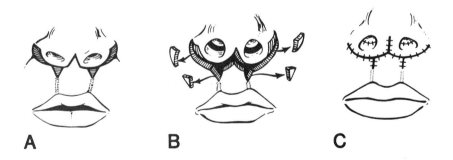

Figure 3.11 V–Y columella lengthening.

mined to the nasal tip (Figure 3.11B). The nostrils are rotated and the ala advanced medially and superiorly. The skin incisions are closed with 7-0 chromic sutures (Figure 3.11C).

The forked flap technique of Millard (1958) can be used in either primary or secondary columella lengthening. As seen in Figure 3.12, bilateral vertical flaps are outlined based on the columella and incorporating lip closure scars. A wedge of tissue is removed from the nostril floor (Figure 3.12A). The nasal tip is elevated, the membranous columella is separated from the cartilaginous septum, and the forked flaps are brought together to provide columella length. At the time of this procedure, continuity of the orbicularis oris muscle can be reestablished through the prolabial segment if this has not been done in the original lip repair. The removal of the forked flap tissue often improves the appearance of the lip in which there is a wide prolabium (Figure 3.12B).

Abbe Flap

A tight and deficient upper lip may result when excess tissue has been discarded at the time of primary lip repair. The tight upper lip is more frequent following bilateral cleft lip repair, although the problem of the very tight upper lip is becoming rare with current techniques of lip repair. Robert Abbe in 1898 was the first to use a cross lip flap to correct a tight lip following cleft lip repair. The technique can produce a philtrum of excellent appearance and achieve a balance between the

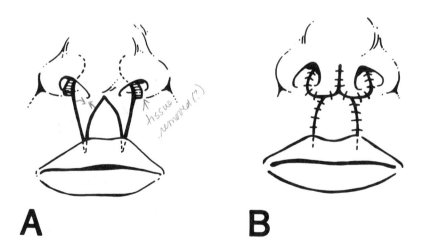

A   **B**

Figure 3.12 Forked flap columella lengthening.

bulk of the upper and lower lips. Minor revisions are occasionally necessary in the area of flap inset. The muscle segment of the flap becomes integrated into the orbicularis oris muscle functional unit of the upper lip.

As shown in Figure 3.13, the flap is outlined in the midline of the lower lip. A shield-shaped design is created that is approximately 1 cm wide at the vermillion border and approximately 6 mm wide at its inferior extent. The flap should be inserted in the midline of the upper lip, regardless of the position of scars. Although it is tempting to replace an irregular scar at the lateral portion of the prolabium with the flap, asymmetrical placement of the flap produces an unattractive appearance (Figure 3.13A). A full-thickness flap of the lower lip tissue is raised and supported on the labial vessels. A small mucosal bridge is maintained (Figure 3.13B). The flap is inserted and sutured in layers to reestablish continuity of the lateral lip muscle segments with the muscle layer of the flap (Figure 3.13C). The pedicle is divided 10 to 12 days later.

Palatal Fistula

A palatal fistula, the result of incomplete healing of a primary repair, should usually be surgically closed. Prosthetic obturator closure of the defect is an alternative; however, in most patients, this represents a less satisfactory approach. Successful closure of a palatal fistula is often more difficult than it appears. Large, well-vascularized flaps must be developed, and provision must be made for both lining and an oral surface. Frequently, closure of a small fistula will require nearly a complete repeat of the primary operation. Large anterior defects in the densely scarred palate may be difficult to close with local tissue due to previous

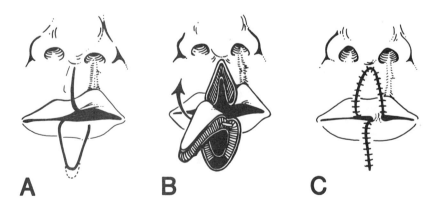

A   **B**   **C**

Figure 3.13 Abbe flap.

operative procedures. A tongue flap has been described for use in such cases (Jackson, 1972). An anteriorly placed flap is raised from the dorsum of the tongue and sutured to the anterior palate defect. The pedicle is divided 21 days later, and the tongue donor is closed primarily.

A standard fistula closure technique is shown in Figure 3.14. A lateral palatal fistula is illustrated with a two-layer closure. The nasal lining is created from turnover flaps of tissue immediately surrounding the defect. The oral lining is provided by a transposition flap.

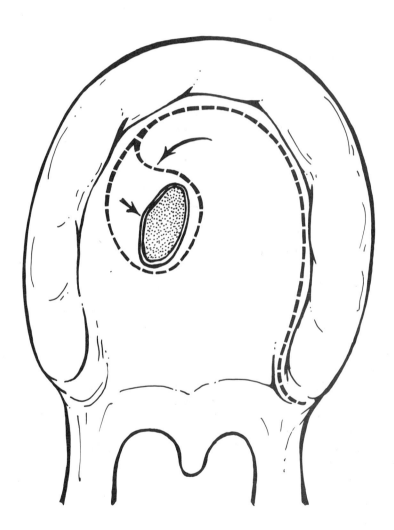

Figure 3.14 Palatal fistula closure.

SUMMARY

I have outlined some of the important surgical issues and surgical techniques in the continuum of care of the patient with cleft lip and/or palate. Again, the surgical considerations are only one component in the interdisciplinary management of this patient.

ACKNOWLEDGMENT

The artwork for this chapter was drawn by Mary Albury Noyes.

REFERENCES

Abbe, R. (1898). A new plastic operation for the relief of deformity due to double harelip. *Medical Record, 53,* 477–478.

Bardach, J., Morris, H. L., & Olin, W. H. (1984). Late results of primary veloplasty: The Marburg Project. *Plastic and Reconstructive Surgery, 73,* 207–215.

Bauer, B. S. (1989). Alveolar bone grafting: Early. In J. L. Marsh (Ed.), *Current therapy in plastic and reconstructive surgery* (pp. 189–192). Toronto: Decker.

Boo-Chai, K. (1966). An ancient Chinese text on cleft lip. *Plastic and Reconstructive Surgery, 38,* 89–91.

Brauer, R. O. (1971). General aspects of bilateral cleft lip repair. In W. C. Grabb, S. W. Rosenstein, & K. R. Bzoch (Eds.), *Cleft lip and palate* (pp. 265–281). Boston: Little, Brown.

Brown, J. B., & McDowell, F. (1945). Simplified design for repairs of single cleft lips. *Surgery, Gynecology and Obstetrics, 80,* 12–26.

Clodius, L. (1964). Maxillary orthopedia by means of extraoral forces. In R. Hotz (Ed.), *Early treatment of cleft lip and palate.* Bern: Hans Huber.

Cronin, T. D. (1957). Surgery of the double cleft lip and protruding premaxilla. *Plastic and Reconstructive Surgery, 19,* 389–400.

Desai, S. N. (1983). Early cleft palate repair completed before the age of 16 weeks: Observations of a personal series of 100 children. *British Journal of Plastic Surgery, 36,* 300–304.

Dorf, D. S., & Curtin, J. W. (1982). Early cleft palate repair and speech outcome. *Plastic and Reconstructive Surgery, 70,* 74–81.

Franco, P. (1561). *Petit traite contenant une des parties principalles DeChirurgie.* Lyons, France: Thibault Payan.

Furnas, D. W. (1984). Straight line closure: A preliminary to Millard closure in unilateral cleft lips. In M. E. Schafer (Ed.), *Clinics in plastic surgery 11* (No. 4, pp. 701–737). Philadelphia: W. B. Saunders.

Georgiade, N. G. (1972). Improved technique for one stage repair of bilateral cleft lip. *Plastic and Reconstructive Surgery, 48,* 318–324.

Georgiade, N. G., & Latham, R. A. (1975). Maxillary arch alignment in the bilateral cleft lip and palate infant, using the pinned coaxial screw appliance. *Plastic and Reconstructive Surgery, 56,* 52–60.

Grabb, W. C. (1971). General aspects of cleft palate surgery. In W. C. Grabb, S. W. Rosenstein, & K. R. Bzoch (Eds.), *Cleft lip and palate* (pp. 373–392). Boston: Little, Brown.

Hagedorn, M. (1884). Uber ein modifikation deshasenchartenoperation. *Zentralblatt fur Chirurgie, 11,* 756.

Hagerty, R. F., Mylin, W. K., & Hess, D. A. (1969). The prosthetic closure of cleft palate. In G. Sanvenero-Rosselli & G. Boggio-Robutti (Eds.), *Transactions of the Fourth International Congress of Plastic Surgery, Amsterdam.* Excerpta Medica Foundation, International Congress Series No. 174, pp. 457–461. Amsterdam: Excerpta Medica Foundation.

Hallock, G. G. (1985). In utero cleft lip repair in A/J mice. *Plastic and Reconstructive Surgery, 75,* 785–790.

Hogan, V. M. (1973). A clarification of the surgical goals in cleft palate speech and the introduction of the lateral port control (LPC) pharyngeal flap. *Cleft Palate Journal, 10,* 331–345.

Jackson, I. T. (1972). The use of tongue flaps to resurface lip defects and close palatal fistulae in children. *Plastic and Reconstructive Surgery, 49,* 537–541.

Jackson, I. T., McLennan, C., & Scheker, L. R. (1983). Primary veloplasty or primary palatoplasty: Some preliminary findings. *Plastic and Reconstructive Surgery, 72,* 153–157.

Jackson, I. T., & Silverton, J. S. (1977). Sphincter pharyngoplasty as a secondary procedure in cleft palates. *Plastic and Reconstructive Surgery, 49,* 518–524.

Jolleys, A., & Robertson, N. R. E. (1972). A study of the effects of early bone grafting in complete clefts of the lip and palate—Five year study. *British Journal of Plastic Surgery, 25,* 229–237.

Kahn, S., & Winsten, J. (1960). Surgical approaches to the bilateral cleft lip problem. *British Journal of Plastic Surgery, 13,* 13–27.

LeMesurier, A. B. (1962). *Harelips and their treatment.* Baltimore: Williams and Wilkins.

Lexer, E. (1904). *Malformations, injuries and diseases of the face. Von Bergmann's system of practical surgery.* Philadelphia: Lea and Febiger.

Maier, N. F. (1963). *Problem-solving discussions and conferences: Leadership methods and skills.* New York: McGraw-Hill.

Malgaigne, J. F. (1834). *Manuel de medecine operatoire, fondée sur l'anatomie normale et anatomie pathologique.* Paris: Germer Bailliere.

Millard, D. R. (1958). Columella lengthening by a forked flap. *Plastic and Reconstructive Surgery, 22,* 454–457.

Millard, D. R. (1960). Complete unilateral clefts of the lip. *Plastic and Reconstructive Surgery, 25,* 595–605.

Millard, D. R. (1968). Extensions of the rotation-advancement principle for wide unilateral cleft lips. *Plastic and Reconstructive Surgery, 42,* 535–544.

Millard, D. R., Jr. (Ed.). (1976a). *Cleft craft: The evolution of its surgery. Bilateral and rare deformities.* Boston: Little, Brown.

Millard, D. R., Jr. (Ed.). (1976b). *Cleft craft: The evolution of its surgery. The unilateral deformity.* Boston: Little, Brown.

Mirault, G. (1844). Lettre sur le bec-de-lievre. *Malgaigne Journal de Chirurgie 2,* 257.

Nordin, K. E., & Johanson, B. (1955). *Frei Knochen-transplantation bei Defekten in Alveozarkam nach Kieferortopadischer Enstelluling der Maxilla bei Lippen-Kiefer Gaumenspalten* (Vol. 1). Stuttgart: Thieme.

Owen, E. (1904). *Cleft palate and hare lip: The earlier operation on the palate.* Chicago: W. I. Keerner.

Pare, A. (1575). *Les oeuvres de M. Ambrose Pare.* Paris: G. Buon.

Peet, E. (1961). The Oxford technique of cleft palate repair. *Plastic and Reconstructive Surgery, 28,* 282–294.

Randall, P. (1959). A triangular flap operation for the primary repair of unilateral clefts of the lip. *Plastic and Reconstructive Surgery, 23,* 331–347.

Randall, P. (1965). A lip adhesion operation in cleft lip surgery. *Plastic and Reconstructive Surgery, 35,* 371–376.

Randall, P. (1971). Triangular muscle flap. In J. T. Hueston (Ed.), *Transactions: Fifth International Congress of Plastic and Reconstructive Surgery* (pp. 159–163). Chatsworth, Australia: Butterworth.

Randall, P., & Graham, W. P. (1971). Lip adhesion in the repair of bilateral cleft lip. In W. C. Grabb, S. W. Rosenstein, & K. R. Bzoch (Eds.), *Cleft lip and palate* (pp. 282–287). Boston: Little, Brown.

Randall, P., LaRossa, D., Solomon, M., & Cohen, A. B. (1986). Experience with the Furlow double-reversing Z-plasty for cleft palate repair. *Plastic and Reconstructive Surgery, 77,* 569–576.

Rose, W. (1891). *On hare lip and cleft palate.* London: H. K. Lewis.

Sadove, A. M., Nelson, C. L., & Jones, J. E. (1989). Alveolar bone grafting: Later. In J. D. Marsh (Ed.), *Current therapy in plastic and reconstructive surgery* (pp. 192–197). Toronto: Decker.

Schmid, E. (1955). Die annaherung der kieferstumpfe bei Lippen-Kiefer-Gaumen-Spalten: Ihre Schdelichen Folgen and Vermeidung. *Fortschritte der Keifer-und Gesichts-Chirurgie, 1,* 37–39.

Schweckendiek, W. (1962). Die Ergebnisse der Kieferbildung und die Sprache nach der primaen Veloplastic. *Archiv fur Ohren-Nasen-und Kehlkopfheilkunde, 180,* 541–551.

Skolnick, E. M. (1958). Otologic evaluation in cleft palate patients. *Laryngoscope, 68,* 1908–1949.

Skoog, T. (1969). Repair of unilateral cleft lip deformity: Maxilla, nose and lip. *Scandinavian Journal of Plastic and Reconstructive Surgery, 3,* 109–133.

Tennison, C. W. (1952). The repair of the unilateral cleft lip by the stencil method. *Plastic and Reconstructive Surgery, 9,* 115–120.

Thompson, J. F. (1912). An artistic and mathematically accurate method of repairing the defect in cases of hare lip. *Surgery, Gynecology and Obstetrics, 14,* 498–505.

Trier, W. C. (1985). Primary palatoplasty. In W. C. Trier (Ed.), *Symposium on cleft lip and cleft palate.* Philadelphia: Saunders.

Veau, V. (1938). *Bec-de-lievre.* Paris: Masson.

Von Graefe, C. F. (1817). Kurze nachrichten and auszuge. *Journal der Practischen Arzneykunde und Wundarzyneykunst, 44,* 116.

von Langenbeck, B. R. K. (1861). Operation der angeborenen totalen Spaltung des harten Gaumens nach einer neuen methode. *Deutsches Archiv fur Klinische Medizin, 13,* 231.

CHAPTER 4

Oral and Maxillofacial Surgery and the Management of Cleft Lip and Palate

Mohamed El Deeb, Daniel E. Waite, and John Curran

El Deeb, Waite, and Curran discuss the discipline of oral and maxillofacial surgery, review its history, and emphasize the dental and medical training involved. They focus on the concerns and treatment for dental and alveolar problems and upper and lower jaw discrepancies in patients with cleft lip and palate.

1. *Describe the dental anomalies that are frequently seen when the cleft involves the alveolar ridge. Approximately what percentage of patients have clefts that involve the alveolar ridge?*

2. *The authors advocate for repair of the alveolar cleft, but state that the timing of bone grafting has been controversial. Why? When do they prefer to repair the alveolar cleft, and what data are used to support this decision?*

3. *Describe the role of the orthodontist prior to bone grafting and why orthodontic manipulation can be helpful to the oral and maxillofacial surgeon.*

4. *The authors point out the importance of careful and systematic analysis of records through the growth and developmental years. What are the three planes where jaw discrepancies can occur? Although surgical correction of jaw discrepancies most often is deferred until more complete growth and development, what is the rationale for early surgical correction of severe cranial and skull base deformities?*

5. *Discuss the possible speech benefits and speech problems following a maxillary advancement.*

The cleft lip and palate deformity includes a variety of defects, ranging from minor notching of the lip to complete unilateral or bilateral involvement of the soft and hard palate, dental alveolar ridges, and lip. Habilitation of the patient with cleft lip and palate involves careful consideration for the patient's dental–oral function, appearance, speech, hearing, deglutition, and social and emotional well-being. For treatment to be optimal, several disciplines need to be involved in the long-term planning and clinical decision making. The oral and maxillofacial surgeon plays an important part in this process as a member of the cleft palate team.

In the United States, the oral and maxillofacial surgeon has been treating abnormalities and diseases of the mouth since the middle 1800s. The organized specialty of oral and maxillofacial surgery had its beginning in 1918 under the name of the American Society of Exodontists. In 1921, the name was changed to the American Society of Oral Surgeons, and subsequently to the American Society of Oral and Maxillofacial Surgeons in 1977. In 1955, the educational requirement for oral surgery was established as 3 years of advanced study and training following completion of a dental degree from an accredited dental school. As of 1989, all accredited programs in oral and maxillofacial surgery require 4 years of training after a Doctorate of Dental Surgery degree.

Although training programs in oral and maxillofacial surgery are sponsored largely by dental schools, and certainly arise out of the dental profession, a major part of the training is in hospitals. A typical training program in oral and maxillofacial surgery today requires a resident (graduate student) to spend a significant amount of time on services in medicine, anesthesia, and general surgery. In many training programs, shorter periods of time may be required in related areas of interest, such as neurosurgery, otolaryngology, and plastic surgery. The greater emphasis in training, however, is within the surgical discipline, where residents treat patients with problems relating to the oral cavity and related structures of the head and neck. Training in oral and maxillofacial surgery also encompasses basic research, leading to the acquisition of higher academic qualifications. This emphasis on research has acted as a catalyst for the development of new ideas.

The development of computerized axial tomography, magnetic resonance imaging, and three-dimensional image reformation has significantly increased the oral surgeon's diagnostic and treatment planning capabilities. These developments have promoted considerable progress in the fields of orthognathic surgery, surgery on the temporomandibular joint, cleft palate surgery, and preprosthetic surgery. The broad scope of oral and maxillofacial surgery is now defined as that part of dental practice that deals with the diagnosis and surgical and adjunctive treatment of diseases, injuries, and defects of the oral and maxillofacial regions.

THE ORAL AND MAXILLOFACIAL SURGEON'S ROLE ON THE INTERDISCIPLINARY CLEFT PALATE TEAM

The oral and maxillofacial surgeon has a sound appreciation of the dental and surgical needs of the patient with cleft palate and can provide a variety of surgical services at various stages in the growth and development of patients with skeletodental malformations, including cleft palate. The need for consultation with an oral and maxillofacial surgeon regarding treatment will occur early in the patient's life. Developing jaw discrepancies, supernumerary teeth, impacted teeth, poor quality of dentition, cleft defects in the alveolar ridges, and velopharyngeal problems are only a few of the conditions that will require the input and expertise of an oral and maxillofacial surgeon. Patients may benefit from a variety of oral and maxillofacial surgical procedures associated with growth and development. These procedures may be interrelated with treatments provided by other medical disciplines, such as otolaryngology and plastic and reconstructive surgery, and have the common goal of providing optimal functional and aesthetic dentofacial configuration. Ideally, this goal is achieved as the patient reaches physical maturity.

The wide acceptance of the interdisciplinary team approach for the habilitation of patients with cleft palates has not eliminated controversy concerning approaches to treatment. It has, however, encouraged the coming together of a group of professionals who can, through their mutual concern for the patient, establish realistic goals for treatment. Such scientific curiosity, often stimulated by the inadequacies perceived in current treatment modalities, will bring about improvements in future treatment for patients.

The majority of patients may present to the oral and maxillofacial surgeon with the lip and palate already repaired, but with a variety of residual problems requiring assessment, diagnosis, and treatment during the patient's growing years. Problems in which the oral and maxillofacial surgeon should participate during treatment of patients with cleft palates may include the following: dentoalveolar problems, repair of alveolar clefts in patients with unilateral or bilateral cleft palates with or without repositioning the premaxillae, surgical reconstruction of the resorbed and/or missing premaxillae, management of teeth erupting through a grafted alveolar cleft defect, surgical reconstruction of resorbed maxillary or mandibular arches, and management of dentofacial (jaw discrepancy) problems.

DENTOALVEOLAR PROBLEMS IN PATIENTS WITH CLEFT PALATES

The primary and secondary dentitions are very important, both functionally and aesthetically. Care of the dentition is carefully monitored and managed by the family or pediatric dentist. Regular visits with a dentist will ensure an emphasis on prevention of dental disease and maintenance of oral health. Approximately 75% of clefts involve the alveolar ridge or that portion of the upper jaw that houses the teeth. However, despite advances made in the surgical correction of cleft lip and palate and the development of the interdisciplinary team, many such patients continue to present with residual alveolar cleft defects and associated oronasal fistulae (Figures 4.1A and 4.1B). In the patient with a unilateral cleft, the lack of bony support to the alar base contributes to deformities of the nose, lip, and face (Figures 4.2A and 4.2B). When the cleft is bilateral, the nasal base is further distorted and the deformity enlarged. It is advisable to graft (with bone) the alveolar cleft defect before the final correction is made on the alar base and lips. This will provide continuity of the underlying bone, which will subsequently support the final revised soft tissue.

Many dental anomalies may be present in a patient with cleft palate, especially in the area near the alveolar cleft (Jordan, Kraus, & Neptune, 1966). These anomalies include congenitally missing teeth (most often the lateral incisor), early loss of deciduous teeth, and altered patterns of calcification and eruption. It is also common to find supernumerary or extra teeth in the cleft region (Figure 4.3); they may be peg-shaped

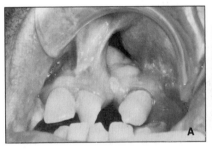
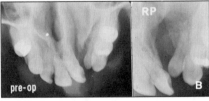

Figure 4.1 (A) Clinical photograph showing a large buccal oronasal fistula and communication in a patient with unilateral cleft palate. (B) Occlusal (left) and periapical (right) radiographs showing a large alveolar cleft defect associated with oronasal communication.

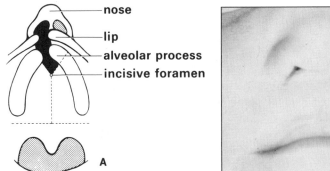

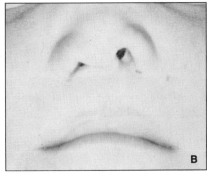

Figure 4.2 (A) Schematic drawing showing unilateral alveolar cleft defect (marked by dark color). Note the lack of bony support related to the alar base of the nose. (B) Clinical photograph showing flaring of the alar base on the side with the alveolar cleft defect, due to the lack of bony support.

or conical, with short roots that diminish their usefulness as supporting teeth for future dental reconstruction. These teeth may also obstruct the eruption of normal permanent teeth, especially the permanent incisors (Primosch, 1981). Thus, early identification of supernumerary teeth and their removal at the appropriate time are important. The decision to remove impacted or supernumerary teeth prior to their eruption should be carefully considered because certain disadvantageous results may occur, including possible injury to permanent tooth buds and loss of alveolar bone. Scarring and fibrosis following surgery may also interfere with normal eruption of the permanent teeth. Certainly, the fewest possible surgical entries into the area near the alveolar cleft defect provide the best end result.

Permanent teeth that erupt into the dental arch adjacent to a cleft are often deficient in bony support along with root surface on the cleft side. They frequently become loose and associated with periodontal disease (Figures 4.4A and 4.4B). If these teeth are needed to assist in providing long-term support for a fixed or removable prosthesis, then the provision of additional bone through bone grafting in the cleft area will greatly improve the prognosis. Premature loss of any teeth may complicate and compromise a patient aesthetically and functionally. In unilateral cleft defects, unstable segments tend to move under masticatory force. Thus, the long-term use of a fixed prosthesis in the unrepaired cleft is less than successful and often contributes to early loss of abutment teeth (Figure 4.5). Removable appliances may be less likely to fail, but are less aesthetic and place demands on the patient for additional oral hygiene and maintenance.

Poor alignment of adjacent teeth near the alveolar cleft may be related to the absence of one or more teeth, or may be due to the pres-

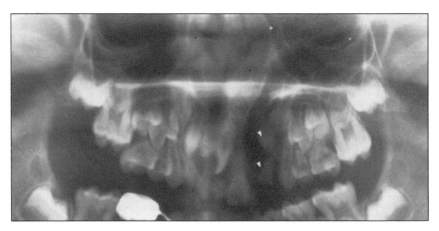

Figure 4.3 Panoramic radiograph showing supernumerary teeth (marked by arrows) in the area of the alveolar cleft defect.

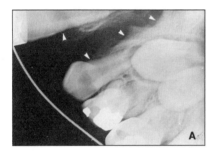 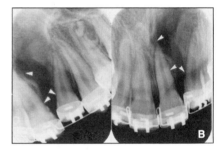

Figure 4.4 Periapical radiograph showing alveolar cleft defects in two different patients (A and B). Note the lack of bone in the area (marked by arrows), which jeopardizes adjacent teeth.

ence of supernumerary teeth in the cleft area. The permanent central incisors generally will erupt into a reasonable position and will, therefore, need only minimal orthodontic and surgical assistance. The permanent canine is usually either situated at the distal margin of the residual alveolar cleft or displaced superiorly along the bony defect (Figure 4.6). This tooth will often erupt into the cleft defect, and, due to lack of adequate bony support, periodontal breakdown may lead to premature loss of this tooth. It has been demonstrated that the canine on the cleft side shows a tendency for delayed eruption compared with canines on the non–cleft side (El Deeb, Messer, Lehnert, Hebda, & Waite, 1982; Fishman, 1970). The lateral incisor is very often missing in cleft patients; however, if it should be present, it also is predisposed to perio-

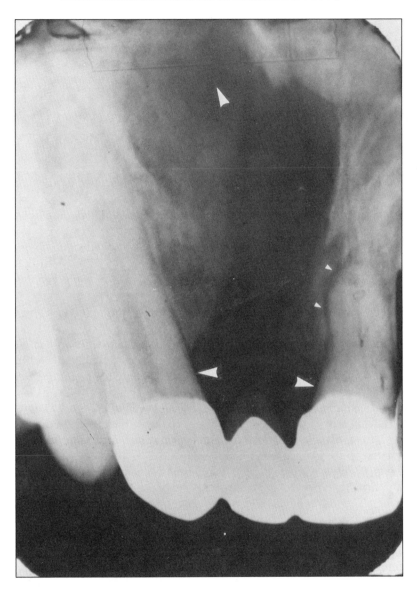

Figure 4.5 Periapical radiograph showing unrepaired alveolar cleft defect. Note the
lack of bony support (marked by large arrows), which may lead to periodontal involvement of the adjacent teeth. Note the widening of the periodontal
involvement of the adjacent teeth. Also note the widening of the periodontal ligament space (marked by small arrows). The lack of bone may lead
to unstable segments, which may jeopardize the bridge.

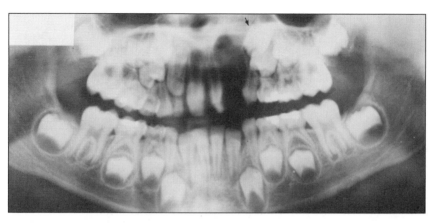

Figure 4.6 Panoramic radiograph showing the upper canine situated high in the alveolus, superior to the area of the alveolar cleft defect. Note there is initial formation of the root. This represents an ideal timing for bone grafting in the cleft.

dontal breakdown and ectopic or maleruption because of the inadequate bony support adjacent to the cleft.

Fishman (1970) found that a group of patients with bilateral cleft lip and palate demonstrated the highest incidence of delayed eruption of teeth, followed in order by those with posterior clefts, unilateral clefts of the lip and palate, and clefts of the lip and alveolus. Delayed eruption of teeth adjacent to each side of the cleft was also found by Ranta (1971). Delayed eruption may reflect lack of eruptive direction for teeth in cleft areas due to disruption of the normal gubernacular epithelial relationship to the primary predecessor teeth, either by the defect or by surgical intervention (Carollo, Hoffman, & Brodie, 1971). In bilateral cleft palate involving the alveolar bone, the premaxilla and its associated dentition become separated from the posterior maxillary arches. In the majority of cases, the premaxilla becomes mobile and displaced. This could create a problem to the orthodontist who is preparing a patient for surgery. If the premaxilla is in good alignment with the maxillary and mandibular arches, then surgical grafting is needed to stabilize the premaxilla and provide a continuation with the posterior maxillary arches (Figures 4.7A and 4.7B). If the premaxilla is displaced in relationship to the mandibular arch, then surgical repositioning of the premaxilla and grafting are needed.

Speech may be influenced by the contour of the dental arch, the alveolar cleft, oronasal communication, and the type of appliance used for replacing missing teeth (Kent & Schaaf, 1982). As a general rule, the labial oronasal fistula (Figure 4.1) causes fewer speech complications than a palatal fistula (Figure 4.8). Nonetheless, to approach nor-

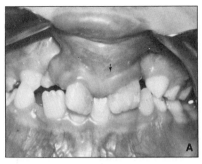
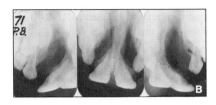

Figure 4.7 (A) Clinical photograph showing unrepaired bilateral alveolar cleft defects. The premaxilla (marked by arrow) is mobile and presents a difficult problem for the orthodontist. (B) Periapical and occlusal radiographs showing unrepaired bilateral alveolar cleft defects. Note the lack of bony support. This represents a high risk to the erupting teeth, and the premaxilla may become mobile.

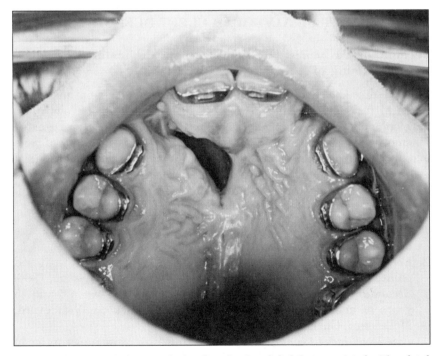

Figure 4.8 Intraoral photograph showing alveolar cleft defect associated with palatal oronasal communication (fistula).

mality in speech, it would be best to have no defect at all and normal dentition. An oronasal fistula is a source of inconvenience to patients and may lead to nasal secretion entering the mouth and fluid being regurgitated from the oral cavity to the nose. This communicating cavity contributes to unsightly crusting of the nostrils and to uncontrollable odors. Although patients can usually adapt to its presence, most are grateful if the surgeon can restore the anatomical barrier between the oral cavity and the nose, enhancing normal oral and nasal functions.

Inadequate orthodontic treatment and ungrafted alveolar cleft defect(s) may lead to a collapse in the affected posterior maxillary segment(s). When this occurs, usually each affected segment is collapsed medially and superiorly (Figure 4.9). When a problem of malocclusion is evaluated, it is important to evaluate the relationship between the upper and lower jaw as well. If there is a considerable discrepancy between the jaws, then future surgery may be needed to align the basal bone in a good relationship, enabling the orthodontist to align the teeth in a normal and acceptable position. Skeletodental malrelationships can occur anteroposteriorly, horizontally, and vertically, as discussed later in this chapter.

MANAGEMENT OF ALVEOLAR CLEFT DEFECTS

Terminology, Historical Background, and Indications for and Timing of Repair of Alveolar Clefts

Surgical procedures to repair clefts should aim toward an optimal physiological function, leading to minimal interference with growth and development of the maxillofacial complex. Clinicians have been attracted for many years to the idea that early restoration of continuity of bone across the alveolar defect would be advantageous to subsequent facial growth and development; however, the timing of bone grafting for the alveolar cleft has been a continuing controversy. The following terminology has been utilized in the literature.

1. *Primary osteoplasty*—Early bone grafting simultaneously with closure of cleft lip (Nylen, 1966)
2. *Early secondary osteoplasty*—Bone grafting after repair of the lip and palate and after complete eruption of deciduous teeth (Nylen, 1966)
3. *Secondary osteoplasty*—Bone grafting performed between 6 and 15 years of age (Boyne & Sands, 1972, 1976: Jackson, Vandevard, McLennan, Christie, & McGregor, 1981)
4. *Late secondary osteoplasty*—Bone grafting after complete eruption of permanent teeth (Nylen, 1966; Pickrell & Quinn, 1967) and after completion of the growth (Boyne & Sands, 1976)

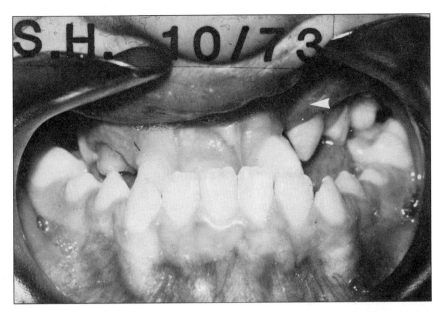

Figure 4.9 Intraoral photograph showing skeletofacial malrelationship in patient with bilateral cleft palate. Note the collapsed posterior segment, medially and superiorly (marked by arrow). Also note that there is a lingual crossbite between the maxillary and mandibular teeth.

The first attempts at grafting bone in growing patients with clefts were performed by von Eiselberg (1901) and by Lexer (1908). Drachter (1914) reported closure of a cleft with tibial bone and periosteum. Skoog (1965a, 1965b) reported on the correction of the alveolar cleft defects without bone grafting by utilizing periosteal flaps, and named the procedure "boneless bone grafting." Since then, opinions continue to differ on the indications for, timing of, and management of grafts of maxillary alveolar clefts (Berkowitz, 1978). Schmid (1955), Nordin (1957), and, more recently, Rosenstein and colleagues (Rosenstein, Jacobson, Monroe, Griffith, & McKinney, 1972; Rosenstein et al., 1982) reported favorably on bone grafting during infancy. The deleterious effects of early intervention on the subsequent growth of the maxillary complex, however, have now been well documented (Jolleys & Robertson, 1972; Koberg, 1973; Pickrell, Quinn, & Massengill, 1968; Rehrmann, Koberg, & Koch, 1970; Robertson & Jolleys, 1968, 1983). Bone grafting delayed until the eruption of the secondary dentition is now a more widely accepted procedure (Boyne & Sands, 1972; Broude & Waite, 1974; El Deeb et al., 1982; Hogeman, Jacobsson, & Sarnas, 1972; Johanson, Ohlson, Friede, & Ahlgren, 1974; Stenstrom & Thilander, 1963).

The indications for closure of alveolar clefts depend upon the size, the location, and the type of cleft. Indications cited in the literature include the following:

1. To improve deficiency of a firm bony base (Drachter, 1914)
2. To increase stability of the maxillary components in the corrected position and decrease the incidence of relapse, if grafting is associated with maxillary osteotomies (Backdahl & Nordin, 1961; Backdahl, Nordin, Nylen, & Strombeck, 1963; Johanson et al., 1974; Stenstrom & Thilander, 1963)
3. To stabilize the mobile premaxilla in patients with bilateral cleft palate (Pickrell et al., 1968)
4. To elevate the nasal alar base and to improve the lip line and enhance cosmetic appearance (Epstein, Davis, & Thompson, 1970; Hall & Posnick, 1983; Petrovic, 1971; Pickrell et al., 1968; Turvey, Vig, Moriarity, & Hoke, 1984)
5. To prevent collapses of the posterior maxillary segments (Epstein et al., 1970)
6. To improve passage of air through the nose (Jackson, Scheker, Vandervord, & McLennan, 1982; Matthews, Broomhead, Chir, Grossman, & Goldin, 1970)
7. To create a new alveolus for the eruption of teeth in the cleft area (Boyne & Sands, 1976; El Deeb, Hinrichs, Waite, Bandt, & Bevis, 1986; El Deeb et al., 1982; Enemark, Sindet-Pedersen, & Bundgaard, 1987; Jolleys & Robertson, 1972)
8. To decrease the incidence of malpositioned teeth in the anterior maxillary region (Waite & Kersten, 1980)
9. To improve status of the patient's oral hygiene by separating the nasal cavity from the oral cavity (Kwon, Waite, Stickel, Chisholm, & McParland, 1981; Waite & Kersten, 1980)
10. To accomplish closure of oronasal fistulae more easily (Jackson et al., 1982)
11. To augment and repair edentulous and missing premaxillae (El Deeb et al., 1982)

Secondary osteoplasty is usually carried out close to, or after completion of, lateral growth of the maxilla. One of the primary reasons for bone grafting in alveolar clefts is to provide a bony base for the eruption of the canine tooth (Figure 4.10). Therefore, an important issue is to place the graft at the time appropriate to allow for this normal eruption. The chronologic age of the patient is not as important in selecting the time for secondary osteoplasty as the patient's dental age. The stages of tooth development and tooth eruption determine dental age. The ideal time for grafting the alveolar cleft is when the permanent canine tooth bud is high and formation of the root has commenced and is between

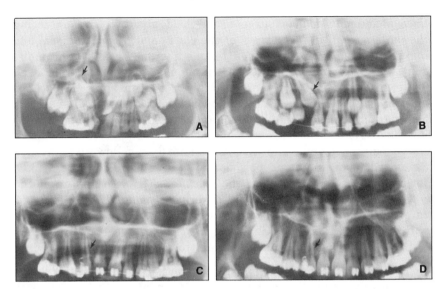

Figure 4.10 Panoramic radiographs showing (A) preoperative view with erupting canine (marked by arrow), demonstrating initial formation of tooth root and unrepaired alveolar cleft defect; (B) canine erupting into the grafted area; (C) canine erupting into full occlusion; and (D) position of the erupting canine following completion of orthodontic alignment.

one-fourth and one-third complete (Figure 4.6). The lateral incisor is usually missing from the cleft side, but when it is present, consideration should be given to earlier bone grafting to facilitate its eruption into normal position. The permanent teeth usually erupt through the bone graft without difficulty; however, orthodontic management is usually necessary for final positioning of teeth (El Deeb et al., 1982).

El Deeb et al. (1982) evaluated 46 patients with cleft palate who had 64 canines that erupted into the grafted alveolar cleft defect. The conclusions were that (a) the ideal time for performing alveolar bone grafting for patients with a cleft of the alveolos varies slightly from patient to patient; (b) the canine will erupt through the autogenous bone graft; (c) canines in the cleft area will subsequently have normal root development provided there are no developmental disturbances in growth; (d) the canine will erupt later than normal into the grafted alveolar defect, and a longer time is required for the eruption to occur through the bone graft; (e) surgical uncovering and orthodontic intervention may be required for complete eruption; (f) grafting is highly successful in patients from 9 to 12 years old when the canine root is one-fourth to one-third formed; and (g) the postoperative observation period is very important and requires complete cooperation between the orthodontist, the oral and maxillofacial surgeon, and the dentist involved in treating the patient. Within the context of the cleft palate team, the oral and maxillofacial surgeon coordinates treatment with the pediatric or family dentist and the orthodontist so that problems created by the cleft and its dentition are dealt with appropriately. Serial intraoral radiographs and clinical observation usually allow the correct decision to be made for the timing of removal or maintenance of teeth and the timing of grafting for alveolar cleft defects.

Utilizing these seven principles, a long-term follow-up study was developed to evaluate the periodontal status of 34 canines erupted through grafted alveolar clefts in 26 patients (18 with unilateral and 8 with bilateral clefts). The results were compared with those for 58 canines that erupted through normal alveolus in 29 control patients without clefts (El Deeb et al., 1986; Hinrichs, El Deeb, Waite, Bevis, & Bandt, 1984). The conclusions from this study were the following:

1. The plaque index was statistically higher for canines erupting through normal alveolar bone in the non–cleft side in patients with unilateral cleft lip and palate than in control patients. This suggested that grafted patients with clefts had poorer habits of oral hygiene than did controls.
2. There was no statistically significant difference between the overall periodontal status of controls and that of patients with unilateral or bilateral grafted alveolar clefts.
3. The use of autogenous bone grafting for treatment of alveolar cleft defects resulted in erupting canines that had more than 90% of their possible clinical attachment intact.
4. Grafting of alveolar cleft defects resulted in a clinically satisfactory periodontium to support these canines.

The longevity of the canines erupting through grafted alveolar clefts depends not only on their periodontal status, but also on the status of the pulp. In another study, El Deeb, El Deeb, and Bevis (1989) used the analytical pulp-tester (APT) to evaluate the pulpal response of canines that had erupted through grafted alveolar clefts in 16 patients with unilateral clefts. The results of this experiment revealed that 31% of canines that erupted in the grafted unilateral cleft palate did not respond to APT, whereas all contralateral canines in the non–cleft side responded to APT. The conclusion from this study was that the clinician should follow these patients, as these teeth may later show other signs of pulpal degeneration that might require endodontic intervention.

The early management of the premaxilla in the patient with bilateral clefts has presented another area of controversy that must be considered. Hayward (1983) advocated a conservative approach to the management of the premaxilla, delaying any surgical repositioning until after the age of 7. At this time, repositioning can be combined with alveolar bone grafting if needed. This view is supported by Bishara and Olin (1972) and by El Deeb and colleagues (El Deeb et al., 1982; El Deeb, Lehnert, & Waite, 1983).

Presurgical Considerations for Repair of Alveolar Clefts

Dentition.   Dental decay and periodontal disease may ravage the adolescent dentition and complicate later orthodontic, surgical, or fixed prosthodontic procedures. The necessity for good and ongoing dental care and a high standard of oral hygiene must be reemphasized as an essential precursor to the initiation of orthodontic and surgical treatments. As a rule, the removal of permanent teeth from the maxilla should be avoided. Premature loss of any teeth may complicate and compromise achievement of the objectives of bone grafting in an alveolar cleft and of eruption of teeth, and may lead to further resorption of bone. The timing of the removal of redundant supernumerary teeth in the cleft is an important consideration. We believe these teeth should be left in position as long as possible and, ideally, removed during surgery at the time the graft is placed. Our opinion is based on the principle that the presence of teeth (even supernumerary teeth) may give rise to the preservation of alveolar bone. Supernumerary teeth should be removed only if they interfere with the eruption of the permanent teeth.

Orthodontic treatment.   Orthodontic treatment is instituted to correct existing anterior or posterior crossbites and to establish optimal form in the arch with proper overbite and overjet, when possible. This is easier to accomplish prior to bone grafting (Koch, 1977). The orthodontist sometimes performs an early orthopedic treatment. This treatment may be successful at the beginning, but will not be efficient in the long run unless it is closely coordinated with adequately timed, conservative, and gentle surgery (Hotz, Gnoinski, Nussbaumer, & Kistler, 1978). This treatment also widens the cleft and gives a more accurate indication of the true bony deficiency. It also improves surgical access to the cleft area, which frequently has a coexisting oronasal fistula. Surgical repositioning of maxillary segments can also provide good results, but this will substantially increase the operative time required and may not allow the same precision in coordinating maxillary and mandibular dental arches as does orthodontics. The orthodontist also plays an important role in moving the teeth surrounding the alveolar cleft defect away from this area to provide the surgeon with adequate alveolar bone, mesial and distal to the cleft defect. Placing the bone graft in direct contact with teeth, rather than with bone, may interfere with the final resulting outcome.

Treatment planning. The presurgical record should include a complete review of the patient's medical history, casts for study, and photographs and radiographic studies (cephalograph and maxillary occlusal, periapical, and panoramic radiographs). The periapical X-ray is helpful in verifying the quantity of bone on the tooth surface adjacent to the cleft (Figures 4.4A and 4.4B). The alveolar height of this bony shelf will determine the ultimate bony level of the graft. It is important to note that chronologic age and dental age are not necessarily coincident, and the stage of tooth development is most important in selecting the time for the surgery. Tooth development can be determined from a panoramic radiograph. Three-dimensional computerized reformation may give an accurate picture to determine the size of clefts. This does not usually vary according to the degree of magnification, as is the case with panoramic radiographs.

The patient and family require careful, compassionate consideration, as well as supportive preparation for the surgery. This will enhance their level of understanding and cooperation with the surgical team before, during, and after the surgical period. It is also helpful for the entire cleft palate team to review the patient's status prior to surgery, not only to emphasize the interest of all clinicians in the patient's progress, but also to ensure that other areas of need are not overlooked.

The Surgical Procedure and Technique for Repair of Alveolar Clefts

Although the procedure is carried out under general anesthesia, patients are usually admitted to the hospital on the day of surgery. Young children, especially patients with clefts, are prone to rapid onset of upper respiratory infections and to exacerbations of chronic ear infections. It is prudent, therefore, to ensure that they have had a physical examination by their pediatrician a week prior to hospitalization so that unnecessary cancellations of surgery do not occur. These are very unsettling for both the patient and the family who have been psychologically prepared for the event, as well as wasteful of expensive medical resources.

The patient will also undergo a rigorous physical examination after admission to the hospital. This will include laboratory investigations and additional radiographic examination, if indicated, and a careful assessment by the anesthesiologist. Patients with cleft palate occasionally have additional congenital anomalies—for example, existing or previously repaired cardiac defects—that require special consideration during anesthesia and surgery. Prophylactic antibiotics are usually utilized during and after surgery to protect the grafted site from infection.

Nasotracheal intubation is employed to maintain the airway during surgery, for the delivery of oxygen and anesthetic agents. Intubation should be inserted through the nares on the non-cleft side in unilateral clefts, whenever possible. In bilateral clefts, either nares may be acceptable. If it is impossible to place the tube in either nostril due to obstruction or to the presence of a pharyngeal flap, an oral endotracheal tube is necessary.

In the unilateral cleft palate, the palatal mucosa along the margin of the cleft is incised and two flaps are reflected nasally to form the nasal floor (Figures 4.11A, 4.11B, and 4.11C). The dissection is carried forward through the alveolus and into the vestibule and around the oronasal fistula. These flaps are turned toward each other and sutured, forming the new nasal floor (Figures 4.11C and 4.11D). The sutures are individually placed with the ties toward the nasal side. The bone graft is usually placed against the suture line, and must be free of nasal contamination. For that reason, adequate suturing in a watertight, sealed fashion is needed.

Once the nasal floor is established, the bone graft can be inserted (Figure 4.11E). The most successful results will be obtained using fresh chips of autogenous bone marrow, usually from the iliac crest. Flint (1964) described a simple method of obtaining substantial amounts of cancellous bone from the iliac crest with minimal postoperative discomfort and disability for the patient. The procedure is suitable for most cases of bone grafting for alveolar clefts. If stability of maxillary segments is needed, then a block of corticocancellous bone is shaped to fit the alveolar defect and is wedged into place. The closure of soft tissues is then completed using sliding mucogingival and palatal flaps (Figure 4.11F). Sutures on the oral side must also provide a tension-free, watertight closure. Figure 4.12 shows schematic drawings of the frontal view of the alveolar cleft defect before (A) and after (B) grafting with bone.

In bilateral alveolar clefts, the surgical approach for grafting is similar to that in repair of the unilateral cleft, with a few exceptions. Care must be exercised in the reflection of tissues along the premaxillary segment. The premaxilla is usually mobile and attached to the vomer and the cartilaginous nasal septum. The blood supply is from the pedicle of the labial mucosa and the nasal septal mucosa. Therefore, the labial reflection of tissue on the premaxillary segment should be avoided. Palatal flaps are raised bilaterally and reflected medially to close the alveolar cleft and to cover the exposed vomer (Figures 4.13A and 4.13B). Following closure of the nasal floor (Figure 4.13C), the previously obtained autogenous bone graft is condensed and inserted bilaterally, and posterior to the premaxilla (Figure 4.13D). The soft tissue flaps are

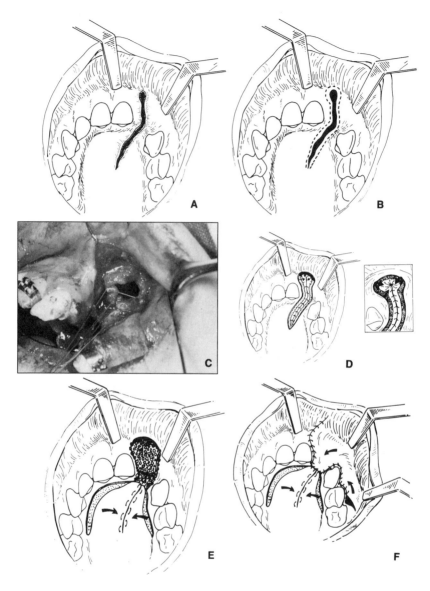

Figure 4.11   (A) Schematic drawing showing a labiopalatal alveolar cleft defect with oronasal communication. (B) Schematic drawing showing the incision line (indicated by the dotted line) on the buccal and palatal mucosa along the margin
of the cleft defect. Intraoral photograph (C) and schematic drawing (D) showing medial reflection of the flaps and suturing of the flaps toward each other
to create the new nasal floor. (E) Schematic drawing showing grafting of
the alveolar cleft defect with autogenous cancellous bone, and suturing of
the palatal mucosa. (F) Schematic drawing showing rotation of the buccal
mucogingival flap and suturing of the flap to the palatal mucosa to close
the alveolar cleft defect.

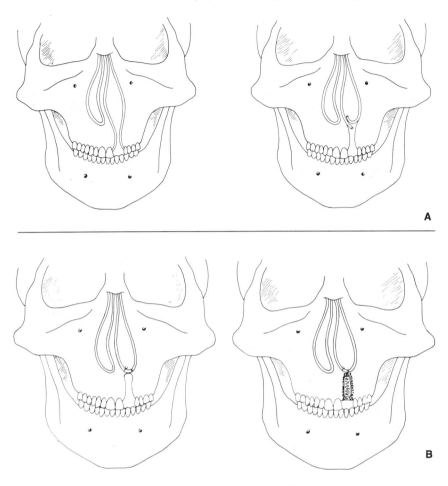

Figure 4.12 Schematic drawings demonstrate steps in closure of unilateral cleft and placement of bone grafts. (From "Residual Alveolar and Palatal Clefts" by D. E. Waite and R. B. Kersten, in W. H. Bell, W. R. Proffit, & R. P. White, *Surgical Correction of Dentofacial Deformities,* Vol. 2, Philadelphia: W. B. Saunders Co. Reprinted with permission.)

then advanced into position and sutured (Figure 4.13E). If the premaxilla requires surgical repositioning, then it is positioned simultaneously with the bone graft.

Once the soft tissue flaps are developed, as described previously, a curved osteotome is inserted palatally and a vertical osteotomy is carried to the level of the nasal septum. The premaxilla is then mobilized with digital pressure and rotated labially. This allows direct visualization for removal of any bone or cartilage interfering with proper repositioning of the segment. Closure of the nasal floor is greatly facilitated

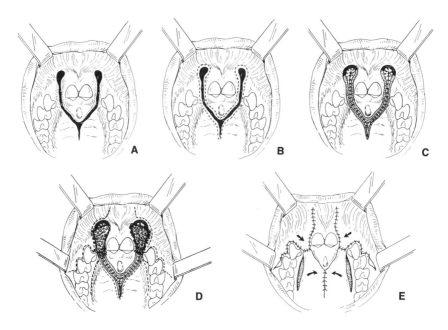

Figure 4.13 (A) Schematic drawing showing bilateral alveolar cleft defects. (B) Schematic drawing showing initiation of bilateral buccopalatal flaps (marked by dotted lines). (C) Schematic drawing showing reflection of the flap upon itself to create the new nasal floor bilaterally. (D) Schematic drawing showing augmentation of the alveolar cleft defect bilaterally with autogenous bone grafting. (E) Schematic drawing showing closing of the buccal and palatal flaps in a bilateral case.

by rotation of the premaxilla labially to allow direct visualization. The premaxilla is then positioned in the desired location and secured to a preconstructed stent. The bone graft is inserted and labial closure is accomplished as previously described. A heavy labial orthodontic wire and occlusal stent are sometimes used to stabilize the premaxilla to the posterior maxillary segments.

Postsurgical Aspects

Surgical considerations.   Adhering to basic surgical principles for handling tissues and closure of wounds will result in a minimum of problems with wound healing and will contribute to a high rate of success. Sutures are removed after 10 days. Careful attention to oral hygiene and use of saline nasal drops to moisten the nasal mucosa, of liquid diet, and of antibiotics and decongestive medications should provide optimal conditions for early healing. A secondary vestibuloplasty may be required to reposition the redundant tissue in the vestibular depth that may have resulted from rotating the flaps into the area around the grafted alveolar cleft defect to cover the graft.

Dental and orthodontic considerations. Postsurgical orthodontic treatment is usually necessary to align the teeth more precisely. Unerupted teeth, particularly the canine in the cleft region, may require orthodontic guidance to bring the tooth into its correct position. El Deeb et al. (1982) studied a total of 64 canines erupting through grafted alveolar cleft defects. They found that 27% of the canines erupted spontaneously, 17% required surgical uncovering, and 56% required both surgical uncovering and orthodontic assistance to accomplish eruption. All 64 canines erupted and were positioned in the oral cavity, where they provided normal function. All 46 patients required orthodontic treatment to accomplish final alignment of the dental arch.

MANAGEMENT OF MAXILLARY/MANDIBULAR DISCREPANCIES

Dentofacial Growth and Development

Following the bone graft, dentofacial growth and development should be closely followed by the cleft palate team, with emphasis on the need to plan for a possible treatment involving a combination of orthodontic and surgical treatment (orthognathic), especially treatment related to the patient's social, psychological, and intellectual well-being. Despite the team's best efforts to predict growth, evaluate patient progress, and recommend timely and sequential treatment, late problems with growth and development may still occur. The essential nature of this congenital anomaly is a deficiency of tissue. As completion of growth approaches, this deficiency of tissue, especially in bilateral clefts (Banks, 1983), frequently presents a noticeable underdevelopment of the mid-facial region. The eventual severity of mid-facial deformity is affected not only by the extent of the initial clefting, but also by the surgical timing, type, impact on growth, and success of any earlier corrective procedures.

Mid-facial deficiency may present as nasal distortion, particularly in the region of the alar base corresponding to the cleft. Buccal and anterior crossbites, overclosure in centric occlusion, dental midline shifts, and anterior or lateral open bite are additional problems. Mandibular growth relative to maxillary growth must also be followed over time to ensure optimal treatment planning. Mandibular deformity may also be present, but frequently the mandible is normal and the apparent prognathism is due to the deficient maxilla.

A systematic approach to the collection and analysis of records, along with a careful clinical assessment, is necessary for all patients with dentofacial deformities. Cleft patients, however, require particular evaluation with standard methods of analysis. Treatment may require modification in light of the special problems that this deformity may present. Scar tissue from several operations may adversely affect speech as well as dentition. The limited blood supply associated with scar tissue may interfere with additional planned procedures.

The team should obtain careful history and clinical examination, models for study, and lateral and posteroanterior cephalographs and panoramic, intraoral occlusal, and periapical dental roentgenograms. Facial and intraoral photographs, analysis of patterns of speech, cinefluoroscopy or videofluoroscopy, and nasoendoscopy are also important. Regular team evaluations are desirable, and presurgical orthodontics is usually necessary. The most common finding in lateral cephalometric analysis is maxillary retrusion; however, a skeletal Class III deformity (prognathism), with or without a high gonial angle, may also be present. This may indicate the presence of a coexisting mandibular deformity that may also require correction.

Presurgical orthodontics is for the purpose of aligning the dental arches prior to surgical repositioning of the jaws. Aligning of teeth is essential for postoperative stability of the arch and for subsequent decrease in the incidence of relapse. The inherently small maxilla, or the presence of scar tissue of the palate, may seriously limit the orthodontic treatment, making surgical expansion of the maxilla necessary. Closure of residual oronasal fistulae, if present, should also be included in the treatment plan. Careful note of velopharyngeal function and the effect of surgical advancement of the maxilla on speech must also be of concern to the surgeon (Schendel, Oeschlaeger, Wolford, & Epker, 1979).

The primary goal of maxillary and mandibular surgery is to correct any anteroposterior, vertical, and transverse discrepancies. For that reason, evaluation of any skeletodental malformations should be accomplished in these three planes (Figure 4.14). Thorough evaluation of facial aesthetics, including the facial contour and proportions of the mid-facial area, with particular emphasis on the infraorbital and nasolabial areas, is needed. Dividing the face using various lines along the midsagittal plane and the Frankfurt horizontal plane might help the clinician in the evaluation. The lines will divide the face into two halves laterally and four quadrants frontally (Figures 4.15A and 4.15B). The clinician can then evaluate those sections of the face that appear to be abnormally proportioned.

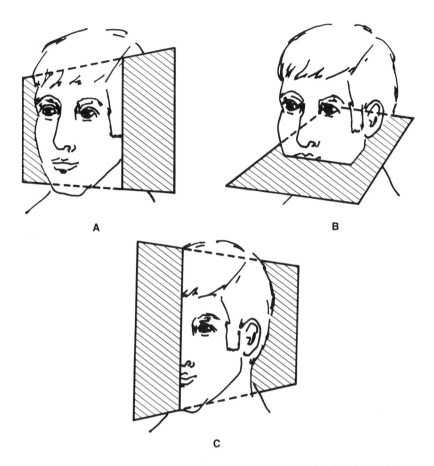

Figure 4.14 Schematic drawing showing examination of the facial deformity in three
dimensions: vertically (A), horizontally (B), and anteroposteriorly (C). (From
"Maxillary Asymmetry" by W. Bell, W. R. Proffit, and R. P. White, 1980,
in *Surgical Correction of Dentofacial Deformities*, Vol. 2, Philadelphia: W. B.
Saunders Co. Reprinted with permission.)

Timing of Maxillary and Mandibular Osteotomies

The timing of facial osteotomies in patients with and without clefts
remains a controversial issue. However, there appears to be agreement
in the recent literature that osteotomies of the skull and the cranial
base should be performed early. When discussing the timing of facial
osteotomies, Freihofer (1982) stated,

> There is no doubt that in severely deformed patients, important psycholog-
> ical, functional, and even vital indications exist to decide on a very early

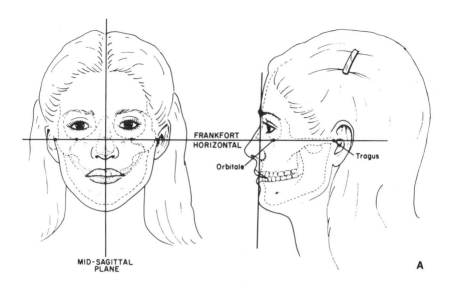

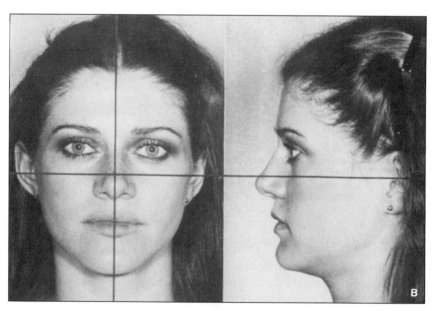

Figure 4.15 Schematic drawing (A) and photograph (B) showing division of the face into two halves laterally, each represented in equal size, by two lines drawn perpendicular to each other along the midsagittal plane and along the Frankfort horizontal line. This will facilitate detection of any abnormalities when the normal is compared with the abnormal quadrant.

operation even at the price of the necessity of correcting a secondary deformity that develops during growth. One should be careful not to try to treat minor aberrations from normal too early because patience on the part of the patient and the surgeon reduces the probability that a second operation will be needed. (pp. 452–453)

Mandibular advancement. Obwegeser (1957) reported marked relapse in mandibular sagittal split advancement. In seven young patients, Freihofer (1977) reported 6% relapse with the same surgical technique in growing children. Wolford, Schendel, and Epker (1979) reported less than 5% relapse in a group of 12 actively growing children. Paulus and Steinhauser (1981) reported 18% relapse on the average. Reichenbach (1966) advocated correction of mandibular deficiency after 12 years of age.

Mandibular repositioning. Many follow-up studies on the treatment of adult prognathic patients can be found in the literature. Cook and Hinrichsen (1973) found that all patients with significant relapse were under 19 years of age. The reported incidence of marked relapse is between 5% and 15% (Egyedi, 1980; MacIntosh, 1981; Stea, 1971).

Maxillary advancement. Freihofer (1977) reported that severe sagittal pseudo-relapse of occlusion occurred in 35% of 20 maxillary advancements after a Le Fort I osteotomy in adolescents (see Note 1). In fully grown patients, the results are far better. Kufner (1971) reported 7% relapse, whereas Nissen and Schmidseder (1981) reported 0% relapse. Incidence of relapse in cleft palate patients treated with maxillary advancement is usually much higher than in patients without clefts. Willmar (1974) found an average relapse of 0.6 mm in patients without clefts and 1 mm in patients with clefts.

Similarly, Stenberg (1986) evaluated the long-term stability of the Le Fort I osteotomy in 14 patients with cleft palate and 8 control patients without clefts. She found that the mean advancement recorded for the control group was 4.4 mm, with a 0-mm posterior relapse. In the group with cleft palate, the mean advancement was 5.4 mm, with a 0.6-mm relapse. There was no significant difference between the results in patients with cleft palate followed for the long term (2 to 15 years) and those followed for the short term (up to 2 years). Twenty-three percent of condylar growth was observed in 5 of the 15 cases. The mean age at the time of surgery for those patients who had evidence of growth was 16 years.

When maxillary and mandibular surgery is required, maxillary osteotomy usually is performed first. Final adjustment of the occlusion and profile is carried out when the maxilla is firm. This may be accomplished by surgical procedures directed at the mandibular position, such as subapical osteotomy, a mandibular setback, or genioplasty. Relapse following maxillary osteotomies has been greatly reduced since the development and utilization of rigid fixation.

In summary, maxillomandibular surgery should be postponed in cases of moderate deformity until growth is complete. When early surgery is considered as a necessity for aesthetic, social, or psychological reasons, the possibility of a second surgery should be presented to the patients and parents.

Presurgical Planning and Speech Considerations

Maxillary advancement surgery usually involves Le Fort I osteotomy of the maxilla with appropriate movement of the osteotomized units into predetermined positions. The surgery is first simulated on models prepared from current dental impressions and mounted on a special anatomical articulator (Figure 4.16A). An accurate wax "bite" and recordings from the face-bow transfer will permit the models to be mounted so as to simulate related movements of the patient's jaws. Repositioning of one model or the other, or of segments of the models, can then be assumed to reflect similar jaw movements at the time of surgery (Figure 4.16B).

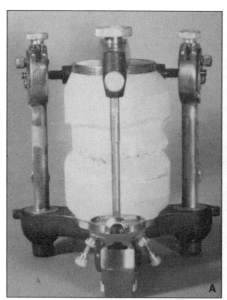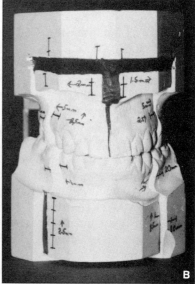

Figure 4.16 (A) Photograph showing maxillary and mandibular casts mounted on a Hanau semiadjustable articulator. (B) Surgical model for a maxillomandibular osteotomy case. Notice that surgical movement could be measured from the presectioned and postsectioned study model lines.

A recent lateral cephalograph is used to trace the skeletal and soft tissue facial profile and to analyze it using established norms as baselines. This enables the clinician to measure on a linear scale the distances through which the skeletal components must be moved at the time of surgery to arrive at a balanced soft tissue profile and acceptable skeletal and dental relationships. These analyses and predictions must be coordinated, and all changes and predictions are tested by "surgery" on the model. Occasional full-face photographs of the patient are also used to test the proposed movements. A realistic appearance for that patient is then simulated and may also serve as helpful information for the patient and related persons.

As mentioned earlier, a specific concern with procedures for maxillary advancement is their possible adverse effect on speech as a result of compromise to velopharyngeal closure (Schendel et al., 1979; Witzel & Munro, 1977). The patient with cleft palate often fails to achieve, or only marginally achieves, closure in normal circumstances. Such patients have little or no compensatory reserve, and there is a greater risk of hypernasal speech occurring after maxillary advancement (Mason, Turvey, & Warren, 1980). Those who already exhibit hypernasal speech may not noticeably worsen; however, those who are not so affected before maxillary advancement are at risk of having increased hypernasality after surgery. Although the risk is small and may be only temporary, it is often alarming to the patient. Consultation with speech pathologists, including appropriate recording and documentation, is essential preoperatively. This also should be followed up postoperatively as needed.

Surgical Procedures—General Considerations

Patients are admitted to the hospital and prepared for a major surgical procedure. For the young patient with cleft palate, special anesthetic considerations are necessary. It is common practice today for the anesthesiologist to induce controlled hypotension during major orthognathic surgical procedures to the maxilla. This aids in reducing blood loss, which otherwise may be considerable, and greatly improves visibility of the surgical site. The surgeon will also employ specific local measures, such as the infiltration of local anesthetic solutions containing low concentrations of epinephrine ($\frac{1}{200,000}$) into the soft tissues to be incised, and the judicious use of electrocautery and packs to minimize blood loss. Despite such careful attention to blood loss, patients may require blood transfusion. Interocclusal acrylic stents may be required to provide stability of the dental occlusion during the postsurgical fixation period, and these should be made immediately prior to surgery and checked against the patient's dentition. Prophylactic antibiotics and steroids are used during and after surgery to prevent infection and reduce postoperative swelling.

The most commonly used surgical procedure for correction of maxillary deficiency is the Le Fort I osteotomy. The basic procedure described here may be modified when unilateral or bilateral alveolar bone grafts and closure of a fistula are carried out simultaneously (Henderson & Jackson, 1975; Tideman, Stoelinga, & Gallia, 1980). Bone grafting is usually indicated, as described earlier in this chapter, and, although allogenic materials are available, autogenous bone is superior and enhances healing and early consolidation of the osteotomized maxilla. The usual locations for bone grafts are posterior, between the pterygoid plates and the posterior maxillary bone (Araujo, Schendel, Wolford, & Epker, 1978) (Figures 4.17A and 4.17B). When sufficient vertical height of bone exists to permit a step-osteotomy as described by Bennett and Wolford (1985), then the bone graft is tailored carefully to fit into the step. This is very helpful in preventing relapse. Interpositional grafts are used, when necessary, to augment the vertical height of the maxilla. Tailored onlay grafts are used to augment deficient molar areas. The use of bone grafts in alveolar clefts has been discussed earlier and, when indicated, are used in conjunction with maxillary osteotomies.

Maxillary Osteotomies

A detailed description of this procedure and its applications can be found elsewhere (Bell, 1973), but a brief description of the surgical approach is in order. The entire maxilla is mobilized in a manner that allows direct visual access to the nasal and antral surfaces, as well as the pterygoid region. This has been shown to be a biologically sound surgical procedure (Bell, 1973). Nelson, Path, Ogle, Waite, and Meyer (1977) and

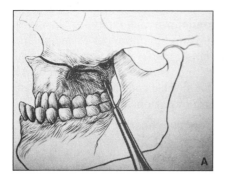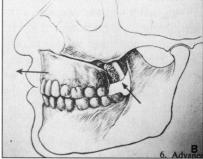

Figure 4.17 (A) Schematic drawing showing cutting the lateral maxillary bone with a surgical drill. Notice the maxilla in a retruded position as related to the mandible. (B) Schematic drawing showing advancing the maxilla into the desired occlusion and placing bone graft between the posterior maxillary surfacial and the pterygoid plate (marked by posterior arrow).

El Deeb, Waite, and Meyer (1981), in animal experiments relating to blood flow, demonstrated that good circulation is maintained in the osteotomized maxilla. Normal healing of the soft tissues and bone will occur provided adequate blood supply is maintained. This blood supply usually has been provided by the palatal and labiogingival tissue. Therefore, detachment and disturbance to these tissues should be avoided.

In unilateral cleft palate patients, the maxilla is divided into a large segment (the non-cleft segment) and a lesser segment (the cleft segment). The skeletodental deformity usually affects the clefted segment more often than the non-cleft segment. If adequate orthodontic follow-up is not provided, usually the small posterior maxillary segment is constricted medially, superiorly, and posteriorly. If the larger segment is in good alignment with the mandibular arch, then posterior maxillary osteotomy is usually indicated to correct the constricted lesser segment. This is usually accomplished by a vestibular incision that is modified near the cleft area (Braun & Sotereanos, 1981) if the alveolar cleft defect is previously unrepaired (Figure 4.18A).

Once the tissue around the alveolar cleft is resected and the vestibular incision is made superiorly, the lateral bony cut in the maxilla is performed above the apices of the teeth utilizing a surgical drill (Figure 4.18B). The medial wall in most cases does not exist due to the presence of the cleft and does not need to be osteotomized. A pterygoid osteotome is then introduced between the posterior segment of the maxilla and the pterygoid plate, and the posterior maxilla segment is then separated from the pterygoid plates (Figure 4.18C). Once this is accomplished, the posterior segment is advanced into the predetermined position utilizing the occlusal acrylic stent for guidance. The maxilla usually is moved downward anteriorly and buccally (Figure 4.18D). Then the nasal floor is closed utilizing the resorbable-type suture. The gap created between the zygomatic maxillary segment and the repositioned maxillary alveolar segments are grafted with autogenous corticocancellous bone (Figure 4.18E). The alveolar cleft defect is also grafted with autogenous cancellous bone.

The segments are either stabilized utilizing an intraosseous wiring or a miniplate for rigid fixation (Figures 4.18E and 4.18F). The mobilized maxillary segment can also be moved to close the gap created by the presence of the alveolar cleft defect. This can be accomplished only if the gap is not more than 5 mm. In this case, no bone grafting to the alveolar cleft area is needed. Additional bone may be added superiorly, toward the nasal side where the alveolar cleft area is usually present. If the gap is larger than 5 mm, it is usually very difficult to move the lesser segment more than that amount because of the possibilities of traumatizing the soft tissue pedicle, as well as the presence of palatal

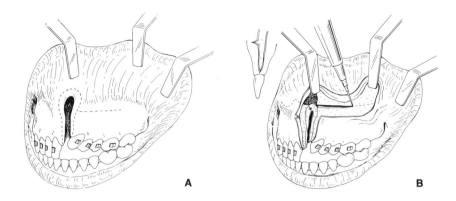

Figure 4.18 (A) Schematic drawing showing an unrepaired alveolar cleft defect and a collapse of the posterior maxillary segment in the cleft area medially, superiorly, and anterioposteriorly. Notice the flap design modification around the oral–nasal fistula. (B) Schematic drawing showing the flap being reflected medially to create the nasal floor. The osteotomy procedure has been performed above the apices of the teeth and through the lateral wall of the maxilla utilizing a surgical drill. (C) Schematic drawing showing sectioning of the pterygoid plate (a) from the maxillary segment (b) utilizing a curved pterygoid osteotome (c). (D) Schematic drawing showing repositioning of the posterior maxillary segment into an occlusal stent (s) and wiring the teeth into a predetermined position. The nasal mucosa is also closed. (E) Schematic drawing showing repositioning of the collapsed posterior maxillary segment into a predetermined position to a preconstructed occlusal stent. Notice placement of the bone graft between the lateral maxillary cut (a) into the alveolar cleft defect area (b) and into the pterygoid plate (c). (F) Schematic drawing showing movement of the posterior maxillary segment into the cleft area forward, as indicated by the arrow, to close the alveolar cleft defect area. Also, notice the lateral and maxillary cut with the bone graft marked by the a's. The maxillary segment is fixed in place utilizing many plates after the maxilla is placed into the preconstructed stent. The schematic drawing also shows the design of the flap (b) to cover the grafted osteotomy area. (G) Schematic drawing showing closing of the various incisions. (H) Schematic drawing showing complete unilateral cleft. Notice the lateral osteotomy cut indicated by the dotted line. (I) Schematic drawing showing the separation of the nasal septum utilizing a nasal septal osteotome. (J) Schematic drawing showing bilateral vestibular incision along the clefted and nonclefted segments. Notice also that insising the nasal mucosa in the clefted area is needed by utilizing a sharp blade. (K) Schematic drawing showing fracturing of the maxilla in down-fractured position and suturing of both nasal and oral mucosa in the clefted side. (L) Schematic drawing showing retruded maxilla. Notice the arrows showing the movement of the clefted and nonclefted segments anteriorly, buccally, and downward. The osteotomy cut is marked by a dotted line. (M) Schematic drawing showing movement of the maxilla into the desired position. Notice placement of bone along the lateral maxillary segments (a), along the alveolar cleft defect area (b), and between the pterygoid plate and the posterior maxillary segment.

(Figure continues)

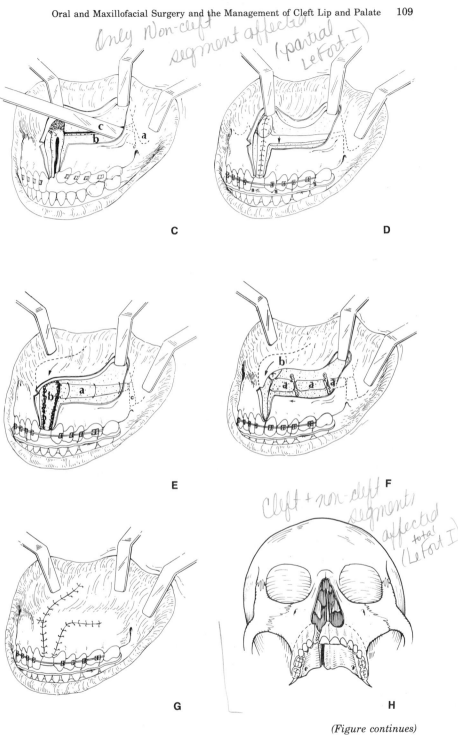

(Figure continues)

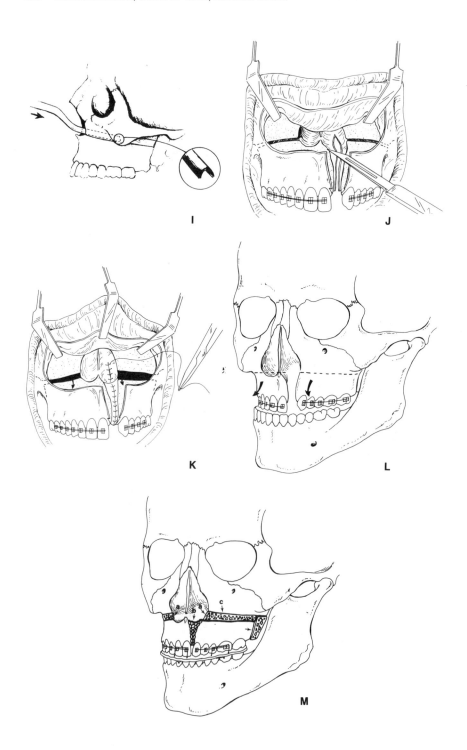

scar tissue from previous surgeries. The maxillary segment can be stabilized by intraosseous wiring (Figure 4.18E), miniplates with rigid fixation (Figure 4.18F), or suspension wire. Rigid fixation will enhance healing, and decrease the degree of postoperative relapse. A modified vestibular flap is then reflected from the superior portion of the vestibule to close the incision area (Figure 4.18G).

If both the nonclefted segment and the clefted segment are affected, then the total Le Fort I maxillary osteotomy is needed. Figure 4.18H shows a schematic drawing that depicts the osteotomy cut with the dotted line. The incision and the maxillary osteotomy are similar to those previously described, except that the nasal septum needs to be sectioned and separated from the maxilla utilizing a nasal septal chisel (Figure 4.18I). The maxilla is pressed inferiorly by applying steady force in the anterior nasal floor. As the maxilla tilts downward, the soft tissues attached to its nasal surface are carefully detached, and sometimes a sharp dissection is needed to free the maxilla from the nasopalatal scar into the down-fracturing position (Figure 4.18J).

Because complete mobilization of the maxilla is very difficult to accomplish manually, raw disimpacting forceps sometimes is used for this purpose. The forward movement of the maxilla in patients with cleft palate may be limited by residual scar tissue from previous palatal surgery, or the presence of a pharyngeal flap that makes this movement more difficult to accomplish than in the patient without cleft palate. The mobilized maxilla, which more frequently consists of two (in unilateral cases) or three (in bilateral cases) segments, is repositioned and wired to the mandible using, if necessary, a previously constructed interocclusal stent. If there is any tear of the nasal or oral mucosa, this should be sutured with the maxilla in the down-fracture position (Figure 4.18K). The bone graft is then placed between the lateral walls of the maxilla, the posterior pterygoid plate area, and the alveolar cleft defect area as described earlier (Figures 4.18L and 4.18M).

The incision line is then closed. The repositioned maxillary bony segments are secured as described earlier by means of direct intraosseous wire ligatures and/or "mini" bone plates. A suspension wire from the piriform operative and/or the zygomatic buttresses might be needed. Intermaxillary fixation may be used for 6 to 8 weeks. Soft tissue wounds are closed without tension. Figures 4.19 through 4.23 show photographs of a cleft palate patient treated with Le Fort I osteotomy.

The Le Fort II or III osteotomies may be considered in patients with marked nasomaxillary hypoplasia, where the Le Fort I osteotomy with bone grafting does not correct the essential aesthetic deformity (Epker, Fish, & Paulus, 1978; Epker & Wolford, 1976).

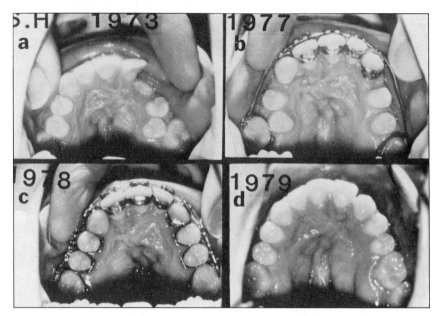

Figure 4.19 (a) Occlusal view for the maxillary arch. Preoperative view at age 9. Notice the multiple dental irregularities. (b) The canine (arrow) erupted through the alveolar cleft defect. (c) Post–alveolar cleft defect graft shown at age 14. The canine erupted into the alveolar cleft defect area. The orthodontist aligned the teeth in segments preoperatively. (d) Post–maxillary Le Fort I osteotomy. Notice good arch alignment. Age of patient: 16.

Mandibular Surgery

As mentioned earlier, a relative or even a slight degree of true prognathism may be present in patients with mid-face hypoplasia. We choose to defer any mandibular surgery that involves setting back the mandible until at least a year after the maxilla has been advanced. Any relapse that occurs can be compensated for by a mandibular setback. This will enable a stable functioning, aesthetic occlusion, and pleasant profile.

Postsurgical Care of the Patient with Repaired Cleft

The topic of patient postsurgical care is well covered in surgical texts, but it should be emphasized here that patients who have undergone a major maxillofacial surgery procedure require specialized nursing care to ensure that a satisfactory airway is maintained and that intraoral wounds are kept clean. Carefully controlled irrigation of intraoral surgical sites, nasogastric tube feeds, and gentle massage of mucosal flaps to reduce congestion and enhance the flow of oxygenated blood into their

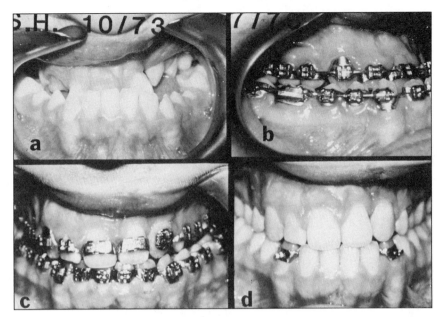

Figure 4.20   (a) An intraoral occlusion view for both maxillary and mandibular arches. Notice the lingual crossbite for both the anterior and the posterior maxillary teeth preoperatively. Age of patient: 9. (b) Preoperative Le Fort I osteotomy occlusion. The orthodontist aligned both the maxillary and the mandibular arches before the osteotomy. Age of patient: 16. (c) Immediate postoperative maxillary advancement and mandibular setback occlusion. Notice improved alignment of teeth. Age of patient: 16. (d) Intraoral view representing the final occlusion following completion of orthodontic treatment. Age of patient: 20.

extremities, should be carried out at regular intervals. Medications to control pain, prevent infection, and reduce swelling; humidification of the nasal passages; chest physiotherapy; and supervised gradual return to physical activity are part of the routine postoperative program for most patients who are encouraged to assume responsibility for their oral hygiene and food intake while still in the hospital so that when discharged they will maintain adequate standards of hygiene and nutrition.

Postoperative X-rays, consisting of cephalometric, panoramic, and laminographic views, are normally used to evaluate the surgical sites prior to the patient's discharge from the hospital. Weekly outpatient visits are made to evaluate wound healing, fixation, and general progress, and the maxillomandibular fixation is usually released between 6 and 8 weeks, when clinical union is evident. However, the use of night elastics should be utilized. Postsurgical orthodontic treatment, when indicated, should commence as soon as possible after release from surgical fixation. Speech evaluation may be carried out after

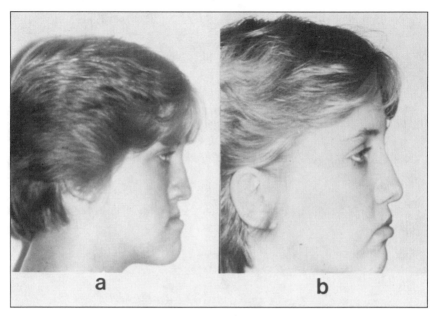

Figure 4.21 Extraoral lateral photographs showing preoperative and postoperative mandibular setback and maxillary advancement procedure. Notice the aesthetic improvement of the patient's facial profile. (From "Maxillary Asymmetry" by W. Bell, W. R. Proffit, and R. P. White, 1980, in *Surgical Correction of Dentofacial Deformities*, Vol. 2, Philadelphia: W. P. Saunders Co. Reprinted with permission.)

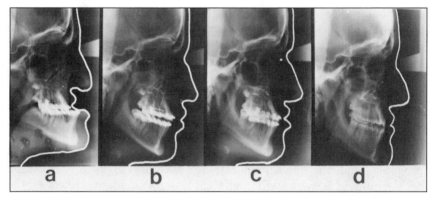

Figure 4.22 Series of lateral cephalometric radiographs: (a) immediately preoperative, (b) immediately postoperative, (c) 2 years postoperative, and (d) 6 years postoperative.

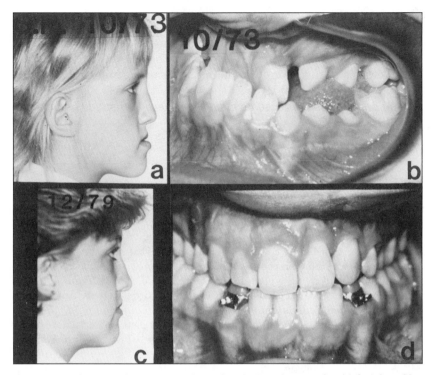

Figure 4.23 Facial profile photographs and occlusion photographs: (a) facial profile—age 8, (b) occlusion—age 8, (c) facial profile—age 20, and (d) occlusion—age 20.

3 months, and if deterioration has occurred, further evaluation should be recorded after 1 year to assess whether velopharyngeal compensation has occurred. In patients with persistent hypernasal speech, correction with a pharyngeal flap or prosthesis should be considered.

SUMMARY

The oral and maxillofacial surgeon's contributions to the treatment of the patient with cleft lip and palate are long term. Such treatment takes place during various stages of the patient's growth and development. Surgical interventions, when properly planned and executed, can greatly enhance the quality of function and the aesthetic result. It is clear that the consultative process among all members of the cleft palate team greatly benefits the patient and should be a part of providing care for the patient with dentofacial anomalies.

NOTE

1. Le Fort I refers to a level of the cutting line as described and classified by Rene Le Fort in 1901. Typically, three levels are described: Le Fort I is at the floor of the nose; Le Fort II is higher in the midfacial area; and Level III is at the level of the eyes. For more complete descriptions of these levels, the reader is referred to Rowe and Williams (1985).

REFERENCES

Araujó, A., Schendel, S. A., Wolford, L. M., & Epker, B. N. (1978). Total maxillary advancement with and without bone grafting. *Journal of Oral Surgery, 36*, 849–858.

Backdahl, M., & Nordin, K. E. (1961). Replacement of the maxillary bone defect in cleft palate. A new procedure. *Acta Chirurgica Scandinavica, 122*, 131.

Backdahl, M., Nordin, K., Nylen, B., & Strombeck, J. (1963). *Transactions of the International Society of Plastic Surgery* (p. 193), 3rd Congress. Amsterdam: Excerpta Medica Foundation.

Banks, P. (1983). The surgical anatomy of secondary cleft lip and palate deformity and its significance in reconstruction. *British Journal of Oral Surgery, 21*, 78–93.

Bell, W. H. (1973). Biologic basis for maxillary osteotomies. *American Journal of Physical Anthropology, 38*, 279–289.

Bennett, M. E., & Wolford, L. M. (1985). Maxillary surgery technical considerations. In W. H. Bell (Ed.), *Surgical correction of dentofacial deformities* (Vol. 3, pp. 45–52). Philadelphia: W. B. Saunders.

Berkowitz, S. (1978). State of the art in cleft palate orofacial growth and dentistry: A historical perspective. *American Journal of Orthodontics, 74*, 564–576.

Bishara, S. E., & Olin, W. H. (1972). Surgical repositioning of the premaxilla in complete bilateral cleft lip and palate. *Angle Orthodontist, 42*, 564–576.

Boyne, P. J., & Sands, N. R. (1972). Secondary bone grafting of residual alveolar and palatal cleft. *Journal of Oral Surgery, 30*, 87–92.

Boyne, P. J., & Sands, N. R. (1976). Combined orthodontic–surgical management of residual palato–alveolar cleft defects. *American Journal of Orthodontics, 70*, 20.

Braun, T. W., & Sotereanos, G. C. (1981). Orthognathic surgical reconstruction of cleft palate deformities in adolescents. *Journal of Oral Surgery, 39*, 255–263.

Broude, D. J., & Waite, D. E. (1974). Secondary closure of alveolar defects. *Oral Surgery, 37*, 829–840.

Carollo, D., Hoffman, R., & Brodie, A. (1971). Histology and function of the dental gubernacular cord. *Angle Orthodontist, 41*, 300–307.

Cook, D., & Hinrichsen, G. (1973). The mandibular sagittal split osteotomy: A clinical and cephalometric review. *Transactions of the Congress of the International Association of Oral Surgery, 4*, 252.

Drachter, R. (1914). Die Gaumenspalte und deren operative Behandlung. *Deutsche Zeitschrift fur Chirurgie, 131,* 1–89.

Egyedi, P. (1980). Overcorrection in mandibular advancement. *Journal of Maxillofacial Surgery, 8,* 266.

El Deeb, M. E., El Deeb, M., & Bevis, R. (1989). Canine erupted through grafted alveolar cleft defects in patients with alveolar cleft: A pulp testing evaluation study. *Cleft Palate Journal, 26,* 100–104.

El Deeb, M. E., Hinrichs, J. E., Waite, D. E., Bandt, C. L., & Bevis, R. (1986). Repair of alveolar cleft defects with autogenous grafting: Periodontal evaluation. *Cleft Palate Journal, 23,* 126–136.

El Deeb, M. E., Lehnert, M. W., & Waite, D. E. (1983, May). *Surgical management of missing and edentulous premaxilla in cleft palate patients.* Paper presented at the annual meeting of The American Cleft Palate Association.

El Deeb, M. E., Messer, L. B., Lehnert, M. W., Hebda, T. W., & Waite, D. E. (1982). Canine eruption into grafted bone in maxillary alveolar cleft defects. *Cleft Palate Journal, 19*(1), 9–16.

El Deeb, M. E., Waite, D. E., & Meyer, M. W. (1981). Evaluation of local blood flow after total maxillary osteotomy. *Journal of Oral Surgery, 39,* 249–254.

Enemark, H., Sindet-Pedersen, S., & Bundgaard, M. (1987). Long-term results after secondary bone grafting of alveolar clefts. *Journal of Oral Maxillofacial Surgery, 45,* 913–918.

Epker, B. N., Fish, L. C., & Paulus, P. J. (1978). Surgical orthodontic correction of maxillary deficiency. *Journal of Oral Surgery, 46,* 171–205.

Epker, B. N., & Wolford, L. M. (1976). Middle-third facial osteotomies—Their use in the correction of acquired and developmental dentofacial and craniofacial deformities. *Journal of Oral Surgery, 34,* 324–342.

Epstein, L. J., Davis, W. B., & Thompson, L. W. (1970). Delayed bone grafting in cleft palate patients. *Plastic and Reconstructive Surgery, 46,* 363–367.

Fishman, L. S. (1970). Factors related to tooth number, eruption time, and tooth position in cleft palate individuals. *Journal of Dentistry for Children, 37,* 303–306.

Flint, M. (1964). Chip bone grafting of the mandible. *British Journal of Plastic Surgery, 17,* 184–188.

Freihofer, H. P. M. (1977). Results of osteotomies of the facial skeleton in adolescence. *Journal of Maxillofacial Surgery, 5,* 267–297.

Freihofer, H. P. M. (1982). The timing of facial osteotomies in children and adolescents in clinics. *Plastic Surgery, 9,* 445–456.

Hall, H. D., & Posnick, J. C. (1983). Early results of secondary bone grafts in 106 alveolar clefts. *Journal of Maxillofacial Surgery, 41,* 289–294.

Hayward, J. R. (1983). Management of the premaxilla in bilateral clefts. *Journal of Oral Maxillofacial Surgery, 41,* 518–524.

Henderson, D., & Jackson, I. J. (1975). Combined cleft lip revision, anterior fistula closure and maxillary osteotomy: A one stage procedure. *British Journal of Oral Surgery, 13*(1), 33–39.

Hinrichs, J. E., El Deeb, M. E., Waite, D. E., Bevis, R. R., & Bandt, C. (1984, January). A periodontal evaluation of canines erupted through alveolar cleft defects in unilateral cleft. *Journal of Oral and Maxillofacial Surgery, 42*(11), 717–721.

Hogeman, K. E., Jacobsson, S., & Sarnas, K. V. (1972). Secondary bone grafting in cleft palate: A follow-up of 145 patients. *Cleft Palate Journal, 9*, 39–42.

Hotz, M. M., Gnoinski, W. M., Nussbaumer, H., & Kistler, E. (1978). Early maxillary orthopedics in CLP cases: Guidelines for surgery. *Cleft Palate Journal, 15*, 405–411.

Jackson, I. T., Scheker, L. R., Vandervord, J. G., & McLennan, J. G. (1981). Bone marrow grafting in the secondary closure of alveolarpalatal defects in children. *British Journal of Plastic Surgery, 34*, 422.

Jackson, I. T., Vandervard, J. G., McLennan, J. G., Christie, F. B., & McGregor, J. C. (1982). Bone grafting of the secondary cleft lip and palate deformity. *British Journal of Plastic Surgery, 35*, 345.

Johanson, B., Ohlson, A., Friede, H., & Ahlgren, J. (1974). A follow-up study of cleft lip and palate patients treated with orthodontics, secondary bone grafting, and prosthetic rehabilitation. *Scandinavian Journal of Plastic and Reconstructive Surgery, 8*, 121–135.

Jolleys, A., & Robertson, N. R. E. (1972). A study of the effects of early bone grafting in complete clefts of the lip and palate—Five year study. *British Journal of Plastic Surgery, 25*, 229–237.

Jordan, R., Kraus, B., & Neptune, C. (1966). Dental abnormalities associated with cleft lips and/or palate. *Cleft Palate Journal, 3*, 22–25.

Kent, K., & Schaaf, N. S. (1982). The effects of dental abnormalities on speech production. *Quintessence International, 12*, 1353–1362.

Koberg, W. R. (1973). Present view of bone grafting in cleft palate (review of the literature). *Journal of Maxillofacial Surgery, 1*, 185–198.

Koch, L. (1977). State of the art, section IV, surgical aspects and management. *Cleft Palate Journal, 14*, 302–312.

Kufner, J. (1971). Four year experience with major maxillary osteotomy for retrusion. *Journal of Oral Surgery, 29*, 549.

Kwon, H. J., Waite, D. E., Stickel, F. R., Chisholm, T., & McParland, F. (1981). The management of alveolar cleft defects. *Journal of the American Dental Association, 102*, 848–853.

Lexer, E. (1908). Die Verwendung der freien Knochenplastik nebst versuchen uber Gelenkversteifung und gelenk Transplantation. *Klinische Chirurgie, 86*, 939–954.

MacIntosh, R. B. (1981). Experience with the sagittal osteotomy of the mandibular ramus: A 13 year review. *Journal of Maxillofacial Surgery, 9*, 151–165.

Mason, R., Turvey, T. A., & Warren, D. W. (1980). Speech considerations with maxillary advancement procedures. *Journal of Oral Surgery, 38*, 752–758.

Matthews, D., Broomhead, M., Chir, J., Grossman, W., & Goldin, H. (1970). Early and late bone grafting of cleft lip and palate. *British Journal of Plastic and Reconstructive Surgery, 23*, 115–129.

Nelson, R. L., Path, M., Ogle, R., Waite, D. E., & Meyer, M. W. (1977). Quantification of blood flow after Le Fort I osteotomy. *Journal of Oral Surgery, 35*(1), 10–16.

Nissen, G., & Schmidseder, R. (1981). Spatergebnisse nach operativer behebung von dysgnathian im Oberkiefer. *Fortschritte der Kiefer-und Gesichtschirurgie, 26*.

Nordin, K. D. (1957). Treatment of primary total cleft palate deformity. Preoperative orthopedic correction of the displaced components of the upper jaw in infants followed by bone grafting to the alveolar process clefts. *Transactions of the European Orthodontic Society* (pp. 333–339). The Hague: European Orthodontic Society.

Nylen, B. (1966). Surgery of the alveolar cleft. *Plastic and Reconstructive Surgery, 37*, 42–46.

Obwegeser, H. (1957). The surgical correction of mandibular prognathism and retrognathia with consideration of genioplasty. *Journal of Oral Surgery, Oral Medicine and Oral Pathology, 10*, 677–687.

Paulus, G. W., & Steinhauser, E. W. (1981). Vergleichende langzeituntersuchung von alveolaren und sagittalen osteotomien zur distalbisskorrektur. *Fortschritte der Kiefer-und Gesichtschirurgie, 26*, 39–41.

Petrovic, S. (1971). Unsere erfahrungen mit sekundaren knochenplastiken bei der therapie der spalten deformation des ober diefers und des gebisses. *Deutsche Zahn-Mund-und Kieferheilkunde, 57*, 230.

Pickrell, K., & Quinn, G. (1967). Primary, secondary and tertiary bone grafts in clefts of the lip and palate. *Panminerva Medica, 9*, 402.

Pickrell, K., Quinn, G., & Massengill, R. (1968). Primary bone grafting of the maxilla in clefts of the lips and palate. A four year study. *Plastic and Reconstructive Surgery, 41*, 438–443.

Primosch, R. E. (1981). Anterior supernumerary teeth—Assessment and surgical intervention in children. *Pediatric Dentistry, 392*, 204–215.

Ranta, R. (1971). Eruption of the premolars and canines and factors affecting it in unilateral cleft lip and palate cases. An orthopantomographic study. *Suomen Hammaslaakariseuran Toimituksia, 67*, 350–355.

Rehrmann, A. H., Koberg, W. R., & Koch, H. (1970). Long-term postoperative results of primary and secondary bone grafting in complete clefts of lip and palate. *Cleft Palate Journal, 7*, 206.

Reichenbach, E. (1966). Uber den zeitpunkt kiefer chirurgisch-orthopadischer. *Eingriffe. Deutsche Zahn-Mund-und Kieferheilkunde, 47*, 305.

Robertson, N. R. E., & Jolleys, A. (1968). Effects of early bone grafting in complete clefts of the lip and palate. *Plastic and Reconstructive Surgery, 42*, 414–421.

Robertson, N. R. E., & Jolleys, A. (1983). An 11 year follow-up of the effects of early bone grafting to infants born with complete clefts of the lip and palate. *British Journal of Plastic Surgery, 36*, 438–443.

Rosenstein, S. W., Jacobson, B. N., Monroe, C., Griffith, B. H., & McKinney, P. (1972). A series of cleft lip and palate children five years after undergoing orthopedic and bone grafting procedures. *Angle Orthodontist, 42*, 1.

Rosenstein, S. W., Monroe, C. W., Kernahan, D. A., Jacobson, B. W., Griffith, B. H., & Bauer, B. S. (1982). The case for early bone grafting in cleft lip and cleft palate. *Plastic and Reconstructive Surgery, 70*, 297–309.

Rowe, N. L., & Williams, J. L. (1985). *Maxillofacial injuries* (Vol. 1). London: Churchill Livingston.

Schendel, S. A., Oeschlaeger, M., Wolford, L. M., & Epker, B. N. (1979). Velopharyngeal anatomy and maxillary advancement. *Journal of Maxillofacial Surgery, 7*, 116–124.

Schmid, E. (1955). *Die Annaherung der Kieferstumpfe bie Lippen-Kiefer-Gaumen spalten.* Stuttgart: George Theime Verlag.

Skoog, T. (1965a). The management of the bilateral cleft of the primary palate (lip and alveolus): Part I. General considerations and soft tissue repair. *Plastic and Reconstructive Surgery, 35,* 34–44.

Skoog, T. (1965b). The management of the bilateral cleft of the primary palate (lip and alveolus): Part II. Bone grafting. *Plastic and Reconstructive Surgery, 35,* 140–147.

Stea, G. (1971). Notre experience dans le traitement du prognatisme. *Revue de Stomatologie et de Chirurgie Maxillo-faciale, 72,* 559.

Stenberg, D. J. (1986). *Long-term facial changes with maxillary advancement in cleft and non-cleft patients.* Unpublished master's thesis, University of Minnesota, Minneapolis.

Stenstrom, S. J., & Thilander, B. L. (1963). Bone grafting in secondary cases of cleft lip and palate. *Plastic and Reconstructive Surgery, 32,* 353–360.

Tideman, H., Stoelinga, P., & Gallia, L. (1980). Le Fort I advancement with segmental palatal osteotomies in patients with cleft palates. *Journal of Oral Surgery, 38,* 196.

Turvey, T. A., Vig, K., Moriarity, & Hoke, J. (1984). Delayed bone grafting in the cleft maxilla and palate: A retrospective multidisciplinary analysis. *American Journal of Orthodontics, 86,* 244–256.

von Eiselberg, F. W. (1901). Zur Technik der Uranoplastik. *Archiv Klinische Chirurgie, 64,* 509.

Waite, D. E., & Kersten, R. B. (1980). Residual alveolar and palatal clefts. In W. H. Bell, W. R. Proffit, & R. P. White (Eds.), *Surgical correction of dentofacial deformities* (Vol. 2, p. 1329). Philadelphia: Saunders.

Willmar, K. (1974). On Le Fort osteotomy: A followup study of 106 operated patients with maxillofacial deformity. *Scandinavian Journal of Plastic and Reconstructive Surgery, 12,* 5–68.

Witzel, M., & Munro, I. (1977). Velopharyngeal insufficiency after maxillary advancement. *Cleft Palate Journal, 14,* 176–180.

Wolford, L. M., Schendel, S. A., & Epker, B. N. (1979). Surgical–orthodontic correction of mandibular deficiency in growing children. *Journal of Maxillofacial Surgery, 7,* 72.

CHAPTER 5

Orthodontic Diagnosis and Treatment Procedures

Richard R. Bevis

In addition to describing the discipline of orthodontics and the education and training required, Bevis outlines some general principles of orthodontic treatment for patients with cleft lip and palate. The orthodontist needs to closely monitor each patient's facial, dental, and jaw growth and development because this can directly affect what can and cannot be accomplished with appliance therapy alone. Bevis discusses the phases of orthodontic treatment dependent upon dental and skeletal development and the phases of treatment from infancy to adulthood.

1.   *Bevis emphasizes the importance of minimizing time spent in orthodontic treatment phases and the value of coordinating effort with other disciplines. Defend his views.*
2.   *Bevis cites some research indicating good facial form and development of the maxilla when clefts have gone unrepaired for several years. What information would persuade you to encourage early palatal closure?*
3.   *Define cephalometry. Why is it important to orthodontists in diagnosis and treatment planning?*
4.   *Describe the rationale for presurgical orthopedics and early bone grafting. What are the disadvantages? In what situation does Bevis appear to support presurgical orthopedics?*
5.   *What are the treatment goals and objectives in the early mixed dentition stage? Later mixed dentition stage? Permanent dentition?*

Edward Angle (1907), the father of edgewise orthodontics, defined orthodontics as the correction of the malocclusion of teeth, whereas Noyes
(1911) called orthodontics "a study of the relation of the teeth to the
development of the face and the correction of arrested and perverted
development" (p. 69). Graber (1972) stated that any definition "must
include the aspects of preventive, interceptive, and corrective orthodontics" (p. 10). A definition of the dental specialty of orthodontics and
its role in the treatment of persons with cleft lip and palate must include
all the previously mentioned definitions, plus a special interest, knowledge, and commitment to close follow-up of facial form and functional
development. Treating patients with clefts is similar to treating patients
without clefts, but there can be several limitations and restrictions.

The required training for the specialty of orthodontics beyond the
Doctorate of Dental Surgery (DDS) degree includes several thousand
hours of didactic instruction and supervised clinical orthodontic treatments. The orthodontic resident must master all the anatomical sciences,
including embryology, histology, head and neck anatomy, and cellular
biology. Other courses typically include biometry, surgical orthodontics
(orthognathic surgery), mechanics of tooth movement, and cephalometry (measurement of head radiographs or X-rays). The resident must
become proficient in the prediction and altering of facial–dental growth
and development, as well as at cephalometry as it applies to head and
neck anatomy. Training also encompasses aspects of abnormal development, including syndromes of the head and neck, discrepancies of
facial and jaw growth, and psychological concerns associated with facial
disfigurement. The orthodontist must master all aspects of tooth movement, including the mechanical and physical response of the bone to
tooth (root) pressure.

The disorder of cleft lip and palate and the challenges it presents
to the orthodontist should also be an integral part of training. The
orthodontist must learn to work with the cleft palate patient and family
in close association with the other health care professionals as a part
of a cleft palate team. Each team member should have some knowledge of the general treatment principles of other team specialties,
including the response of bone to healing, transplantation, bone grafting,
soft tissue flaps, and grafts, as well as speech concerns and timing
of treatment.

The orthodontic concerns and treatment of cleft palate patients
are well documented in the literature (Aduss, 1971; Berkowitz, 1977;
Burston, 1958; Graber, 1949, 1954; Jacobson & Rosenstein, 1986; Olin,
1966; Pruzansky, 1953; Ross, 1987; Subtelny, 1966; Vargervik, 1981;
Vig & Turvey, 1985). Successful management demands a team effort,
with the timing of various treatments closely correlated with the
patient's growth and development. Based on over 20 years of team

participation, it is clear to me that each patient is unique. Even among identical twins (Figure 5.1), although there are similarities, there are important differences. The variety and severity of the cleft malformations make planning and treatment challenging, but gratifying. The team with which I work continues to learn from treatment of each patient. We modify our plans to meet each patient's needs, but attempt to consistently apply the knowledge generated over many years to achieve the goals of normal form and function. The best learning tool in stimulating innovative and constructive treatment goals is to be an active member of a cleft palate team. The team approach assures not only the most favorable treatment timing, but also the expeditious and effective achievement of the overall treatment goals.

GENERAL PRINCIPLES OF ORTHODONTIC TREATMENT

Although each patient has a unique need for orthodontic intervention, some general principles or guidelines can be applied to all patients with cleft lip and/or palate:

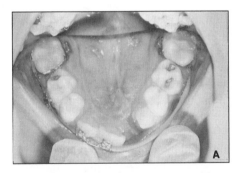

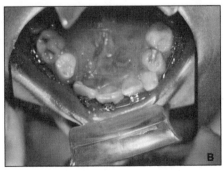

Figure 5.1 A comparison of the anterior oral view and palatal view of identical twins with unilateral cleft lip and palate. Although similar in tooth size and appearance, the clefts are different, and each requires a unique treatment plan.

1. Minimize the patient's time spent in fixed orthodontic appliances.
2. Coordinate the timing of orthodontic treatment with other treatments to yield stable, long-lasting results.
3. Monitor the stages of interceptive treatment, as well as dental and skeletal growth and development.
4. Coordinate orthodontic treatment to the most favorable growth and development stages, including the development of speech.

Each treatment phase should be as short as possible to minimize the effects of appliance wear on the patient's dental health, speech and oral function, physical comfort, and future cooperation. Unwarranted retreatments and prolonged orthodontic therapy can create an attitude of disinterest and burnout on the part of the patient. Furthermore, everyone involved with the patient becomes frustrated when a once-optimal result slowly evaporates as a patient grows out of his or her early treatment a few years later. A principle that holds for treatment of all patients, but is especially applicable to the orthodontic management of a patient with cleft palate, is to never treat too early when the treatment may interfere with normal growth or be completed before the pubertal growth spurt is realized.

Helpful short-term orthodontic therapy can be performed in the very young (i.e., newborns), throughout the mixed dentition, and into adulthood with dramatic and rewarding results. Both removable and fixed orthodontic appliances are useful in obtaining the treatment goals established by the interdisciplinary team. Comprehensive pretreatment records and periodic treatment planning conferences are required with all the professionals who are, or will be, involved with the patient's dental and medical care.

Finally, specific orthodontic procedures must be formulated with other team members who have to deal with the direct consequences of any orthodontic therapy. For example, early removable orthodontic appliances may present short-term hazards for speech, but be very beneficial for speech articulation in the long run. Therefore, specific treatment plans and timing of treatment must be coordinated with other disciplines to yield the optimal outcome.

THE ORTHODONTIST'S ROLE ON THE CLEFT PALATE TEAM

It is important that the orthodontist and the pediatric dentist meet early in the patient's treatment regarding tooth guidance and bone support in or near the maxillary alveolar cleft. Subsequently, the orthodontist is involved with the oral surgeon in determining the benefits and timing of alveolar bone grafting and labionasal fistula closure. Reconstructive surgery is involved with both soft and hard tissue alterations in the lip, palatal, and pharyngeal areas, as well as with nasal modifications. The majority of these procedures occur early and affect arch form and development to some degree; however, with advancements in surgical techniques, severe deviations in dental and jaw growth and development are infrequent. Timing is important for all the team members, and the orthodontist's treatment procedures can be crucial for the rest of the team. Orthodontic decisions as the child is growing can affect later treatments, such as prosthodontic management of missing teeth and bony defects where tooth replacement and tooth longevity must be considered. The speech pathologist can provide important input about the timing and effect on speech of either removable or fixed appliance treatment. The social worker and/or psychologist needs to be involved in decisions regarding early versus late treatment options. The psychological health and cooperation of both the patient and the family must be considered before treatment can begin. Of utmost importance in final treatment outcome is the patient's overall oral and dental health. Without excellent cooperation and support of the dentist and a rigorous home program, treatment will be compromised.

The orthodontist's major role on the team is to follow the facial and dental growth and development of each cleft palate patient with a best estimate of final outcome from an aesthetic and functional occlusion standpoint. The final aesthetic and functional occlusion is based on the additive effects of multiple treatment planning sessions from the early years to the adult years. The individual growth and development of each patient is an ever-changing composite of the soft and hard tissue changes with multiple tooth and arch variables. The team must rely on the orthodontist for periodic evaluation and prediction of growth and development and for providing direct treatment that is appropriately associated with the patient's physical and behavioral growth and development.

GROWTH AND DEVELOPMENT IN THE CLEFT PALATE PATIENT

Chapter 2 discusses in more detail the embryology and formation of the primary and secondary palate. The discussion in this chapter is more superficial. Growth in the primary palate (upper lip, premaxilla) starts embryologically with a proliferation from the first branchial arch, called the maxillary process. The process grows medially from lateral to the stomodeum to near the medial nasal process. Veau (1938) proposed that cleft lips are the result of failure of mesodermal penetration of the epithelial walls formed during the uniting of facial processes. Tondury (1961) similarly explained cleft formation as a disturbance and incomplete formation of the epithelial wall based on defective growth of a nasal swelling (e.g., of the lateral nasal process). Stark (1954) felt that clefting is the result of reduced amounts of mesoderm in the tissue within the cleft area.

Whereas the primary palate begins development from 4 to 5 weeks in the embryo, the secondary palate (hard and soft palate) begins formation at 7 to 8 weeks. The secondary palate develops in three stages after a medial extension of the maxillary process grows vertically into two palatal shelves. The three stages involve a movement of the shelves from a vertical to horizontal position by (a) shelf growth, (b) shelf elevation, and (c) shelf merging.

A failure of any of the three stages or a combination of effects will cause various degrees of clefting in the palate. For example, four injections of 2.5 mg of cortisone into pregnant Ajax strain mice at 11½ to 12½ days postconception will cause offspring with cleft lips and palates to rise from the expected 10% to 100% (Isaacson & Chaudhry, 1962).

The maxilla is further altered with continuing growth after birth. According to Latham and Scott (1970), unless early intervention occurs with removable molding appliances immediately after birth, arch collapse and asymmetrical deviations occur in the premaxilla, posterior maxillary segments, and nasal septum. Early surgical intervention will stabilize the maxilla and round out the upper arch form, but may constrict and slow down future anterior–posterior growth. A study from Sri Lanka of 28 unoperated males with cleft lip and palate over age 13 reported similar maxillary growth compared with normal Sri Lankan children of the same age group (Mars, James, & Lamabadusuriya, 1990). However, in another report, these same adolescents were found to have severely disordered speech (Sell & Grunwell, 1990).

To establish an approach for overall patient management, each team must weigh the benefits and costs of early presurgical orthodontic intervention and timing of initial palatal repair on facial–dental growth and development against behavioral aspects, such as speech and psychological concerns.

MONITORING AND RECORDING GROWTH AND DEVELOPMENT

Skeletal Patterns

Future arch discrepancies requiring orthognathic surgical treatment may become apparent as early skeletal patterns are evaluated in the young patient. The skeletal relationships in the early phase of the mixed dentition must be noted and documented because this will aid in future treatment planning. If the patients are being treated in a rural setting, the complete diagnostic record set takes on even more significance. In many settings, members of the interdisciplinary teams, including the orthodontist, must communicate findings and treatment plans to other health professionals in the patient's local community. They, in turn, need to base their treatment decisions on the records available for each patient.

Records

The first set of records obtained may not be a complete or ideal set. However, it is very important that an attempt be made to obtain at least a portion of the records in the very young patient. Early information, such as number, status, and position of developing teeth, is important not only to the orthodontist, but to other members of the team in planning future treatment.

Figure 5.2 demonstrates a complete set of records, including

1. Full-face and profile photographs of the right and left sides of the face
2. Complete set of intraoral photos, including occlusals
3. Lateral and posterior–anterior (PA) cephalometric (head) radiographs (tomographic radiographs may also be helpful)
4. Full-mouth and/or panographic-type intraoral radiographs
5. Plaster casts or models of each arch with good peripheral extension onto basal bone (registration is made in centric relation, or when the patient bites [occludes] with the mandible in the most retruded position)
6. Full medical–dental history in conjunction with complete intraoral and functional examination of the patient

Accurate models and standardized radiographs, as the child grows and develops, are essential in sound planning and treatment. Models or impressions of the teeth in the upper and lower arches should be obtained periodically. Care should be exercised in extending the peripheries on basal bone to allow for more accurate model surgery later, if needed (see Chapter 4). High-periphery styrofoam disposable trays have proved to be excellent in the production of good models. Errors in predicting the type and extent of surgery can occur when the wrong occlusal registration is either taken or used. Only those familiar with the importance of the occlusion in treatment planning should be allowed to record it. The occlusal centric relation bite can be checked later with good intraoral photos, and finally at the second clinical examination.

Cleft palate patients or craniofacial patients with canted or asymmetrical occlusal planes, facial asymmetries, or open bites are definite candidates for face-bow transfers to a jaw movement articulator. Checking bites and remounting are very important in certain orthognathic surgical procedures, and are described in more detail in Chapter 4.

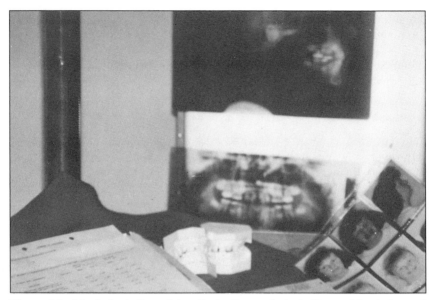

Figure 5.2 A typical set of complete orthodontic records, including models, photos, and full-mouth and cephalometric radiographs.

As mentioned previously, cephalometry is an art that both orthodontists and oral surgeons must understand. Taking the cephalometric radiographs can be as important in the final analysis as making the actual tracing and predicting the postsurgical tracing. The most commonly used is the lateral cephalometric radiograph in centric occlusion. Centric occlusion is defined as the place where the teeth first touch in the natural bite. The following is a checklist for making sure the radiograph is taken properly:

1. Properly position the head in a head-holding device called a cephalostat.
2. Make sure the head is in a normal position without strain on the spinal column.
3. Standardize the distance from the source and adjust the film cassette to the fixed distance.
4. Use the proper radiographic settings to ensure the proper contrast for accurate tracing.
5. Have the patient relax the facial muscles and hold the centric occlusion for the duration of the procedure.

Once a satisfactory lateral radiograph has been obtained in centric occlusion, other radiographs can be added for specific information. For example, important information may be obtained in surgical mandibular advancement cases by taking a lateral radiograph with the lower jaw in the advanced position.

PA cephalometry has gained renewed importance with recent advancements in orthodontics and oral surgery. This dimension gives more insight into problem analyses in facial asymmetry and maxillary repositioning. The checklist for attaining consistent radiographs holds for PA radiographs as well as for lateral head radiographs.

Frontal tracing will show a balance of detail in the eye orbits (sockets), the nasal septum (partition), and the maxillary and mandibular central incisors and molars. Soft tissue is more difficult to evaluate because of the limited amount shown on the perimeter of the radiograph. Frontal tracing may prove to be important for evaluating asymmetrical orthognathic surgical cases where special emphasis is on soft tissue planning.

Tomography is a radiographic procedure that results in a radiograph showing detail of a specific layer or section of tissue. In orthodontics, it usually delineates certain sections of the maxilla or mandible. (Laminagraphy or planography are synonymous terms.) Tomograms have been helpful not only in diagnosis and treatment planning, but also in postoperative evaluations of mandibular and maxillary surgical corrections sometimes needed for the cleft palate patient. PA tomograms of the nasal septum also have proved to be very useful in maxillary surgery. They have become a routine diagnostic aid in all premaxillary subapical and full maxillary impaction procedures (Figures 5.3 and 5.4). A deviated septum found prior to surgery can be shown visually to the patient in the diagnosis and treatment planning sessions or immediately prior to the surgical procedure.

Temporomandibular joint (TMJ) radiographs have found a place in all phases of maxillofacial treatment planning and postsurgical evaluations, and can be useful for the cleft palate patient when mandibular surgery is needed. Tomograms are useful follow-up radiographs a day or two following surgery for a final check on condylar position.

Other techniques are under development in many craniofacial centers. The use of a cephalostat to consistently position the head and of serial radiographic studies will certainly lend more credibility to such studies. Also, the use of digital computerized tomography for TMJ and midface deviations gives added useful information to the surgeons and orthodontists for workups and postsurgical evaluation of the cleft palate patient.

Other radiographs, such as panoramic radiograph, serve as an excellent screening film for tooth development in the mandible and maxilla. The maxillary sinuses and the mandibular rami are especially in good view. One must not be tempted to read specific dental details from the panogram, however. Detailed dental diagnosis and evaluation requires other dental radiographic projections, such as bitewings, occlusals, and periapicals. Recently, three-dimensional computerized reconstruction of

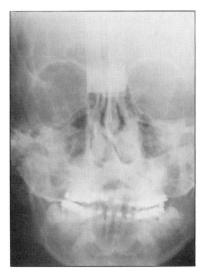

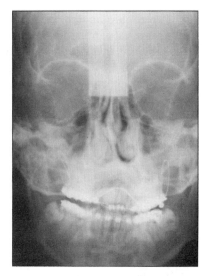

Figure 5.3 Posterior–anterior tomogram showing severely deviated nasal septum prior to maxillary surgery.

Figure 5.4 Posterior–anterior tomogram following maxillary surgery.

computerized tomography scans and magnetic resonance imaging have provided the orthodontist and craniofacial surgeon with excellent views of the craniofacial structures for more definitive treatment planning.

ORTHODONTIC TREATMENT PHASES

Although the orthodontist can provide important information regarding overall clinical management for persons with craniofacial anomalies throughout the growing years, there are times when active orthodontic treatment can be considered. As mentioned previously, the team's treatment philosophy will dictate certain orthodontic intervention times consistent with the orthodontic principle of coordinating treatment to growth and development. Active orthodontic treatment can be considered at the following times or phases of dental development: presurgical orthopedics and early bone grafting (infancy to age 2), early mixed dentition, later mixed dentition, permanent dentition (adolescent), and adult (nongrowing). Although each of these is discussed separately, there are important transitional relationships that are unique for each patient.

Presurgical Orthopedics and Early Bone Grafting

Much discussion and debate has occurred over many years regarding the benefits of early presurgical orthopedics (orthodontically positioning the maxillary segments prior to lip and palatal repair) and bone grafting (placing bone in the alveolar cleft area). The two can be separate issues, and doing one (e.g., presurgical orthopedics) does not necessitate doing the other (e.g., early bone grafting) (Gruber, 1990). For a more complete discussion of the history, rationale, and procedures, the reader is referred to sources that favor presurgical orthopedic procedures (Burston, 1958; Gruber, 1990; Hotz, Gnoinski, & Perko, 1986; Huddart & Crabb, 1977; Huebner & Marsh, 1990; McNeil, 1956; Rosenstein, 1990) and those that do not (Aduss & Figueroa, 1990; Berkowitz, 1977; Pruzansky, 1964; Ross, 1987; Subtelny, 1990).

The rationale for presurgical orthopedics and early bone grafting in most cases is to normalize, as much as possible, the position of maxillary segments before and/or following the molding effect of lip repair. Without attempts to control the segments, there can be some collapsing of the lateral maxillary segment on the cleft side(s). The primary rationale for early bone grafting following presurgical orthopedics is to stabilize the more optimally positioned maxillary segments. The rationale for not doing premaxillary orthopedics and early bone grafting is that any crossbite that occurs can be corrected later. Early intervention does not eliminate the need for future orthodontic treatment or facilitate more favorable growth, and early bone grafting may actually inhibit normal maxillary growth. The important questions are what the most efficient and effective treatment is for each patient to ensure the best outcome in the long run, and whether the benefits outweigh the costs (time, effort, discomfort, family cooperation and frustrations, etc.).

Based on the evidence available at this time, the team I work with does not believe that presurgical orthopedics or early bone grafting should be standard procedure for all patients. In our judgment, the benefits are not significant enough, in most cases, to justify the procedure. However, it is helpful for the reader to understand the procedure. The following text is from Rosenstein (1990), and Figures 5.5 through 5.8 are based on personal communication with Dr. Rosenstein.

1. In the patient with a complete unilateral cleft of the lip, alveolus, and palate, the action of the repaired lip will usually mold the greater segment to a butt alignment with the lesser segment if the latter is held immobile with a prosthesis [see Figure 5.5].
2. With the segments thus aligned, the integrity of the arch form can be fixed with a bone graft, and later the palate can be repaired without undue distortion of the alveolar ridge.
3. In the patient with a bilateral complete cleft of the lip, alveolus, and palate, if both lateral segments can be held from collapse and the premaxilla positioned favorably through lip action, it is conceivable that the butting can occur here, too [see Figure 5.6] . . . . This alignment can occur during a period of anywhere between 3 and 9 months. Stabilization of the bony segments by bone graft is definitely contraindicated in the complete unilateral cleft when the segments are overlapped and, simi-

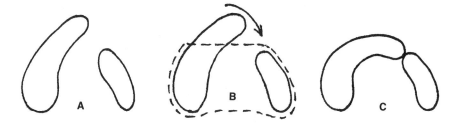

Figure 5.5 Diagrams showing (A) the relationship of the greater and lesser maxillary bony segments before lip surgery; (B) the prosthesis in place (dotted lines), holding the lesser segment stable (the arrow shows the direction of movement of the greater segment following lip repair); and (C) the butt alignment of the segments.

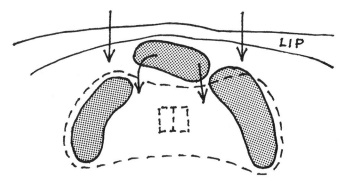

Figure 5.6 Diagram showing the direction of force of the repaired lip, the movement of the premaxilla, and the prosthesis (dotted lines) designed to hold the lateral segments stable.

> larly, in the bilateral complete cleft when both lateral segments approximate each other and block the premaxillary segment anteriorly [see Figures 5.7 and 5.8]. (p. 120)

If the team is faced with an early treatment although the newborn stage of development was not treated (especially for severe malpositioning of the premaxilla), a number of options are available for orthodontic treatment. Figure 5.9 demonstrates one possibility—the combined treatment with a removable maxillary appliance connected to high-pull J-hook headgear for traction—to reduce and impact a protruberant premaxilla. The surgical treatments at this stage are limited to soft tissue grafting to stabilize the premaxilla. This removable appliance restricts the premaxilla and guides the proximal apposition to its counterpart edges in the posterior segments of the maxilla. The success of the technique relies heavily on cooperation, and the family must be trained not only to place the appliances, but also to encourage a few

Should not do bone grafts

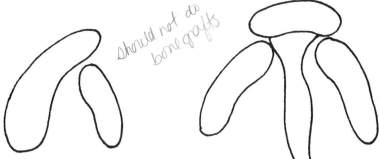

Figure 5.7 Diagram showing overlapping of the bony maxillary segments in unilateral cleft lip and palate.

Figure 5.8 Diagram showing the collapse of the lateral maxillary bony segments and blocking of the premaxilla anteriorly.

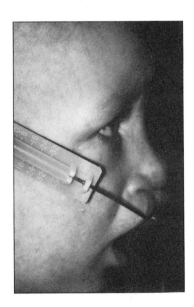

Figure 5.9 Removable high-pull traction appliance to reduce excessive premaxillary protrusion.

hours of long-term wear. Daytime wear is preferable, to avoid potentially dangerous nighttime wear (dislodgement may be harmful to adequate breathing, with possible suffocation).

Early Mixed Dentition

Posterior-lateral expansion-type appliances can be very helpful in correcting palatal width problems in the early mixed dentition. Cooperation is always a consideration in the effectiveness of removable appliance therapy. Not enough wear would result in inadequate expansion, whereas too much expansion, which sometimes is the result of an overzealous home appliance activation program, results in a loose appliance and relapse to original collapsed positions. Fixed palatal expansion devices can also be very important in the early mixed dentition for molar and cuspid width correction. Although cooperation is usually not a problem with fixed expansion, continuous wear can be a hazard for speech articulation.

Partially erupted teeth, cooperation, and the patient's speech needs can present limitations to the effectiveness of removable appliance use in the mixed dentition phase. For example, in one patient, a removable split-palate device to expand the maxillary segments was not effective and the optimal time for a bone graft was approaching (as seen in the panogram in Figure 5.10). A fixed appliance (see Figure 5.11) was utilized to more rapidly expand the anterior maxilla in preparation for bilateral bone grafting for premaxillary stabilization (age 10 years). A combination of unerupted molars and fibrous gum tissue often results in poor retention for the first insertion and progressive activation of a removable appliance. Fixed posterior bands with undercuts can be effective in increasing retentiveness.

Most patients with cleft lip and palate in the mixed dentition stage require some preliminary tooth alignment to condense spaces and prepare for surgery. Surgical treatment about this time may involve removal of supernumerary teeth, fistula closure, and alveolar bone grafting. Because the alveolar bony defect may result in deficient bone support for teeth in the cleft area, care has to be taken with even the most limited tooth movement. Anterior brackets with large amounts of angulation incorporated in the slot must be avoided to prevent moving the root into the cleft void. Due to the alveolar cleft, the patient may have malformed, impacted, displaced, or missing permanent teeth. Such cases need a careful evaluation to determine not only the appropriate treatment, but also the timing of a coordinated effort with other team members.

The timing of alveolar bone grafting or premaxillary stabilization is critical in relation to both the dental and the chronological age of the patient. Bone grafting must be accomplished in time to assure the appropriate eruption of the developing permanent teeth. The best grafting age is between 7 and 8 years of age if the lateral incisor is missing or is judged not to be a usable tooth for the long term. If a lateral incisor is developing and considered to have a good long-term prognosis, the alveolar bone graft is done a few years earlier to provide increased bone support for that tooth. The rationale for timing of alveolar bone grafting is discussed in Chapter 4. When severe skeletal discrepancies exist between the maxilla and the mandible, bone grafting may be delayed until the completion of facial growth.

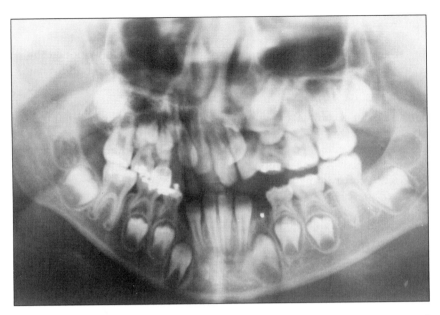

Figure 5.10 Panoramic radiograph of a 10-year-old patient with bilateral cleft lip and palate. Poor cooperation and speech difficulties were associated with removable appliance wear.

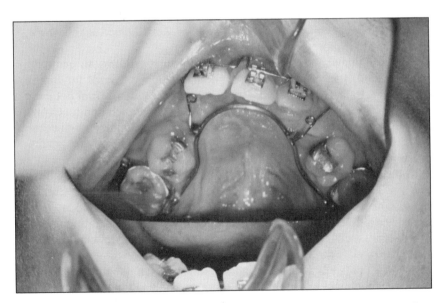

Figure 5.11 Photograph of the maxillary arch with a fixed orthodontic appliance in place for the same patient represented in Figure 5.10. The fixed appliance was necessary to accomplish maxillary expansion.

Later Mixed Dentition

Later mixed dentition treatment includes placing full appliances on the existing teeth, generally in both arches to align the teeth and arches to one another. Five main areas of treatment focus of orthodontic and possible orthognathic treatment are common in the mixed dentition patient: (a) condensing of spaces where missing teeth will require future partial or fixed bridgework; (b) correction of midline asymmetry and overjet versus underjet problems associated with a small maxilla and shifting premaxilla due to the clefting; (c) Pseudo Class III or full Class III malocclusion requiring space for erupting teeth in intermaxillary elastics; (d) posterior crossbite (unilateral or bilateral) requiring rapid or slow expansion; and (e) mixed dentition orthognathic situations requiring future surgery, but involving preliminary alignment of teeth and arches for that surgery.

Permanent Dentition—The Teenage Years

Although partial fixed or removable appliances are sometimes used for teenagers, full fixed orthodontic appliances are usually necessary in the 12- to 13-year-old cleft palate patient to align the erupting cuspids and bicuspids, as well as to coordinate the upper and lower arches to each other. The goals for orthodontic treatment in young adults are to finalize the treatment plan and to establish a good working occlusal pattern, as well as a balanced facial appearance.

The orthodontist is concerned not only with guiding an erupting cuspid, but also with positioning a supernumerary lateral for future prosthetic reconstruction. The orthodontist also makes a final determination of the patient's growth pattern to determine arch and tooth size versus profile fullness and basal bone support. Additionally, final determination can be made in the teenage years whether to extract permanent teeth in borderline extraction situations.

The orthodontist is also concerned with the maxillary and mandibular jaw relationship at this stage because the maximum pubertal growth spurt occurs around age 12 to 13 in girls and 14 to 15 in boys. The orthodontist must maintain, if possible, an overjet relationship in the anterior tooth region at a time when growth is somewhat diminished in maxillary cleft area and maximized in the lower jaw due to pubertal growth (Figure 5.12). Class III elastics, lower bicuspid extractions, and expansive flaring of upper anterior teeth can be used to maintain overjet in Pseudo Class III underjet patients. Surgical management may be necessary in some cleft patients in whom a forward-growing mandible is found to create extreme underjet in a deficient maxilla.

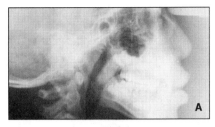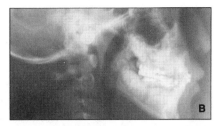

Figure 5.12 Lateral cephalometric radiographs showing (A) the anterior crossbite before treatment with a Frankel III appliance and (B) the crossbite after treatment. The appliance was designed to control mandibular growth while promoting maxillary growth.

Orthodontic treatment may be required to correct asymmetry of the jaws and face, especially in unilateral cleft situations. The asymmetry can be demonstrated in the upper and lower dental midlines and their comparison with the facial midlines. Also associated with the dental and facial asymmetry may be unilateral crossbites and unequal right and left molar relationships. In underjet situations, the first attempt made with orthodontic appliances is to expand the cleft area to bring the upper midline on center with the face. Open coils and arch bar sheaths can be effective in opening space for midline shifting (Figure 5.13). Care must be exercised in close evaluation of periodontal tissue and bone support over the anterior teeth, especially in the area of the cleft. Too much expansion and tooth torque may expose excessive root structure. Consideration must also be given to upper and lower facial balance and to optimal position of the upper lip.

A tightly scarred upper lip may cause a significant, and in some cases a total, relapse following anterior expansion. The team must be involved in final treatment options available to teenage patients. It is the orthodontist's role to present the various options to the team for consideration of future plastic and oral surgical procedures, as well as future prosthetic options. It is disconcerting to both the patient and the team members when 2 or 3 years of orthodontic expansion mechanics is overcome by abnormal growth and a modified treatment plan has to be formulated.

A common focus for orthodontists in cleft palate treatment is guidance of the cuspids. A frequent technique is the initial bonding for an unfavorably erupting cuspid with an attachment button. Traction mechanics on one or two teeth is employed with memory chains and elastic rope ties (Figure 5.14). Labial expansion with arch wires and transpalatal expansion arches is also common. Unilateral cross-elastics can also be useful to gain overjet in a posterior upper segment.

If teeth are missing in a teenager, serious consideration should be given to extraction of permanent teeth on the nonaffected side of the

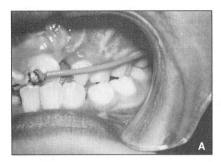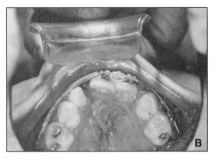

Figure 5.13 (A) Facial view and (B) palatal view of expansion tubes and a partial upper fixed appliance used to gain space and overjet in a patient with a cleft palate.

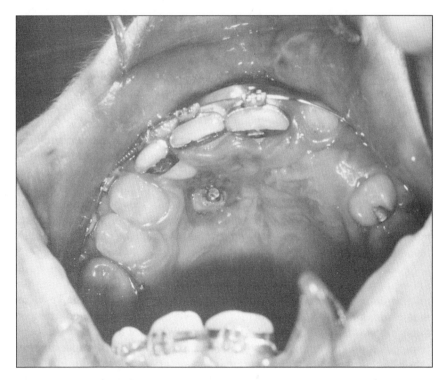

Figure 5.14 Photograph of maxillary arch showing palatally erupting cuspid being guided to normal tooth position with a traction elastic.

maxilla to reduce the length of, or necessity for, fixed bridgework. A completed set of progress records, perhaps with team consultation, is usually reserved for the extraction decision. Cuspids can sometimes be used as laterals, and midline shifts can be achieved to attain facial alignment with the extraction of one bicuspid on the unaffected side (Figure 5.15). However, final decisions are best made by the prosthodontist, orthodontist, and patient and family.

Surgical intervention must be considered even in the early teenage years if the growth and facial disfigurement are severe and psychosocial issues are apparent. The periodic team evaluations and treatment planning sessions, with input from the patient's school speech pathologist, psychologist, social worker, and so forth, are very important. The teasing of classmates and neighborhood children can be reduced considerably and the patient's self-esteem can be enhanced by various orthodontic and combined surgical procedures to balance facial asymmetries and correct a variety of jaw discrepancies (Figure 5.16).

Adult (Nongrowing) Orthodontic Treatment

The time at which the cleft palate patient reaches full maturity and facial growth is essentially completed varies between males and females. Growth of the female patient tends to slow at a much earlier age (16 to 17 years of age) than that of the male patient (18 to 19 years of age). Therefore, the adult patient who presents to a cleft palate treatment center with severe skeletal problems that have gone without orthodontic or surgical intervention well into the adult age group is much more likely to have a compromised treatment result with *only* orthodontic treatment, or to need extensive assistance from the various surgical techniques. Untreated malpositioned teeth usually have been in traumatic occlusion and have associated mobility, bone loss, and shortened root structure. A combined orthodontic and surgical-assisted plan to correct collapsed segments, Pseudo Class III as well as Class III malocclusions, multiple missing teeth, and impacted cuspids is usually the treatment of choice for patients having limited previous contact with interdisciplinary care. For the cleft palate patient who has been followed regularly for interdisciplinary treatment planning over many years, the outcome is much more favorable and the combined treatments less extensive. Exceptions have occurred. As noted earlier in this chapter, teams in other countries (Mars, 1990) have reported on cleft palate patients who have been seen as adults with unoperated clefts, but who have favorable segmental position and little collapse of segments. However, these unoperated adults usually have unintelligible speech or very poor speech aesthetics (Sell & Grunwell, 1990). Clearly, patients can benefit from early treatment of malpositioned teeth and

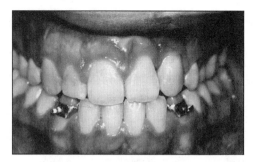

Figure 5.15 Occlusal photograph showing the cuspid in lateral incisor position (patient's left side) and restored with aesthetic resin to appear more like a lateral incisor.

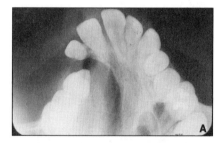

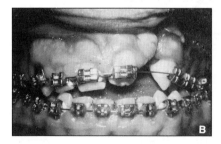
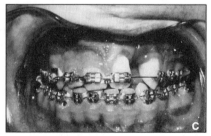

Figure 5.16 (A) Maxillary occlusal radiograph of a teenage patient showing malposition of the anterior teeth and posterior crossbite (patient's left side). (B) Anterior occlusal photograph of the same patient showing start of fixed appliance treatment. (C) Anterior occlusal photograph of the same patient as treatment progresses to accomplish better alignment of teeth and more normal arch form.

collapsed segments so that when the permanent teeth erupt, they have a good eruptive position and there is adequate bone to accommodate them.

In the adult patient, the treatment of collapsed segments can be successfully accomplished with surgically assisted maxillary widening and rapid maxillary expansion orthodontic techniques. The widening allows for a prosthodontic replacement of the missing and malformed dental units (Figure 5.17). The prosthodontic treatment not only gives a favorable aesthetic appearance to the dental arch, but also can give better support to the upper lip. The upper lip will appear to be more full and contribute to improved aesthetics from both a full-face and profile view. Chapter 6 discusses prosthodontic treatment for patients with cleft lip and palate in more detail.

Adult multiple-facet treatments are common on all cleft palate teams. Many adults are interested in maximizing their function and facial form, especially after completing facial and dental growth and development.

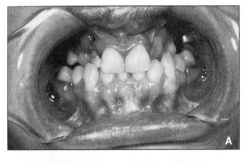

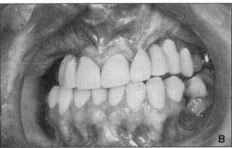

Figure 5.17 (A) Anterior occlusal photograph of an adult patient before treatment. (B) Anterior occlusal photograph of the same patient following surgically assisted correction of the crossbite. The treatment involved coordinated efforts of the orthodontist, oral surgeon, and prosthodontist.

SUMMARY

Restoring the patient with cleft lip and palate to the best possible form and function is the common goal underlying orthodontic general principles. These principles include minimizing the patient's time in fixed appliances, coordinating the orthodontic treatment with the other team treatments, maximizing the long-term stability and results, staging the treatments, and maximizing development of the dentition and face. A wide range of orthodontic procedures and treatments are available, from the early intervention removable appliances, to preparing the posterior and anterior maxillary segments for surgery, to adult treatments where fixed appliances and surgical widening techniques are required to restore normal arch form. The expectation is that, following orthodontic treatment, the patient will have restored confidence and a new awareness of symmetry in the mouth when the tongue performs its movements in the process of chewing, swallowing, and speech. Facial appearance is also very important psychologically. The orthodontist plays a key role in the team evaluation, deliberation, and decision making for each patient to achieve optimal facial form and function.

REFERENCES

Aduss, H. (1971). Craniofacial growth in complete unilateral cleft lip and palate. *Angle Orthodontist, 41,* 202–213.

Aduss, H., & Figueroa, A. (1990). Stages of orthodontic treatment in complete unilateral cleft lip and palate. In J. Bardach & H. Morris (Eds.), *Multidisciplinary management of cleft lip and palate.* Philadelphia: Saunders.

Angle, E. H. (1907). *Treatment of malocclusion of teeth* (7th ed.). Philadelphia: S. S. Wick.

Berkowitz, S. (1977). Cleft lip and palate research: An updated state of the art. Section III: Orofacial growth and dentistry. *Cleft Palate Journal, 14,* 288–301.

Burston, W. R. (1958). The early treatment of cleft palate conditions. *Dental Practitioner, 9,* 41–52.

Graber, T. M. (1949). Craniofacial morphology in cleft lip and cleft palate deformities. *Surgery, Gynecology and Obstetrics, 88,* 359–369.

Graber, T. M. (1954). The congenital cleft palate deformity. *Journal of the American Dental Association, 48,* 375–395.

Graber, T. M. (1972). *Orthodontics: Principles and practice.* Philadelphia: Saunders.

Gruber, H. (1990). Presurgical maxillary orthopedics. In J. Bardach & H. Morris (Eds.), *Multidisciplinary management of cleft lip and palate.* Philadelphia: Saunders.

Hotz, M., Gnoinski, W., & Perko, M. (Eds.). (1986). *Early treatment of cleft lip and palate.* Bern, Switzerland: Hans Huber.

Huddart, A. G., & Crabb, J. J. (1977). The effect of presurgical treatment on palatal tissue area in unilateral cleft lip and palate subjects. *British Journal of Orthodontics, 4,* 181–185.

Huebner, D. V., & Marsh, J. L. (1990). Alveolar molding appliances in the treatment of cleft lip and palate infants. In J. Bardach & H. Morris (Eds.), *Multidisciplinary management of cleft lip and palate.* Philadelphia: Saunders.

Isaacson, R. J., & Chaudhry, A. P. (1962). Cleft palate induction in strain A mice with cortisone. *The Anatomical Record, 142,* 479–484.

Jacobson, R., & Rosenstein, S. (1986). Cleft lip and palate: The orthodontist's youngest patient. *American Journal of Orthodontics and Dentofacial Orthopedics, 90*(1), 63–66.

Kernahan, D. A., & Rosenstein, S. W. (1990). *Cleft lip and palate—A system of management.* Baltimore: Williams and Wilkins.

Latham, R. A., & Scott, J. H. (1970). A newly postulated factor in the early growth of the human middle face and the theory of multiple assurance. *Archives of Oral Biology, 15,* 1097–1100.

Mars, M., James, D., & Lamabadusuriya, S. (1990). The Sri Lankan cleft lip and palate project: The unoperated cleft lip and palate. *Cleft Palate Journal, 27,* 3–10.

McNeil, C. K. (1956). Congenital oral deformities. *British Dental Journal, 101,* 191–198.

Noyes, F. B. (1911). The teaching of orthodontics as Dr. Angle viewed it. *Dental Cosmos, 73,* 802–808.

Olin, W. H. (1966). Cleft lip and palate rehabilitation. *American Journal of Orthodontics, 52,* 126.

Pruzansky, S. (1953). Descriptions, classifications and analysis of unoperated clefts of the lip and palate. *American Journal of Orthodontics, 39,* 590–611.

Pruzansky, S. (1964). Presurgical orthopedics and bone grafting for infants with cleft lip and palate: A dissent. *Cleft Palate Journal, 1,* 164–187.

Rosenstein, S. W. (1990). Early maxillary orthopaedics and appliance fabrication. In D. A. Kernahan & S. W. Rosenstein (Eds.), *Cleft lip and palate: A system of management.* Baltimore: Williams and Wilkins.

Ross, R. B. (1987). Treatment variables affecting facial growth in complete unilateral cleft lip and palate. *Cleft Palate Journal, 24,* 5–77.

Sell, D., & Grunwell, P. (1990). Speech results following late palatal surgery in previously unoperated Sri Lankan adolescents with cleft palate. *Cleft Palate Journal, 27,* 162–168.

Stark, R. B. (1954). The pathogenesis of harelip and cleft palate. *Plastic and Reconstructive Surgery, 13,* 20.

Subtelny, J. D. (1966). Orthodontic treatment of cleft lip and palate—Birth to adulthood. *Angle Orthodontist, 36,* 273.

Subtelny, J. D. (1990). Orthodontic principles in treatment of cleft lip and palate. In J. Bardach & H. Morris (Eds.), *Multidisciplinary management of cleft lip and palate.* Philadelphia: Saunders.

Tondury, G. (1961). On the mechanism of cleft formation. In S. Pruzansky (Ed.), *Congenital anomalies of the face and associated structures.* Springfield: Charles C. Thomas.

Vargervik, K. (1981). Orthodontic management of unilateral cleft lip and palate. *Cleft Palate Journal, 18,* 256.

Vargervik, K. (1983). Growth characteristics of the premaxilla and orthodontic principles in bilateral cleft lip and palate. *Cleft Palate Journal, 20,* 289.

Veau, V. (1938). Hasenschanten menschlicher Keimlinge auf der Stufe. *Zeitschrift fur Anatomie und Entwickelungsgesch, 108,* 459–493.

Vig, K. W., & Turvey, T. A. (1985). Orthodontic surgical interactions in the management of cleft lip and palate. *Clinics in Plastic Surgery, 12,* 735–748.

CHAPTER 6

Prosthodontic Management of Maxillofacial and Palatal Defects

Herbert A. Leeper, Paul S. Sills, and David H. Charles

Leeper, Sills, and Charles discuss prosthodontic issues and procedures applicable not only to persons with cleft lip and palate, but to individuals with other oral problems as well. They define the discipline of prosthetic dentistry, state the training involved to become this type of specialist, and espouse the opportunities for cooperative efforts between speech–language pathologists and prosthodontists. They list several oral and patient factors that influence prosthesis design and detail a physiological systems approach to assessment and management. Finally, the authors focus on specific oral problems and their clinical management.

1. *Define the discipline of prosthodontics. Distinguish between prosthodontist and maxillofacial prosthodontist.*

2. *What do the authors mean by the dual role of the "prosthetic speech appliance"?*

3. *The authors emphasize the importance of prosthodontists and speech pathologists working together. Describe a clinical situation in which cooperative efforts between the speech pathologist and prosthodontist would be ideal.*

4. *What do the authors mean by a physiological assessment of the speech-producing mechanism? How can this be helpful in determining a management strategy?*

5. *In the authors' focus on evaluation of velopharyngeal function, they describe a multidimensional approach. What dimension is readily available to the speech clinician in any work setting?*

6. *What are some of the existing dental hazards to articulation? Anterior appliances? What is known about speakers' adaptations to oral–facial defects and to speech prostheses?*

7. *What are some conditions in which prosthodontic treatment rather than surgical treatment might be indicated for soft palate defects?*

8. *Describe what is meant by a prosthesis reduction program. Describe the procedures typically used.*

9. *How does the palatal lift differ from an obturator?*

Many speech disorders are associated with maxillofacial defects, particularly defects involving maxillary and palatal regions. Etiologies of these defects can be generally classified as developmental (cleft lip and palate) or acquired trauma (oral cancer). Regardless of the cause, the defect may influence speech by changing the resonance properties of the vocal tract through the inappropriate coupling of the nasal cavity (resonation) and by changing the capacity to impound, direct, or constrict the vibrated flow of air (articulation).

In our view, restoration and maintenance of the oral functions of mastication, deglutition, and speech can be practically achieved by close technical interaction and cooperation between the disciplines of speech pathology and prosthodontics. Prosthodontics is a branch of dentistry concerned with restoration and maintenance of a patient's oral function, comfort, appearance, and health. Restoration of the natural teeth and replacement of missing teeth and associated contiguous tissues with artificial substitutes fall within the purview of this dental specialty. A prosthodontist is a dental specialist with advanced training in prosthetic dentistry. Specialty training in prosthodontics generally consists of a 2- or 3-year postgraduate university-sponsored education. Maxillofacial prosthodontics is a subdivision of this specialty that covers the restorative rehabilitation of patients with extensive oral–facial deformities. A maxillofacial prosthodontist requires an additional 1 to 2 years of study, usually acquired in a hospital-based setting. Because of the nature of palatal defects, the planning and fabrication of prosthetic speech appliances usually requires more specialized clinical training and skill than that involved with routine removable partial denture therapy.

Because a great deal of variability exists within the configuration of palatal defects, classification of all possible defects and elucidation of their individual treatment protocols are outside the scope of this chapter. Instead, we limit this discussion to general treatment considerations and those factors influencing speech prosthesis design. We also include management guidelines for patients presenting hard palate defects, soft palate defects, and velopharyngeal competency problems. Although the focus of this chapter is on defects that are common to the cleft palate condition, other congenital and acquired conditions affecting these structures and functions are discussed.

TERMINOLOGY—THE PROSTHETIC SPEECH APPLIANCE

"Prosthetic speech appliance" is a hybrid term describing the dual role of this device in replacing oral structures and assisting in speech rehabilitation. A pure speech appliance, such as a palatal lift, on the other hand, fulfills no prosthetic function. These appliances and removable dentures have similar features. A removable denture replaces both dental and oral tissues and may be inserted or removed from the mouth by the patient. Removable dentures may be partial (replacing some missing teeth) or complete (replacing all of the teeth). Acceptable removable partial dentures must resist (a) functional forces that tend to dislodge them, (b) forces acting on the supporting tissues, and (c) laterally directed forces. Partial denture clasps encircle selected abutment teeth to resist forces that dislodge the denture. Supporting elements (rests and bases) resist forces directed toward the teeth and underlying soft tissues. Vertically oriented denture components known as bracing elements resist laterally directed forces (Henderson & Steffel, 1981) (see Figure 6.1).

Successful prosthetic speech appliances must incorporate these basic features of partial denture design. A maxillary prosthetic speech appliance commonly consists of a palatal base structure to which other components connect. The size, location, and nature of the palatal defect determine the type of component that will attach to the base. For cleft defects limited to the hard palate, the attached obturator usually forms part of the base of the prosthesis. However, posteriorly located defects involving soft palate clefts and velopharyngeal incompetence (VPI)

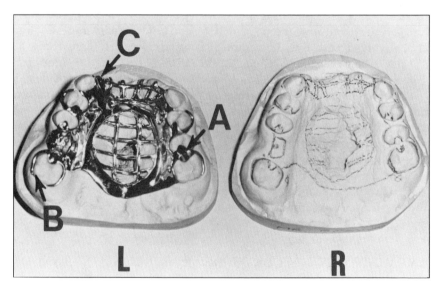

Figure 6.1 Left: Maxillary cast metal partial denture framework on a master model illustrating (A) supporting elements, (B) clasping elements, and (C) bracing elements. Right: Diagnostic model showing proposed framework design.

require a posterior "tail" or pharyngeal section added to the maxillary base. This extension supports either an obturator (bulb) or palatal lift. Thus, the location of the palatal defect directly influences the eventual form or design of the prosthetic speech appliance. The term *obturator* is used in this chapter to suggest complete or partial obturation of an opening. For openings in the hard palate (e.g., as a result of surgical removal of part of the palate or palatal fistulae following cleft palate repair), complete coverage or obturation is required. For velopharyngeal closure problems, partial obturation of the velopharyngeal space is required, and the pharyngeal section has commonly been called a *speech bulb*.

FACTORS INFLUENCING PROSTHETIC THERAPY FOR MAXILLARY DEFECTS

Several factors influence the design of the prosthetic speech appliance and the treatment outcome. These can be divided into oral factors and patient factors.

Oral Factors

A major factor influencing prosthetic therapy is the patient's dental status, which encompasses a variety of tooth-related conditions. These conditions can act alone or together to affect prosthesis design. Healthy mouths pose few problems for construction of prosthetic speech appliances, whereas mouths in poor health complicate therapy and threaten the prognosis for successful treatment. The types of dental conditions and the influence they exert on a prosthetic speech appliance design have been examined in detail elsewhere (Henderson & Steffel, 1981) and are described briefly in the following list:

1. *Number and location of existing teeth.* In a patient with full dentition, multiple tooth surfaces offer a wide range of possible locations for retentive and supporting elements, and in general simplify the speech appliance design. Partial dentition presents more difficult design problems, which increase in complexity when many teeth are missing. Entirely tooth-supported designs generally exhibit greater stability than do those that rely on support from both the teeth and the mucosa. Artificial teeth form a component of all partially edentulous designs, and attention to cosmetics as well as function must be considered.

At times, the original location of the teeth may be unsuitable for function or aesthetics. In many cases, orthodontic treatment improves tooth position and arch alignment to facilitate prosthesis construction (Chierici, 1979; Shiere, Fox, & Perry, 1962).

When all of the teeth are missing, a modified complete denture may be constructed to act as a speech appliance. In these situations, retention of the complete denture may be poor due to an inadequate retentive seal about the peripheral tissues. Denture adhesives may provide the only means for adequate prosthesis retention.

2. *Condition of existing dentition.* Existing teeth must be free of cavities and restored to an acceptable contour prior to instituting prosthetic therapy. Routine alloy and composite restorations are frequently sufficient for treatment of cavities; however, when large tooth defects must be repaired or contour significantly altered, full crown coverage must be employed.

3. *Occlusal relationships.* Occlusal relationships refer to the manner in which the opposing teeth intercuspate (mesh). Close intercuspation may prevent ideal location of rests and clasp units.

4. *Periodontal (gum) condition.* The periodontium consists of the ligamentous tissue attaching teeth to bone, and the mucosa surrounding the teeth. Periodontal disease attacks the tooth–bone attachment and, in its most destructive form, causes tooth loss. Mouths severely affected by this disease may possess teeth unsuitable for prosthesis support or retention. In such cases, the prosthesis design must be modified to avoid overstressing periodontally compromised teeth.

5. *Oral hygiene.* All removable prostheses attract dental plaque, which places teeth and gums at greater risk for cavities and gum disease. Individuals wearing removable prostheses must maintain effective plaque control to ensure a favorable prognosis.

Patient Factors

Patient factors also play an important role in the design of the prosthetic speech appliance and in the treatment outcome. Age and health are particularly important factors.

1. *Age.* Young, immature individuals with incompletely developed oral structures requiring prosthetic speech appliances are best served by transitional types of prostheses. Transitional prostheses differ from permanent designs in that the base is made of acrylic resin instead of cast metal. Although acrylic lacks the strength and long-term stability of the metal casting, its advantages for the young patient include the ease of base modification to accommodate growth and the lower cost of fabrication.

2. *Health.* Patients with physical handicaps require careful evaluation to determine their capacity to insert and remove prosthetic speech appliances. Patients with serious handicaps may require assistance with routine oral hygiene procedures, such as toothbrushing and flossing to prevent the loss of teeth due to gum disease or decay.

TEAM APPROACH TO DEFECT MANAGEMENT

Interdisciplinary Therapeutic Concepts

Any team approach to a complex problem, such as the prosthetic management of individuals with maxillofacial defects, is complex in its own right. Decisions about what is best for the patient, when procedures should be done or redone, and how long the desired effect should take are not simply matters of majority rule by the team. Each team member has input to the decision-making process, but the team members who have the most expertise for a particular segment of management must ultimately make the final decision. In many situations, the prosthodontist and the speech pathologist work together to establish the need for a temporary or permanent prosthesis for speech purposes. The prosthodontist must make the decisions concerning the optimal occlusal relationships of the prosthesis for purposes of proper aesthetics and masticatory function, and must also consider replacement of missing teeth in either a fixed or removable form for each patient.

Although the prosthodontist is trained to make prostheses for a variety of oral functions and for patients who span in age from young infants to the elderly, design of appliances that provide a basis for improved speech production should be done in conjunction with the speech pathologist. The two professionals often share the same dental operatory during the evaluation stages of prosthesis fitting so that subtleties in modification of the prosthesis design for the maxillary–alveolar region will not adversely affect speech sound production. Similarly, based on measurement of the amount of air escaping from the nose and from perceptual judgments of nasal tone, the speech pathologist may advise the prosthodontist to increase the size of an obturator (speech bulb) or add vertical height and/or posterior extension to a palatal lift to improve resonance balance for patients with posterior (soft palate) defects.

It is important that the two professionals do not feel that such an interaction is mandated by virtue of title alone, but rather that each feels respect for the other person's discipline. Because both professionals have basic anatomical, physiological, and aesthetic knowledge about the oral–pharyngeal mechanism, discussions concerning the treatment plan should flow easily. Information gained over time while working together allows each professional to seek additional information using common referents and vocabulary. This process speeds the management of each case and provides an excellent training ground for young preprofessionals who may view the interaction during teaching rounds (Sharry, 1981).

Initial Prosthodontic Assessment

At the initial meeting with the patient, the prosthodontist must conduct a thorough examination of the hard and soft tissues, supported by appropriate radiographs. This diagnostic evidence provides essential information for determining dental factors affecting the prosthetic treatment plan and prognosis. At this appointment, the prosthodontist may make preliminary impressions of both jaws. Plaster diagnostic models are recovered from the impressions (see Figure 6.1, right). The models are then mounted on a dental articulator. Mounted models permit a clear view of tooth relationships, which is a necessary preliminary step in designing the prosthesis. In addition, the prosthodontist studies the maxillary model to choose the optimal location for prosthesis components.

model

Prosthetic Clinical Procedures

Once the treatment plan has been accepted by the patient and the preliminary adjunctive dental treatment is completed, a series of dental procedures must be accomplished to fabricate the prosthetic speech appliance. The following general procedures are involved in the construction of a permanent, metal framework, as well as most types of removable prosthetic speech appliances (see Henderson & Steffel, 1981, for detailed procedures). Specific clinical procedures, associated with the treatment of individual palatal defects, are discussed separately.

1. Teeth are prepared by reshaping their surfaces as necessary to accommodate to the design requirements of the partial denture base.

2. Full arch impressions are made of the prepared teeth and soft tissues. Existing palatal clefts must be temporarily occluded to prevent impression material from flowing into the defect (Figure 6.2A).

3. A master model (cast) made from the impression serves as a base on which the metal framework is constructed (Figure 6.2B).

4. The fit of the metal framework (Figure 6.2C) must be verified in the mouth. Minor adjustments of the framework usually are needed to ensure optimal fit. Once fitted, temporary acrylic resin is adapted to that portion of the metal framework associated with the defect. The acrylic resin forms a base to which other impression materials can be added to capture the anatomic form of the defect. The defect impression is converted to permanent acrylic resin by routine dental laboratory procedures (Figure 6.2D). This step may be delayed until the artificial teeth are set and processed onto the metal framework.

5. Artificial teeth are positioned according to the dictates of aesthetics and function. The prosthodontist must attempt to develop a dental occlusion that contributes to prosthesis stability. With large defects, the objective of a stable prosthesis may be only partially realized. When the criteria of tooth placement are satisfied, the prosthesis is completed by routine dental laboratory procedures (Figure 6.2E).

6. During the delivery of the completed prosthesis to the patient, the prosthodontist must first ensure that the fit is both accurate and

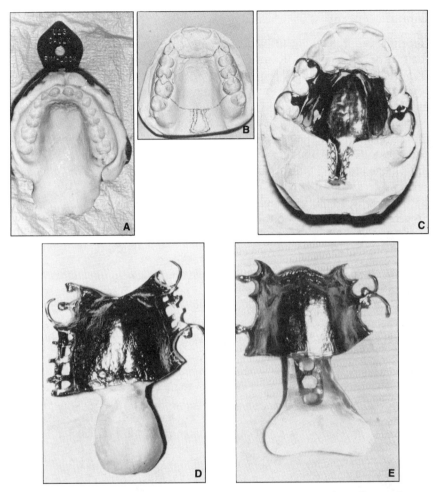

Figure 6.2 Dental procedures for fabrication of prosthetic speech appliances from a variety of patients: (A) full arch impression, (B) diagnostic model, (C) metal framework on master cast, (D) wax technique for functional impression of palatal tissue, and (E) posterior section in permanent acrylic resin as a completed speech prosthesis.

comfortable. Pressure areas on the mucosa must be located and eliminated. The patient must also receive instructions for insertion and removal of the prosthesis and for proper care and use. The importance of ongoing dental care and prosthesis maintenance must be stressed. Several office visits are usually required to correct minor tissue irritations common to all newly made prostheses. Finally, a regular dental recall schedule (e.g., every 6 months) should be arranged.

Dental Implants

Recent advances in dental implantology provide exciting possibilities for treatment of partially and completely edentulous patients requiring prosthetic speech appliances. Dental implants consist of man-made tooth analogues that are surgically implanted into edentulous regions of the jaw to replace missing teeth (Figure 6.3). The clinically proven, biologically acceptable dental implant pioneered by P-I Branemark allows prosthodontists to achieve excellent support and retention for prostheses (Parel, Branemark, & Janson, 1986). This improvement in prosthesis stability minimizes destructive forces associated with most removable appliances, thus reducing the need for remakes. We anticipate reports of clinical investigations regarding implant-supported prostheses for speech rehabilitation.

Principles of Speech Assessment

The speech pathologist's role in the evaluation process generally revolves around estimating the patient's speech output employing perceptual, acoustical, and physiological measurement procedures. As with the prosthetic assessment, the speech evaluation procedures noted within each of the sections that follow are appropriate for defects of the entire oro-

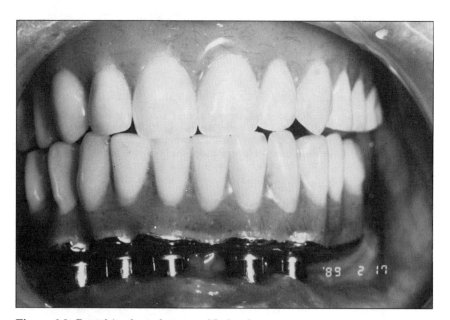

Figure 6.3 Dental implants for a mandibular denture.

facial complex. Systematic evaluation of each speech subsystem (i.e., respiratory, laryngeal, velopharyngeal, articulatory) will allow the clinician to develop a thorough description of the type and severity of the speech problem. Thus, information gained about articulatory precision in patients with primarily hard palate defects (e.g., oral–nasal fistulae) must be tempered with concerns about the airflow through a potentially inadequate velopharyngeal mechanism (posterior defects) before a decision may be made about the primacy of "articulation problems" from anterior anomalies.

Our approach to prosthetic management from a physiological model is based, in general, upon concepts espoused by Netsell and Daniel (1979). Although these authors discuss a system for describing and understanding speech disorders called "dysarthrias," we feel the underlying principles apply equally to peripheral and central nervous system control of the speech-producing mechanism in individuals with disordered anatomical and physiological characteristics, such as cleft lip and palate. As suggested by Rosenbek and Netsell (1984), the goal of a physiological evaluation of an individual's speech-producing mechanism is to determine the severity and type of involvement of each valve in the system and to determine the existence and severity of the cognitive, linguistic, and motor processes interacting within that system. Such an approach should allow the clinician to select and organize a management strategy based on knowledge of what each component in the system is capable of producing.

The functional components (Netsell & Daniel, 1979) are the nine valves employed in the system to produce speech and include, from bottom to top, (a) abdominal area, (b) diaphragm, (c) rib cage, (d) larynx, (e) velopharyngeal port mechanism, (f) posterior aspect of tongue, (g) anterior portion of tongue, (h) jaw, and (i) lips. Evaluation of each component is necessary to detect the efficiency of each valve in the system and to indicate how each valve interacts with the others for conversational speech production. Given the limited size of this chapter and the various areas of management to be covered, only cursory information is given about the first four subsystems (i.e., the respiratory and laryngeal components). Emphasis throughout the chapter is on the velopharyngeal and oral articulatory valves. It is important to reiterate, however, that when evaluating any patient with suspected orofacial problems that may need prosthetic and speech management, each of the nine major functional components must be examined. To assume that difficulty in one area of the orofacial complex affects only that isolated area is unsound in a "systems physiology" approach to multiple actions of the human speech subsystems (Folkins, 1985). Thus, from a speech pathologist's point of view, assessment of respiratory, laryngeal, velopharyngeal, and articulatory control is important for every patient.

Although we emphasize articulatory and resonation features with anterior and posterior appliances, the effects of such appliances may be observed in laryngeal tone and respiratory action for speech utterances. To ignore such "downstream" effects would be to assume independence of each subsystem in a coordinated structure of speech production, and this is simply not the case.

Evaluation processes: Respiratory. Most speech pathologists review the entire speech-producing mechanism during a diagnostic evaluation. Guidelines for evaluating the oral–peripheral system are provided by Kuehn (1982), Mason and Simon (1977), and St. Louis and Ruscello (1981). Often limited in these speech evaluation protocols are methods of examining the respiratory system. Judgments of breathing patterns and rapidity of the respiratory cycle, especially during speech, are made by observing chest wall action. In some cases, static pulmonary function tests, such as tidal volume, inspiratory and expiratory volumes, and vital capacity measures, are obtained with a spirometer. Although the objective measure of partitions of lung volume is valuable as a tool to aid in referral of patients with possible respiratory disease, it does not tell the speech clinician much about the dynamic movement of air directly associated with the speech samples being produced. In the past decade, Hixon and colleagues (Hixon, 1982; Hixon, Goldman, & Mead, 1973; Hixon, Mead, & Goldman, 1976; Hixon & Putnam, 1983), among others, have described details of chest movements for a variety of speakers using noninvasive kinematic analysis techniques, such as magnetometrics and inductance plethysmography. The results of these studies are interpreted as suggesting that commercially available instruments are available to monitor, record, and analyze the respiratory control of components of the chest wall (i.e., rib cage, abdomen) for prosthetic patients during a variety of speech tasks. Furthermore, modifications to any of the articulators upstream (i.e., the velopharyngeal mechanism) should have an effect on the amount and timing action of the respiratory system working to produce breath support for speech (Warren, Dalston, Trier, & Holder, 1985).

Evaluation processes: Laryngeal. Laryngeal activity of the speech system also demands investigation. A growing number of researchers have related physiological and acoustic attributes of voice to the perception of vocal quality. Studies of vocal frequency (f_0) and sound pressure level (SPL) (Coleman, Mabis, & Hinson, 1977), spectral noise level (SNL) (Hanson & Emanuel, 1979), maximum phonation time (MPT) (Eckel & Boone, 1981), and measurements of jitter and shimmer (Horii, 1982) have been reported. In addition, physiological measures of air pressure and airflow activity in voice production have been completed by Isshiki (1964), Mead, Bouhuys, and Proctor (1968), Netsell (1969), and Hollien

(1977). Laryngeal airway resistance measures combining ratios of air pressure and airflow during voiceless consonant /p/ plus vowel /i/ (CV) production have been reported by Smitheran and Hixon (1981) and Leeper and Graves (1984). This measure may be used to estimate changes in opposition of the laryngeal mechanism and upper airway to airflow from the lungs.

Past research suggests that speakers with cleft palate have laryngeal problems (McWilliams, Lavorato, & Bluestone, 1973). Curtis (1968) speculated that hypernasal speakers may expend more vocal effort to attain a given loudness level due to the leak in the system. This increase in respiratory drive through the system to make up for the damping of the partially open velopharyngeal system might cause increased subglottal pressure, laryngeal resistance, vocal frequency, and intensity. This speculation was supported by Hamlet (1973) who, via ultrasonography, investigated vocal fold closure patterns in subjects imitating hypernasal speech. She reported that the "glottal tightness" (a reduced open quotient) she found in nasalized vowels resulted from very strong adductory forces operating on the laryngeal mechanism. This increase in glottal resistance could also affect the pattern of chest wall action that drives the system to overcome the upstream loss of intensity due to the hard palate defect (oral–nasal fistula) or soft palate defect (velopharyngeal incompetence). Similar findings of laryngeal dysfunction in children with VPI have been reported (Zajac & Linville, 1989).

Such interpretations are consistent with the findings of Bernthal and Beukelman (1977) who, employing aeromechanical evaluation procedures, indicated that, as the velopharyngeal orifice area increases, the damping component of the nasal tract increases and sound intensity shunted through the mouth decreases. Extremes in vocal effort also may cause shifts in habitual use of vocal frequency. Our approach is to ask each prosthetic patient to perform a variety of tasks designed to determine the modal frequency and range of vocal frequency and intensity, the MPT, and the aerodynamic measures of average and variability of airflow and laryngeal airway resistance. These measures allow us to document changes in vocal output following placement of a prosthesis that separates the nose and mouth. Clinical experience suggests that some individuals with cleft palate develop unique respiratory and laryngeal operation strategies supraglotally to deal with the loss of oral sound pressure level. One role of the speech pathologist is to delineate which strategies are useful and which are inefficient in the patients' operation of an integrated system comprised of numerous functional valving units. Failure to identify and manage a malfunctioning valve downstream may lead to continued respiratory and laryngeal valving problems (e.g., inadequate phrasing, hyperadduction of the folds) following successful surgery or prosthetic management of the palatal and/or velopharyngeal defect. Conversely, changes in the oral or velopharyngeal structures may have a positive effect on the laryngeal and respiratory system function.

Evaluation processes: Velopharyngeal.   Although the available methods to assess velopharyngeal function are dealt with in more detail in Chapter 9, certain methods are discussed briefly here in conjunction with prosthetic management. The most frequently used method of assessment is perceptual judgments by trained or naive listeners (Moller & Starr, 1984). Support for this approach comes from the work of Schneider and Shprintzen (1980), who surveyed the preferences of speech pathologists concerning procedures for evaluating velopharyngeal competency. In order of preference from most to least, the respondents chose (a) listener judgments of symptoms (93%), (b) oral examinations (88%), (c) articulation tests (92%), (d) lateral-view cine- or videofluoroscopy (72%), (e) lateral cephalometrics (50%), (f) oral manometry (47%), (g) multiview cine- or videofluoroscopy (24%), (h) oral panendoscopy (22%), (i) airflow studies (18%), and (j) nasendoscopy (8%). The fact that the respondents came from a variety of employment centers, not only hospitals or other medical facilities, may account for the low usage of instrumentation. Also, it is important to remember that frequency of use does not necessarily relate to the reliability and validity of the evaluation procedure.

Typically, speech clinicians ask patients with velopharyngeal incompetence to imitate high vowels (e.g., /i/ and /u/) and to produce syllables with consonants exhibiting high air pressures (i.e., /p/, /t/, /s/, /ʃ/, /tʃ/) that are embedded in words, within phrases, or in sentence-length utterances. The patient may also be asked to change rate of speaking and/or stress and effort so that the clinician can evaluate physiological function related to utterance length and phonetic complexity. Articulation testing is performed routinely with a standardized inventory of sounds (e.g., *The Fisher–Logemann Test of Articulation Competence,* 1971; *Goldman–Fristoe Test of Articulation,* 1969; *Templin–Darley Tests of Articulation,* 1969). In most cases, these inventories evaluate sounds in prevocalic, intervocalic, and postvocalic word positions, either through picture naming, imitation, or sentence production. Conversational samples of speech are also elicited via topic or pictures. These samples are recorded graphically from live phonetic transcriptions or electronically on audio- or videotape for later phonetic/phonological analysis and for obtaining reliability measures of scoring sound production.

The most frequently used radiographic techniques include lateral-view cinefluoroscopy or videofluoroscopy or lateral cephalometrics. The use of these techniques has been described by Williams (1971) and Hollien (1976). Lateral X-rays (cephalometrics) have been used in the past, but provide information only about static positioning of the speech structures, usually during sustained vowel or consonant productions (e.g., /u/, /i/, /s/), and thus do not show three-dimensional action of the velopharyngeal mechanism. Lateral-view cine- or videofluoroscopy does show movement and timing features of articulation action associated with connected speech utterances (Shprintzen, Lencione, McCall, & Skolnick, 1974). To note sphincteric action with the appliance in place, the basal view (bottom to top) of the velopharyngeal port is useful. Likewise, to determine the optimal area for placement of the posterior section of the lift or obturator (bulb) along the lateral pharyngeal wall, the anterior–posterior (frontal) view appears best. The speech samples used for dynamic views of the system typically range from simple syllables to phrases or sentences, generally "loaded" with plosive, fricative, or affricative sounds in high-vowel contexts. Often the speech samples chosen reflect the questions being posed by the examiner in an attempt to obtain the best views of the velopharyngeal port and other articulatory valves of interest.

Quantification of the videofluoroscopy procedures clinically means visualization and categorization of closure using descriptive terms such as "touch closure" and "partial blending" (McWilliams & Bradley, 1964; Van Demark, Kuehn, & Tharp, 1975). Linear quantification involving size and distance measurements (Kuehn & Moll, 1976; Shelton & Trier, 1976; Skolnick & Cohn, 1989) was once a tedious technique of hand measurement from projected tracings of each cinefluorographic frame. This has now been made easier by computer digitization of the sampled events. Even videotapes may be digitized with computer scanning techniques. However, these newer methods (including computerized tomography, Moon & Smith, 1987) still rely on several views (lateral, frontal, basal) to indicate what part of the structure is operating most effectively. Kuehn (1982) wrote an excellent summary of these assessment procedures and their strengths and weaknesses. In addition, Stringer and Witzel (1989) recently reported a comparison of videofluoroscopy and nasopharyngoscopy for evaluating VPI.

Direct visualization of the laryngeal and velopharyngeal mechanism is also useful for describing closure prior to and following prosthetic management. Both rigid endoscopes (Pigott, 1969; Taub, 1966) and flexible fiberoptic endoscopes (Croft, Shprintzen, Daniller, & Lewin, 1978; Miyazaki, Matsuya, & Yamaoka, 1975) have been recommended to assess closure patterns in situ via oral or transnasal views. The major advantage of these direct visualization techniques is that they do not employ radiation to explore the structural movement, thus avoiding radiation hazards to the patient. Furthermore, the flexible fiberscope used transnasally allows for the observation of the three-dimensional action of the velopharyngeal sphincter before, during, and after fitting of a palatal prosthesis. As with other observational techniques, descriptions of the type, height, and extent of closure on the lateral, posterior, and frontal aspects of the sphincter are used to adjust dental prostheses or augment surgical procedures (Matsuya, Yamaoka, & Miyasaki, 1979). Speech samples used also typically require the patient to produce high vowels (e.g., /i/, /u/) in conjunction with high-pressure consonants (e.g., /p/, /s/, /t/). These samples are produced at fast and slow rates of speech, to stress the mechanism to account for as many variations in closure styles as possible. Again, quantification of object size presents a problem in distance calibration for the examiner; that is, the further the distance, the smaller the object, but not in a linear fashion. Thus, a graphic description or categorization of size, shape, and function is typically used to note changes in velopharyngeal action during prosthetic fitting. Initial attempts at determining reliability may be seen in the research of Karnell, Ibuki, Morris, and Van Demark (1983) and D'Antonio, Marsh, Province, Muntz, and Phillips (1989). In addition, Golding-Kushner (1990) and colleagues in a working group recently provided a protocol for standardization for reporting nasopharyngoscopy and multiview videofluoroscopy in various patient samples.

Aerodynamic measurements of oral and nasal airflow and pressure, nasal resistance, and estimated velopharyngeal orifice area have also been used by a number of clinicians to document changes in the velopharyngeal mechanism before and after prosthetic management (Wood & Warren, 1971). As an indirect, noninvasive technique for estimating velopharyngeal function, the efficiency of the valve is determined from ratios of differential oral–nasal air pressure and nasal airflow obtained during a variety of speech events. These procedures are not unlike those methods discussed previously with other instrumental approaches to assessment, such as employing high vowels with consonants demonstrating high intraoral air pressure. Correlations of nasal airflow, nasal airway resistance, and differential oral–nasal air pressure to overall velopharyngeal function are high (Allison & Leeper, 1990; Dalston, Warren, Morr, & Smith, 1988; Laine, Warren, Dalston, & Morr, 1988; Morr, Warren, Dalston, & Smith, 1989; Smith, Fiala, & Guyette, 1989; Warren, 1964, 1975, 1982; Warren & DuBois, 1964) and demonstrate reduction in overall articulation intelligibility as nasal air emission increases (Schneiderman & Mann, 1978). In addition, the duration of the onset and offset, the slope of the pressure or airflow pulse, and the total duration of the pressure-flow events are strong aeromechanical correlative measures with articulatory function at either the velopharyngeal or articulatory levels of the subsystem (Warren, 1982; Warren et al., 1985). Correlations with simultaneously recorded acoustic measures of oral–nasal sound energy (Dalston & Warren, 1986) have also been noted as strong. Instrumentation to measure velopharyngeal efficiency suffers, as do other indirect procedures, from the problem that their measures (e.g., estimated velopharyngeal orifice area) may be related to other physiological or psychological factors controlled by the subject and may not reflect absolute size or function of the mechanism during conversational speech or speech under certain stress situations.

Another microcomputer-based instrumental approach that appears to be gaining prominence in assessment of the acoustics of speech is nasometry. The Nasometer is an instrument that assesses the ratio of nasal acoustic energy divided by oral plus nasal acoustic energy (nasalance). Nasalance values range from 0% to 100%. Thus, if a speaker with velopharyngeal inadequacy produces speech phrases without nasal consonants, nasalance scores should increase compared with those of speakers without velopharyngeal inadequacy. Furthermore, if a person who is perceived as hyponasal produces a passage "loaded" with nasal speech sounds (which should produce normally higher nasalance scores), the scores may decrease and fall within the oral range of nasalance values. Studies (Dalston, 1989; Dalston, Warren, & Dalston, 1991a) have evaluated velopharyngeal function and listener judgments of hyper- and hyponasality in persons with suspected velopharyngeal inadequacy. In addition, the Nasometer has been shown to be useful in identifying (screening) subjects with more than mild hypernasality (Dalston, Warren, & Dalston, 1991b). Although normative data are available for nasalance scores in a variety of English dialects (Seaver, Dalston, Leeper, & Adams, 1991), the application of this instrumental approach has only recently been applied to persons wearing prosthodontic appliances for anterior and posterior defects (Molt, 1990). Future research should be forthcoming that describes the relationships between nasalance scores and perceptual judgments of resonance in individuals fitted with a variety of palatal speech appliances.

Undoubtedly, the best approaches for estimating the size of the velopharyngeal orifice derive from the clinician's desire to manage the incompetence correctly and to revise the appliance to suit the patient's needs. Such an approach must be multidimensional and should include physiological, acoustic, and perceptual assessment of speech where possible (Van Demark et al., 1985).

Evaluation processes: Articulatory. Regardless of the patient's oral condition, the speech pathologist must develop an evaluation format that will allow description of the patient's speech patterns before and after prosthetic management. Typically, the approach is to perform a phonetic inventory of sounds using a whole-word format, while looking specifically for perceptual errors of production that signal place, manner, and voicing difficulties. Our experiences have led us to observe articulation in a whole-word or sentence format using the *Templin–Darley Tests of Articulation* (1969), paying special attention to vowels in interconsonantal positions and consonants in the traditional initial, medial, and final positions of words. Depending upon the individual's age, we often use the sentence production format from the same test and evaluate conversational speech from topic- or picture-elicited communication. Particular attention is given to cosmetic and acoustic–perceptual aspects of sound production. An overall rating of articulation effectiveness is also taken from the conversational sample. Often, the dental office staff members are employed to make judgments of the overall effectiveness of the patient's articulation. Audio- and/or videotape recordings of the speech production portion of the evaluation are very useful for comparing changes in speech skills over time or management conditions.

Because many patients seen for treatment have complex orofacial features, we ask them to produce syllables, words, and phrases at normal, slower than normal, and much faster than normal rates of speech. We contend that by "overloading" the speech system with stress on speed, we can evaluate any problems in "targeting" placement of the articulators before and following prosthetic management. With some individuals, both speech and nonspeech oral repetitive movements are used to note changes in sequential and parallel operations of the lips, jaw, tongue, and soft palate during speech production. These methods are particularly useful for noting changes in articulatory activity as the patient adapts to a new or modified prosthetic appliance.

Contexts chosen for evaluation depend upon the site(s) of the defect. Our approach is to first take an overall inventory of defective sounds to lead us toward determining which subset of sounds to further evaluate. We have often found that speech sounds that require the most tongue tip action (e.g., /s/, /ʃ/, /tʃ/, /dʒ/) and the highest intraoral air pressure buildup (e.g., /f/, /p/, /t/, /s/, /tʃ/) in context with high vowel (e.g., /i/, /u/) positions, are the sounds that may serve to evaluate both anterior (hard palate) and posterior (soft palate) anatomical or physiological problems (Van Demark et al., 1985).

Existing Oral or Dental Conditions and the Effects on Speech

For individuals developing speech or attempting speech production following dental alteration of the anterior oral region, the change in size, shape, and position of the oral structures may adversely affect correct production of a number of speech sounds. To ignore the common dental hazards already present in patients with clefts involving the primary palate (e.g., congenitally missing lateral incisors, anterior and posterior crossbite, Class III malocclusion, malpositioned teeth) or to manufacture hazards because of questionable design of anterior intraoral appliances is unprofessional. These problems simply add an additional burden to the patient and to speech clinicians trying to evaluate or teach correct articulatory patterns. Even though emphasis is placed upon the maxillary segments of the oral cavity, the speech pathologist must consider during the speech evaluation mandibular aspects of oral function for prosthetic design, occlusal factors, and cosmesis. Because the lower jaw and tongue are an integral part of the functioning of the oral mechanism, the relationships between the upper and lower jaws must be considered before and following prosthetic management. Variations in design of the maxillary and mandibular components of the prosthesis may have implications for masticatory, deglutory, and articulatory function. Such considerations are consistent with reports from other authors concerning speech and prosthetic design (Bloomer, 1971; Lawson & Bond, 1969; Palmer, 1974; Starr; 1979). Finally, it should be recognized that many of the existing conditions to be discussed below may produce hazards to articulation, but generally do not alone prevent correct articulation from occurring. The adaptability of the human organism to variations in structure is nowhere more apparent than while observing the oral cavity as it functions for eating and speaking.

The anterior palatal portion of the appliance. Following our desire to understand the functional components of the speech-producing mechanism, special emphasis must be given to the anterior aspects of the prosthesis used with individuals with orofacial anomalies. Often, emphasis is placed only upon the posterior or velopharyngeal component. Although many problems we seek to eliminate are related to the oral–nasal coupling through the inadequate velopharyngeal valve, problems of neurological integrity, oral sensation, jaw relationships, tooth alignment, tongue function, abnormal size and shape of the hard palate, and lip deformities may also significantly contribute to the speech characteristics of the patient with cleft lip and palate.

The factors that may affect sound production following the placement of the appliance into the anterior region of the oral cavity include (a) position of the anterior teeth, (b) alterations in the vertical dimension (interdental space), (c) alterations in the occlusal plane level (an imaginary line drawn from the tips of the anterior teeth to the posterior teeth), (d) confinement of intraoral space (thick alveolar ridge of the dental appliance), (e) problems with anterior overbite (excessive overlap of the upper and lower teeth), (f) increased lingual flange size of the appliance (mandibular denture base overextension), and (g) chronic displacement or loosening of the anterior portion of the appliance (noted as appliance dropping or "clattering" against lower teeth). Each of these factors may cause distortions and/or substitutions of speech sound elements (particularly fricative and sibilant sounds) that may be separate problems from the types of sound errors related to posterior velopharyngeal valving problems. In some patients, both anterior and posterior openings between the oral and nasal cavities occur and must be managed concurrently.

Anterior oral–nasal fistulae. Openings between the oral and nasal cavities fortunately occur in only a small percentage of patients with clefts of the lip, alveolus, and/or hard palate. Although they may occur anywhere inside the anterior nares, in the buccal–nasal sulci, or along the hard palate, a large number are found in the area of the incisive foramen (see Figure 6.4). Whereas some can be readily closed surgically, others may be excessively large or the region may be too scarred to give a useful donor site for successful closure. These fistulae may affect speech adversely. Often, these fistulae exist in conjunction with velopharyngeal incompetency. Thus, the clinician is faced with the task of determining the contribution of each orifice (front or back) to speech performance. We have found that closure of the anterior oral–nasal fistula will allow consideration of the effect of the velopharyngeal incompetency with and without the anterior problem present. Several techniques have been offered to assess changes in resonance balance, nasal air emission, and articulatory precision. The first technique (Bless, Ewanowski, & Dibbel, 1980) promotes the use of soft dental wax to cover the anterior opening. Another group of clinicians (Reisberg, Gold, & Dorf, 1985) recommend using a medical-grade adhesive (Hollihesive, from Holister, Inc., Libertyville, IL 60048) to cover the hole and separate the oral and nasal cavities. In situations where these materials are not available, bubble gum or chewing gum may be used to temporarily obturate the fistula. Care must be taken to remove all the gum from the fistula following the examination to avoid subsequent infection and tissue irritation.

A useful test protocol for these assessments incorporates speech sounds produced on the alveolar ridge area (e.g., /t/, /s/, /tʃ/) in conjunction with high vowels (e.g., /i/, /u/) in syllable, word, and phrase contexts. Thus, the examiner can test sounds that provide a seal around the alveolar ridge, are high in intraoral air pressure, and demand tight closure of the velopharyngeal port. The method involves first testing the individual without the fistula covered to note the amount of resonance imbalance and nasal air emission, and to determine the effect of articulation precision. By covering the anterior defect, changes that occur relate to the removal of the anterior component and indicate that any residual problems may be related to incompetence of the posterior (velopharyngeal) region. Shelton and Blank (1984) suggested that even small oral–nasal fistulae can cause significant speech problems. Evaluations employing perceptual and aeromechanical measures of air pressure and airflow are appropriate for these patients.

Once the speech pathologist has determined the significance of the anterior oral–nasal fistula upon speech production, the prosthodontist

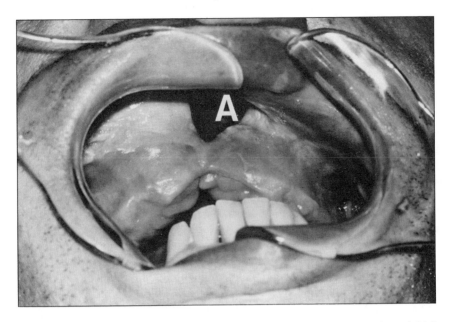

Figure 6.4 An edentulous maxilla with an oral–nasal fistula demonstrating a labial defect (A).

should determine what type of appliance should be used (temporary or permanent; fixed or removable) to close the defect. Testing before and after placement of the anterior prosthesis may be incorporated for appliances designed to aid velopharyngeal closure. Thus, early determination of the effects of the anterior and posterior defects is necessary when designing the total prosthesis. In addition, the patient must then adapt to the alterations of the oral cavity following placement of the dental speech appliance.

Adaptation to the anterior portion of a prosthesis.   Throughout our discussion of the use of prosthetic appliances for "normalizing" speech output characteristics of patients with orofacial defects, we have alluded to changes in articulation related to the anterior oral cavity. As part of the discussion, we feel some time should be spent describing the possible adjustments or adaptations to the placement of prostheses or appliances in the anterior oral cavity. Unfortunately, most available research data have been collected on subjects with normal structures. Thus, we make inferences from these studies regarding individuals with cleft palate or other orofacial defects. Questions typically asked relate to how well a speaker controls articulation if certain dimensions of the vocal tract are altered.

Children obviously have less practice in achieving correct target patterns of speech than adults who have spent many years practicing achievement of articulatory targets that demand knowledge of various shapes and positions of the articulators within the vocal tract. When the oral cavity is suddenly altered by placing an orthodontic-type retainer or palatal template into the upper arch, changes in oral cavity configuration may change learned motor patterns for speech. These changes affect not only size of the oral cavity, but also tactile and kinesthetic feedback for fine coordination of articulation. The result is increased errors in articulation, typically substitutions or distortions of fricatives or affricates (Garber, Speidel, & Siegel, 1980).

Although the primary method for judging adjustments or adaptation to oral–dental appliances has been to assess the phonetic representation of speech, instrumental methods, such as acoustical and biomechanical evaluations, have been applied to normal speaking adults wearing palatal appliances. In a series of studies concerning speech adaptation to palatal prostheses, Hamlet and colleagues (Hamlet, Geoffrey, & Bartlett, 1976; Hamlet & Stone, 1974, 1978; Hamlet, Stone, & McCarty, 1978) have noted the following: (a) more open jaw position after initial adaptation to a dental appliance, (b) formant frequency shifts of the second and third formants with spectral changes for /ʃ/ phonemes following insertion of an appliance, (c) tongue overshoot of targets immediately after insertion of an appliance, (d) rapid readaptation to an appliance after a long period of not wearing the appliance, and (e) rapid oral constriction changes for /s/ sounds and laryngeal devoicing gestures.

A conceptual framework for evaluating speech adaptation to anterior dental prostheses must take into account rapid motor reorganization of speech from the respiratory, laryngeal, and oral articulatory structures (Borden, Harris, Fitch, & Yoshioka, 1979; Fujimura, 1981; Kelso, Tuller, & Harris, 1983). Short- and long-term adjustments to changes in oral cavity size obviously occur to provide a major preprogrammed modification, with finer adjustments probably occurring to enable production of the final utterance output as precisely as that found in "natural" speech. This may occur with the aid of auditory feedback concerning spectral and temporal characteristics of the speech sounds produced. Although it is interesting to review compensation patterns to anterior appliances in normal individuals, the reader should remember that little information is available concerning similar adaptation strategies in individuals with orofacial defects. With oral–sensory, motor, and auditory difficulties being more frequent in the latter individuals, special attention must be given to allowing as much adjustment time as possible for these persons when an anterior prosthesis is inserted.

Clinically, we note adaptation changes in the orofacial patients by reviewing articulation test protocols (*The Templin–Darley Tests of Articulation,* 1969), free field speech samples, and sentences loaded with fricative and affricate sound elements. Because the fitting procedure takes up to 6 weeks of trial, refit, and replacement, the patients have a chance to accommodate over time to the anterior aspects of the appliance.

SPECIFIC DEFECT MANAGEMENT

Anterior Oral Defects (Hard Palate Clefts and Oral–Nasal Fistulae)

Defects of the maxilla may occur as a result of destructive inflammatory conditions, tumors that must be surgically removed, and trauma. Included in this grouping of maxillary defects are clefts of the hard palate and oral–nasal fistulae (see Figure 6.5). Such defects cause fluid and food leakage into the nasal cavity, impaired masticatory function, hypernasality, nasal air emission, and other articulatory problems that contribute to a loss of overall speech intelligibility. Restoration of lost tissues

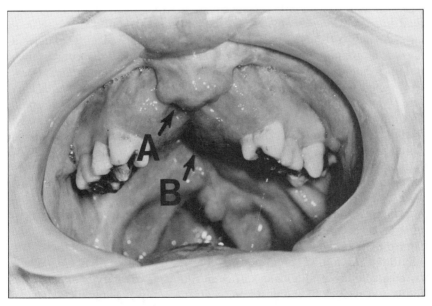

Figure 6.5 An anterior oral–nasal defect showing oral–nasal defect (A) and hard palate cleft (repaired) (B).

by prosthetic appliance obturation can minimize these disabilities. With hard palate defects, prosthetic treatment is directed toward developing an effective seal at the perimeter of the defect at the palatal opening and replacement of missing teeth. Effective obturator coverage will prevent inappropriate transmission of air and fluids between the nasal and oral cavities. In most situations, it is neither possible nor desirable to completely fill the defect. However, obturator extension into the defect may be necessary to obtain the degree of support, retention, and stability ideally required by the prosthesis and that provided by the existing oral structures. The weight of bulky obturators can be significantly reduced by hollowing out its internal mass. In situations where nasal secretions are minimal, the nasopharyngeal surface of the obturator is left open, simulating a "topless box" (Oral, Aramany, & McWilliams, 1979).

The retentive clasps of the prosthesis must be of sufficient strength and number to prevent dislodgement. Tooth contours deficient in retentive capacity may require modification to improve their retentive qualities. Frequently, these contour alterations may be achieved by placing overcontoured fillings on the appropriate tooth surfaces (Sills & Leeper, 1984).

Soft Palate Defects

Methods of treating soft palate defects remain controversial. In most cases, congenital cleft palate defects can be successfully repaired by surgical intervention. However, prosthodontic treatment should be considered where (a) unusually large clefts exist, (b) acquired surgical defects remain, (c) patients present with severe velopharyngeal incompetence and insufficiency, and (d) medical, psychosocial, or religious reasons prohibit surgery (Mazaheri, 1976; Shiere et al., 1962). Patients with this type of defect generally exhibit hypernasality, excessive nasal air emission, and decreased speech intelligibility. Individuals demonstrating good muscular action from the velopharyngeal mechanism usually adapt more readily to the prosthetic speech appliance (Blakeley, 1960, 1964; Wong & Weiss, 1972). Thus, these patients need an appliance that closes the posterior defect area, but allows for maintenance of the anterior oral area for correct articulatory performance.

The prosthetic speech appliance for soft palate defects typically consists of three sections: maxillary, palatal, and nasopharyngeal (see Figure 6.6). In some cases, the complete upper denture serves as the maxillary section of the appliance for the edentulous patient. When the edentulous maxilla lacks sufficient retentive capacity to support the additional weight of the posterior sections, adhesives must be used to augment retention of the prosthesis. Without adhesives, the patient may be unable to chew or speak adequately.

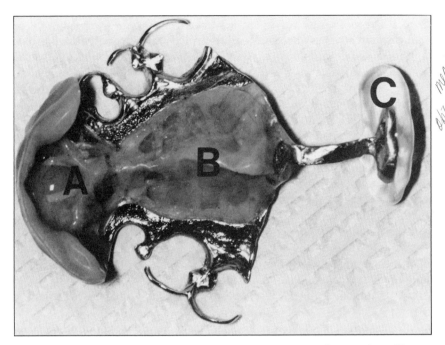

Figure 6.6 Example of a maxillary speech appliance comprising three sections: (A) maxillary section, (B) palatal section, and (C) nasopharyngeal section.

In infants or toddlers, the prosthesis for soft palate defects may serve as a feeding aid and later as an aid for early speech development. Readaptation of these palatal appliances must be accomplished once every month or two to maintain adequate fit and operation. As the oral cavity grows and teeth erupt, additional changes in shape, size, and retention techniques must be accomplished. In older childhood and adolescence, a combination of an orthodontic and palatal obturator may be necessary. As the patient ages, and as dental or occlusal abnormalities may develop for some patients, a palatal prosthesis can be added to partial or full dentures to maintain oral–nasal separation and to provide adequacy of speech production.

Speech considerations. The velopharyngeal mechanism is a three-dimensional valve whose activities serve to separate the posterior oral and nasal passages for deglutition and speech. As a flexible biomechanical valve within the respiratory system, the velopharyngeal port must be sufficiently patent to allow air to pass through it for inspiratory and expiratory function, but must approximate for most speech sounds (except /m/, /n/, and /ŋ/). The primary focus for very young patients with velopharyngeal insufficiency or incompetency is the resultant difficulties with developing oral–nasal contrasts in speech. Continued velopharyngeal incompetence can lead to faulty articulation patterns that may follow an individual from early life through adulthood.

Speech difficulties typically encountered with velopharyngeal incompetency and/or insufficiency include hypernasality (excessive nasal resonance on normally oralized vowels and consonants), nasal air emission, and decreased speech intelligibility from the loss of oral acoustic and aerodynamic power. The articulatory problems generally include (a) substitutions of laryngeal or pharyngeal sounds for lingua–alveolar sounds (Bzoch, 1979); (b) more difficulty producing fricatives, affricates, and plosives than semivowels and vowels (Van Demark, 1974); (c) more difficulty with voiceless than voiced sounds (Moll, 1968); (d) more problems with blends than with singleton consonants (Moll, 1968); and (e) patterns of maladaptive articulation (e.g., glottal stops, pharyngeal fricatives) that remain even after the velopharyngeal port operates within normal limits (Peterson, 1975; Van Demark, Morris, & Vandehaar, 1979).

Although obturators (bulbs) and palatal lift appliances are designed to reduce the size of the velopharyngeal port, their effectiveness may be most useful for increasing the efficiency of the valve. Indirectly, the appliance acts to improve articulation by increasing aerodynamic and acoustic power (Warren, 1986). These changes in velopharyngeal closure should improve listener judgments of hypernasal voice quality (Counihan & Cullinan, 1970) and overall speech intelligibility (Schneiderman & Mann, 1978).

Assessment of the velopharyngeal valve before and after insertion of any speech appliance typically includes perceptual, aerodynamic, radiologic, and/or fiberoptic views of the mechanism. Following a thorough peroral examination of the intraoral structures and their function, most patients being considered for prosthodontic management are carefully evaluated for viability of tissue, size, shape, and function of the velum and the lateral and posterior pharyngeal walls.

Complete soft palate clefts. Cleft size, location, and condition of the tissues surrounding the cleft govern the design of the appliance's velopharyngeal and pharyngeal sections. Obturators for defects of the entire soft palate take their shape from movements generated by the lateral and posterior pharyngeal walls. Impression techniques employing a variety of head and tongue movements help in producing the final obturator form.

The obturator section is constructed in acrylic resin and relies on an internal metal framework for support and connection to the anterior base section. The internal metal frame provides a scaffolding on which impression materials (thermoplastic waxes, light curing resins) are sequentially layered to achieve the most physiologically acceptable obturator form. The obturator should be located at the level of greatest pharyngeal wall movement and need not extend more than 10 mm vertically (Curtis, Beumer, & Firtell, 1979). Soft palate obturators positioned too low may produce gagging and restrict normal tongue movements, whereas those placed too high may occlude the nasopharynx and cause problems of nasal airway patency. Ideally, the nasopharyngeal section should be located in the nasopharynx region at the level of the normal palatal closure (Curtis et al., 1979). Passive contact must exist between the acrylic of the obturator and the mucosa of the velopharynx and pharynx. During swallowing and coughing, the palatal extension and nasopharyngeal section would not be displaced. Nasopharyngeal obturators that incorporate a polished, convex superior surface and a concave palatal surface minimize mucous accumulation and provide adequate tongue space for swallowing and speech purposes.

At the delivery (insertion) stage, movements similar to those used to obtain the impression are used to identify pressure areas where the surfaces of the obturator might impinge excessively on the mucosa. Several postdelivery adjustments must be anticipated after the initial prosthesis placement. At these appointments, clasp adjustments and modification of the obturator may be required to achieve comfort and function.

Partial soft palate clefts. Partial soft palate clefts occur in surgically resected or incompletely repaired palates. Short, taut residual soft palates are common surgical sequelae and, when present, should not be covered by the prosthesis. In these cases, the nasopharyngeal section obturates only the palatal defect and avoids the adjacent tissues. Lifting of the residual soft palate may be required when dealing with long or immobile soft palate tissues (Subtelny, Sakuda, & Subtelny, 1966). Tissues adjacent to the cleft seldom exhibit full movement or elevation. Thus, the obturator should extend from the defect to the opposite lateral pharyngeal wall to prevent palatopharyngeal insufficiency (Curtis et al., 1979). One problem facing some patients is the delay experienced in initiating definitive prosthetic treatment until surgically resected tissues heal: For some patients with oral cancers, radiation therapy may have been recommended as part of the treatment regimen. Radiation therapy prolongs the healing period, sometimes exceeding 6 months. In other respects, treatment of the partial soft palate defect remains similar to that for the total palatal defect.

Procedural considerations with speech appliances. Procedures used by the prosthodontist and speech pathologist to optimize prosthetic speech management are of interest. Rosen and Bzoch (1958) suggested that the posterior portion of the speech appliance be adjusted until the patient can produce voiceless stops, such as /p/ or /t/, or voiceless fricatives, such as /s/, /ʃ/, or /f/, without audible nasal air emission. The patient also must have enough nasal airway patency to produce acceptable /m/, /n/, or /ŋ/ sounds without hyponasal voice quality. High intraoral air pressure oral consonants and high vowels, such as /i/ and /u/, should be combined in syllables or words and placed into a longer context (e.g., phrases). They should be repeated with greater or less stress, and produced at faster and slower than normal speaking rates so that the speech pathologist can evaluate articulatory and phonatory changes following speech appliance fitting.

As an adjunct to the perceptual judgments of change, instrumental measures of velopharyngeal closure may be accomplished via cinefluorography (more recently, videofluoroscopy) (Falter & Shelton, 1964; Shelton, Lindquist, Arndt, Elbert, & Youngstrom, 1971; Shelton et al., 1968; Shelton, Lindquist, Knox, et al., 1971) and aeromechanical evaluations of flow-pressure characteristics of speech (Warren, 1982). In addition, the use of transnasal views of the velopharyngeal port employing flexible fiberscopes (Matsuya, Yamaoka, & Miyazaki, 1979; Osberg & Witzel, 1981) may be useful as a relatively noninvasive technique for observing changes in velopharyngeal function during prosthetic fitting using speech samples noted earlier.

Patient adjustments to the insertion of a speech appliance have been of interest to a number of investigators (Blakeley, 1960, 1964, 1969; Mazaheri & Mazaheri, 1976; Shelton et al., 1968; Shelton, Lindquist, Knox, et al., 1971; Subtelny et al., 1966; Weiss, 1971; Weiss & Louis, 1972; Wong & Weiss, 1972). The underlying premise has been that certain subjects develop posterior and lateral pharyngeal wall action that allows the prosthodontist to reduce the bulb size while still maintaining speech quality within normal limits. Employing a variety of subjective and objective techniques to monitor reduction in nasalization and hypernasality, the researchers noted above reported increased velopharyngeal activity and subsequent reduction in posterior obturator size in selected patients. Wong and Weiss (1972) suggested several factors that appeared to offer stronger prognostication than others: (a) younger patients did better than older patients, (b) females did better than males in reducing nasalization following obturator insertion, (c) family and patient compliance to direction appeared to aid in the development of more velopharyngeal action, and (d) patients with longer veli and greater pharyngeal wall action were more often able to undergo speech bulb reduction. Although the number of patients in each of the listed studies is not large, the findings that one-quarter to one-third of the sampled population could undergo speech bulb reduction speaks well for careful consideration of these procedures.

The important factor in obturation or palatal lift reduction in patients with velopharyngeal incompetence is the ability of the velopharyngeal musculature to adapt to the "foreign body" placed in the defect area. In the case of the lift, the musculature may react by pulling (lifting) away from the object, hence enhancing closure, or in the case of the obturator, there is an increase in lateral–posterior pharyngeal wall and velar closure against the speech bulb. This increased activity by the surrounding musculature allows the speech pathologist to note changes in perceptual, acoustic, and physiological activities associated with speech production, such as reduced hypernasality, reduced nasal air emission, and reduced velopharyngeal port orifice area.

Most appliance reduction programs have focused on the long-term changes in the muscular adaptation of the velopharyngeal complex. Changes in the amount of velopharyngeal closure must be monitored from week to week during an ongoing speech management program. Careful measurement procedures designed to note subtle changes in perceptual, acoustic, visual, or aerodynamic activity are essential in determining how much material may be taken away from the obturator or palatal lift. Reduction of the dental material in the posterior region is usually accomplished by using visual (nasendoscopy), aerodynamic (air pressure/flow), and perceptual judgments (reduced hypernasality, nasal air emission) criteria. Generally, contact paste is placed on the bulb or lift and fitted in the oral cavity by the prosthodontist. A series of speech tasks (syllables, words), including production of high-pressure consonants in high vowel environments produced at slowly increasing rates, seem to satisfy the requirements. Removal of the appliance reveals a "wiping clean" of the portion of the appliance where the most muscle activity has taken place. Reduction of these portions of the prosthesis then allows the musculature to "reach" toward the reduced space while maintaining the general adequacy level of resonance balance. In some cases, patients have been able to withdraw from wearing their lifts or speech bulbs following a "reduction" therapy program. Usually, these adaptations occur over a fairly long period (14 to 16 months) and demand close attention to the subtle alterations in the appliance, as well as the resultant speech output changes.

Consensus regarding the usefulness of these appliance reduction programs still places them in the "experimental therapy" level, although a number of prosthetic–speech clinics have reported reductions in approximately 20% to 30% of patients. New instrumental techniques for analyzing small changes in the acoustic and physiological events associated with speech production in patients wearing prosthetic appliances should provide better information concerning which patients make changes, what the optimal time period is for change, and which speech management programs are most effective.

Design considerations of speech appliances have related primarily to position of the posterior pharyngeal portion of the appliance in the nasopharynx. Early clinical procedures used the area at or near Passavant's ridge as a place of closure. Aram and Subtelny (1959), Fletcher, Haskins, and Bosma (1960), Lloyd, Pruzansky, and Subtelny (1957), and Mazaheri and Millard (1965) reported that, in general, inferior–superior placement of the speech bulb had little or no effect on resonance as long as sufficient closure was present to obtain close approximation. Lateral dimensions appeared as important as vertical dimensions for the maintenance of adequate resonance balance. Other factors considered important in designing posterior speech appliances include (a) maintaining an adequate nasal airway for vegetative breathing and aeration of the nasal passages, (b) placement of the speech bulb in a higher position so that displacement of the appliance by tongue posture or movement does not occur, (c) appropriate balance of forces anterior to posterior to reduce pressure on supporting tooth structure, and (d) development of lateral and posterior tissue tolerance to prevent ulceration and infection in the area of the bulb (Minsley, Warren, & Hairfield, 1991; Shelton & Lloyd, 1963).

Clearly, individual differences in each patient's anatomical defect and physiological action must be considered when fabricating and modifying posterior speech bulb appliances. Functional assessment should include physiological, acoustic, and perceptual measurements of speech performance observed before and after speech appliance insertion. By combining input from both the speech pathologist and the prosthodontist, an appliance that functions properly for masticatory, deglutory, and speech purposes can be successfully developed for the patient.

Velopharyngeal Incompetence in Speakers Without Clefts

General considerations. One important clinical task in human communication disorders is to determine the most effective method of treatment for individuals suffering from velopharyngeal incompetency. These individuals present characteristics of hypernasality, excessive nasal emission of air, and decreased speech intelligibility. These problems may occur as a result of congenital palatal defects, traumatic injuries or cerebrovascular accidents, neuromuscular diseases such as multiple sclerosis, tumors of the brain stem that have been surgically removed, and idiopathic conditions resulting in velopharyngeal incompetence (LaVelle & Hardy, 1979; Mazaheri & Mazaheri, 1976).

The use of a palatal lift prosthesis to reduce hypernasality and nasalization and to increase overall speech intelligibility has been accepted as an effective method of prosthodontic treatment for individuals with velopharyngeal incompetency. This method, first described by Gibbons and Bloomer (1958), employs an oral appliance to elevate the soft palate from a more posterior position to bring the velum close to the posterior pharyngeal wall for speech purposes. By elevating the soft palate, the size of the velopharyngeal valve is decreased and resonance balance and overall intelligibility are increased.

Various procedures have been recommended by researchers for estimating the efficiency of the palatal lift appliance. These procedures include clinical judgments of articulation and voice quality change in speech (Gibbons & Bloomer, 1958), measures of speech intelligibility using a closed-set response paradigm with rhyming words (Kipfmueller & Lang, 1972), lateral X-rays and static breath pressure manometric measures (Marshall & Jones, 1971), combined nasal airflow and differential air pressure measures to estimate velopharyngeal orifice area size (Hardy, Netsell, Schweiger, & Morris, 1969; LaVelle & Hardy, 1979; Shaughnessy, Netsell, & Farrange, 1983), and simultaneous cineradiographic, acoustic, and perceptual measures of speech proficiency (Aten, McDonald, Simpson, & Gutierrez, 1984).

Treatment considerations for palatal lifts. In addition to the patient's dental status, several other factors may affect the dimensions of the lift section of the palatal lift and the individual's accommodation to it. These factors include (a) palatal vault contour, (b) pharyngeal size and form, (c) displacement characteristics of the soft palate, (d) distance between the border of the soft palate and the posterior pharyngeal wall, (e) degree of symmetrical muscular activity of the velum, (f) sensitivity of the gag reflex, and (g) position, size, shape, and activity range of the tongue. Each factor must be considered carefully for the individual with velopharyngeal incompetence; thus, each patient's lift appliance will have a unique design (Leeper & Sills, 1986).

Structural features peculiar to the palatal lift. Tissue pressures exerted on the palatal lift exceed those exerted on simple removable partial dentures. The speech prosthesis must be designed to distribute these forces widely and uniformly to the retaining and supporting structures. To provide the needed strength, the components of the maxillary and palatal sections should be made as a one-unit metal casting. To achieve adequate support for the soft palate, the lift is shaped to resemble a beaver tail, with its broadest dimension positioned close to the palatal boundary (see Figure 6.7). The lift may be augmented by an obturator in those individuals presenting short palates. A clear acrylic resin lift portion

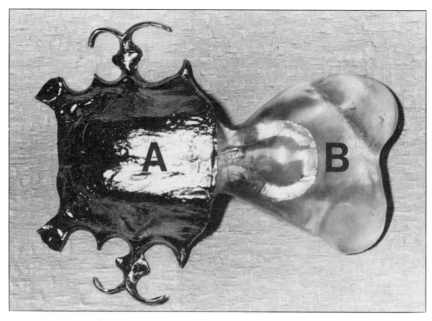

Figure 6.7 Example of a palatal lift speech appliance with (A) maxillary section and (B) palatal section.

nasopharyngeal?   *p169?*   *palatal?*

provides the clinician with good visual access to the underlying tissues, which is helpful when adjusting or modifying the lift (Sills & Leeper, 1984). Palatal lifts may also be used for individuals who have no teeth in the upper arch (Sato, Sato, Yoshida, & Tsuru, 1987).

Meatal obturators.   An older method for treatment of velopharyngeal incompetency employs the use of a meatal obturator (see Figures 6.6 and 6.8). Unlike the palatal lift, which relies on muscular activity of the velopharyngeal structures for effect, the meatal obturator simply impedes nasal airflow in the nasopharynx. Positioned above and behind the hard palate terminus, the meatal obturator acts as a barrier that regulates nasal airflow. Airflow control is achieved by reduction of the lateral borders of the obturator, or by drilling one or more holes through the posterior portion. The remaining components of the meatal obturator resemble those of similar maxillary prosthetic speech appliances. Some prosthodontists prefer meatal obturators because they may weigh less than palatal lifts and are thought to reduce gagging. The nasopharynx impression technique for the meatal obturator is more demanding than that for the palatal lift and requires several sequential impressions to acquire the appropriate configuration (Sharry, 1981).

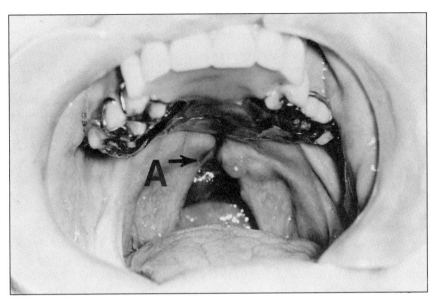

Figure 6.8 Example of a meatal obturator (in situ), partially obscured by terminus of velum.

Prosthetic–speech team management of the patient. Once the appliance framework has been produced in accordance with the treatment plan, acrylic resin tray material is adapted to the lift extension portion of the framework extending onto the soft palate. The lift impression is made initially using a low-fusing thermoplastic material with the soft palate elevated to make contact with the posterior pharyngeal wall. The impression is extended to the degree of lift the palatal tissues require, based upon the objective clinical evaluation of speech production tasks discussed previously, including lateral cephalometrics, videofluoroscopy, nasendoscopic assessment, and aerodynamic information obtained from the patient during speech (Leeper & Sills, 1986; Muntz , D'Antonio, Gay, & Marsh, 1985; Riski, Hoke, & Dolan, 1989). When a desirable amount of velopharyngeal competency is achieved, the tissue surface of the thermoplastic material is reduced approximately 1 mm, and a final wax impression is taken. Often it is prudent to build up the lift portion over several appointments to compensate for functional tissue adaptation, avoid unnecessary tissue irritation, and improve patient tolerance.

During this modification process, the speech pathologist and prosthodontist work together to evaluate the effectiveness of the palatal lift. Lift configuration is influenced by (a) depth of the oropharynx, (b) width of the posterior pharyngeal wall, (c) degree of palatal movement during phoneme production, (d) extent of the lateral pharyngeal wall port openings, (e) degree of hyper- or hypotonic palatal pharyngeal muscles, and (f) sensitivity of the gag reflex.

The prosthodontist must accommodate the lift to the physiological constraints placed on it by tissue displacement, whereas the speech pathologist is interested in obtaining the best resonance balance possible. Clinical speech procedures include assessing resonance balance perceptually with sustained vowel /i/, /a/, and /u/ production in isolation and in conjunction with syllable production of voiceless plosives, fricatives, and affricates. Nasal air emission is assessed perceptually or via air pressure or airflow studies during production of syllables containing high oral pressure consonants and high vowels. As the lift more adequately causes closure of the velar tissue against the posterior and lateral pharyngeal walls, the speech pathologist asks the patient to produce a sustained /m/ or syllable /mʌ/ to note the degree of nasal patency and resonance balance. When too much closure is observed, nasal production becomes oralized (i.e., /m/ becomes /b/) and hyponasal resonance results. At this stage, the prosthodontist reduces the tissue surface of the lift by trimming the thermoplastic material and impresses again with lower viscosity wax. The corrected impression is converted to heat-polymerized clear acrylic resin. Initially, the patient wears the lift continuously except when eating or sleeping. As the patient's experience and confidence increase, the lift can be worn during meals. However, it should never be worn 24 hours a day, as this practice frequently leads to mucosal inflammations, such as papillary hyperplasia. A rest period of 6 to 8 hours per day with the prosthesis out of the mouth is recommended. During this time period, the prosthesis must be stored wet to prevent possible dimensional changes in the acrylic resin created by dehydration.

Assessment of modifications.   Aeromechanical and acoustic measures seem to correlate best with perceptual measures collected during the evaluation period. Sills and Leeper (1984) recently evaluated the records of 14 dysarthric patients with accompanying velopharyngeal incompetence who were each fitted with a palatal lift prosthesis. The results of their evaluation suggested that, on average, significant changes from premanagement (no lift condition) to postmanagement (lift inserted condition) demonstrated decreased nasal airflow, increased respiratory effort (intraoral air pressure, subglottal air pressure), and decreased estimated velopharyngeal orifice areas for plosive and fricative syllable contexts and oral phoneme sentence contexts. These researchers also noted that placement of the palatal lift prosthesis caused their subjects to decrease oral orifice size and to increase the duration of isolated syllable and sentence productions. They also reported that lateral cephalometric X-ray measures confirmed decreased midline velopharyngeal gap size for sustained /u/ and /s/ phonemes. There was also a slight increase in intrinsic length (velar stretch) of the velum following lift placement. These physical findings correlated well with listener judgments of decreased hypernasality and slight improvement in whole-word articulatory precision. These data add support to research concerning palatal lift appliances reported by Gonzalez and Aronson (1970), LaVelle and Hardy (1979), and Aten et al. (1984). These investigators found decreased velopharyngeal port size, decreased hypernasality and nasalization, and slightly improved speech intelligibility following palatal lift management.

Although changes in resonance balance (e.g., decreased hypernasality) or a reduction of nasal air emission should be expected following placement of a palatal lift, certain well-learned, but abnormal articulatory patterns (velar, pharyngeal, or glottal substitutions for tongue fronted sounds) may persist. The clinician should be cognizant of the effects of a palatal lift prosthesis and should continue to manage the articulatory motor skill learning component with other articulators in such a way as to differentiate efficacy of treatment for each speech subsystem (velar, lingual, jaw). Thus, by choosing the optimal combination of speech probes during isolated-syllable, whole-word, sentence, or conversational utterances, the clinician can show differences in acquisition of articulatory skills for lip, jaw, tongue, or velopharyngeal mechanism during production attempts. Reduction in features of nasality and nasalization may also be linked to successful management of the velopharynx, whereas long-term goals for modification of abnormal tongue posturing may be viewed as a separate part of the treatment paradigm.

LONG-TERM MANAGEMENT

Dental

Crucial to the postdelivery success of maxillary prosthetic speech appliance therapy is the requirement for continued dental evaluation (Henderson & Steffel, 1981). Patients wearing such prostheses cannot always be relied upon to monitor their dental status and must therefore return for regular dental examinations. A suitable dental recall schedule based on the individual situation must be determined. A minimum of an annual checkup should be mandatory, with more frequent recalls as required. Of particular concern is the health of the supporting oral structures and of the investing mucosa, and the physical condition of the prosthesis. Typically, with these appliances, the teeth become more prone to caries and periodontal disease. Clasped abutment teeth must be observed for increased mobility and, when present, the cause corrected. Mucosa bordering the acrylic resin portion frequently exhibits inflammation that must be controlled. Finally, prostheses must be inspected for wear and/or damage, and the appropriate adjustment made.

Refitting (relining) of the acrylic resin portion of the prosthetic speech appliance to accommodate changes in the underlying mucosal surfaces must be anticipated. The peripheral seal of obturators must be maintained for effective air and fluid control. Eventually, however, replacement of the prosthesis will be required. Some materials used in its construction have a limited life span, making refabrication of all or a part of the device necessary. Ten or more years of service from one prosthesis should be considered satisfactory.

Speech

Many individuals seen for prosthetic management may be referred from other hospital or rehabilitation units in the area. Because most will return to their "home" unit for ongoing speech therapy, it is imperative that good communication exist between the prosthetic team and that home unit. Communication may be enhanced by providing inservice training for the speech professionals in those units, covering topics such as (a) criteria for admission to the program, (b) technical characteristics of the appliance, (c) modification procedures, (d) timing of modifications, (e) continuing evaluation procedures, and (f) long-term care of the appliance and oral environment. Written progress reports concerning each step in the process should be forwarded to the referring unit or professionals.

Because each prosthetic device described in this chapter is created uniquely for each patient, minor alterations to the anterior and/or posterior components are often necessary. Slight changes in soft or hard tissue environments may cause the appliance to lose its retentive characteristics, or the wearer may begin to adapt to the posterior segment, as evidenced by speech improvement, and need to have some acrylic removed. In any case, information from the home unit may be useful in understanding problems with the appliance. Review by the team's prosthodontist and speech pathologist will allow refitting of the prosthesis following guidelines discussed earlier in the chapter. Important indices of prosthesis fit derive from information regarding speech quality (hypernasality/hyponasality), nasal air emission, aerodynamic activity through the velopharyngeal system (orifice area estimation), structural movement of the velum and the lateral and posterior pharyngeal walls (nasendoscopy, videofluoroscopy), and overall speech intelligibility. Reevaluation using a standard protocol allows the attending professional to note positive and/or negative changes in the patient's performance following appliance alterations. Modifications to the appliance may occur over an 8-month to 2-year period, depending upon the type of insult, the results of various medical and behavioral treatments, and the age and compliance of the individual involved.

SUMMARY

In this chapter, we have attempted to outline procedures for the assessment, fabrication, and modification of prosthetic appliances for anterior and posterior oral defects. Each professional or team of professionals must work together to develop an effective treatment plan that considers oral function and speech performance as equal partners in the rehabilitation process. Through careful record keeping, standardized protocols, and efficient cost–benefit analyses, the team concept in prosthetic care of the orally handicapped individual can work to offer the patient the best opportunity for improved communication.

REFERENCES

Adisman, I. K. (1962, November). Removable partial dentures for jaw defects of the maxilla and mandible. *Dental Clinics of North America*, 849–870.

Allison, D. L., & Leeper, H. A. (1990). A comparison of non-invasive procedures to assess nasal airway resistance. *Cleft Palate Journal, 27*, 40–44.

Aram, A., & Subtelny, J. D. (1959). Velopharyngeal function and cleft palate prosthesis. *Journal of Prosthetic Dentistry, 9*, 149–158.

Aten, J. L., McDonald, A., Simpson, M., & Gutierrez, R. (1984). Efficacy of modified palatal lifts for improving resonance. In M. R. McNeil, M. E. Rosenbek, & A. E. Aronson (Eds.), *The dysarthrias: Physiology, acoustics, perception, management* (pp. 331–342). San Diego: College Hill.

Bernthal, J., & Beukelman, D. R. (1977). The effects of changes in velopharyngeal orifice area on vocal intensity. *Cleft Palate Journal, 14*, 63–77.

Blakeley, R. W. (1960). Temporary speech prosthesis as an aid in speech training. *Cleft Palate Bulletin, 10*, 63.

Blakeley, R. W. (1964). The complementary use of speech prostheses and pharyngeal flaps in palatal insufficiency. *Cleft Palate Journal, 1*, 194–198.

Blakeley, R. W. (1969). The rationale for a temporary speech prosthesis in palatal insufficiency. *British Journal of Disorders of Communication, 4*, 134–139.

Bless, D., Ewanowski, S., & Dibbell, D. (1980). A technique for temporary obturation of fistulae—A clinical note. *Cleft Palate Journal, 17*, 297–300.

Bloomer, H. (1971). Speech defects associated with dental malocclusions and related abnormalities. In L. Travis (Ed.), *Handbook of speech pathology and audiology* (pp. 715–766). New York: Appleton-Century-Crofts.

Borden, G. J., Harris, K. S., Fitch, H., & Yoshioka, H. (1979). *Self monitoring during familiar and less familiar speech events.* Paper presented at the American Speech–Language–Hearing Association Annual Meeting, Atlanta.

Bzoch, K. R. (1979). Categorical aspects of cleft palate speech. In K. R. Bzoch, *Communicative disorders related to cleft lip and palate* (pp. 109–129). Boston: Little, Brown.

Chierici, G. (1979). Cleft palate habilitation. In J. Beumer, T. A. Curtis, & D. N. Firtell (Eds.), *Maxillofacial rehabilitation: Prosthodontic and surgical considerations* (pp. 292–310). St. Louis: Mosby.

Coleman, R. F., Mabis, J. H., & Hinson, J. K. (1977) Fundamental frequency–sound pressure level profiles of adult male and female voices. *Journal of Speech and Hearing Research, 20,* 197–204.

Counihan, D. T., & Cullinan, W. L. (1970). Reliability and dispersion of nasality ratings. *Cleft Palate Journal, 7,* 261–270.

Croft, C. V., Shprintzen, R. J., Daniller, A., & Lewin, J. L. (1978). The occult submucous cleft palate and the musculus uvulae. *Cleft Palate Journal, 15,* 150–154.

Curtis, J. F. (1968). Acoustics of speech production and nasalization. In D. C. Spriestersbach & D. Sherman (Eds.), *Cleft palate and communication.* New York: Academic Press.

Curtis, T. A., Beumer, J., & Firtell, D. N. (1979). Speech, palatopharyngeal function and restoration of soft palate defects. In J. Beumer, T. A. Curtis, & D. N. Firtell (Eds.), *Maxillofacial rehabilitation: Prosthodontic and surgical considerations* (pp. 244–291). St. Louis: Mosby.

Dalston, R. M. (1989). Using simultaneous photodetection and nasometry to monitor velopharyngeal behavior during speech. *Journal of Speech and Hearing Research, 32,* 195–202.

Dalston, R. M., & Warren, D. W. (1986). Comparison of Tonar II, pressure flow, and listener judgments of hypernasality in the assessment of velopharyngeal function. *Cleft Palate Journal, 23,* 108–115.

Dalston, R. M., Warren, D. W., & Dalston, E. (1991a). A preliminary investigation concerning the use of nasometry in identifying patients with hyponasality and/or nasal airway impairment. *Journal of Speech and Hearing Research, 34,* 11–18.

Dalston, R. M., Warren, D. W., & Dalston, E. (1991b). Use of nasometry as a diagnostic tool for identifying patients with velopharyngeal impairment. *Cleft Palate Journal, 28,* 184–188.

Dalston, R. M., Warren, D. W., Morr, K. E., & Smith, L. R. (1988). Intraoral pressure and its relationship to velopharyngeal inadequacy. *Cleft Palate Journal, 25,* 210–219.

D'Antonio, L. L., Marsh, J. L., Province, M. A., Muntz, H. R., & Phillips, C. J. (1989). Reliability of flexible fiberoptic nasopharyngoscopy for evaluation of velopharyngeal function in a clinical population. *Cleft Palate Journal, 26,* 217–224.

Eckel, F., & Boone, D. R. (1981). The s/z ratio as an indication of laryngeal pathology. *Journal of Speech and Hearing Disorders, 46,* 147–149.

Falter, J. W., & Shelton, R. L. (1964). Bulb fitting and placement in prosthetic treatment of cleft palate. *Cleft Palate Journal, 1,* 441–447.

Fisher, H. A., & Logemann, J. A. (1971). *The Fisher–Logemann Test of Articulation Competence.* Boston: Houghton-Mifflin.

Fletcher, S. G., Haskins, R. C., & Bosma, J. F. (1960). A movable bulb appliance to assist in palatopharyngeal closure. *Journal of Speech and Hearing Disorders, 25,* 249–258.

Folkins, J. W. (1985). Issues in speech motor control and their relation to the speech of individuals with cleft palate. *Cleft Palate Journal, 22,* 106–122.

Fujimura, O. (1981). Temporal characteristics of articulatory movements as a multidimensional phrasal structure. *Phonetica, 38,* 66–83.

Garber, S. R., Speidel, T. M., & Siegel, G. M. (1980). The effects of noise and palatal appliances on the speech of five-year-old children. *Journal of Speech and Hearing Research, 23,* 853–863.

Gibbons, P., & Bloomer, H. A. (1958). The palatal lift: A supportive-type aid. *Journal of Prosthetic Dentistry, 8,* 362–369.

Golding-Kushner, K. J. (1990). Standardization for the reporting of nasopharyngoscopy and multiview videofluoroscopy: A report from an international working group. *Cleft Palate Journal, 27,* 337–347.

Goldman, R., & Fristoe, M. (1969). *Goldman–Fristoe Test of Articulation.* Circle Pines, MN: American Guidance Service.

Gonzalez, J. B., & Aronson, A. E. (1970). Palatal lift prosthesis for treatment of anatomic and neurologic palatopharyngeal insufficiency. *Cleft Palate Journal, 7,* 91–104.

Hamlet, S. L. (1973). Vocal compensation: An ultrasonic study of vocal fold vibration in normal and nasal vowels. *Cleft Palate Journal, 10,* 367–385.

Hamlet, S., Geoffrey, V. C., & Bartlett, D. M. (1976). Effect of a dental prosthesis on speaker-specific characteristics of voice. *Journal of Speech and Hearing Research, 19,* 639–650.

Hamlet, S., & Stone, M. (1974). Reorganization of speech motor patterns following prosthodontic changes in oral morphology. In G. Fant (Ed.), *Proceedings of the Speech Communication Seminar.* Stockholm: Royal Institute of Technology.

Hamlet, S., & Stone, M. (1978). Compensatory alveolar consonant production induced by wearing a dental prosthesis. *Journal of Phonetics, 6,* 227–248.

Hamlet, S., Stone, M., & McCarty, T. (1978). Conditioning prostheses viewed from the standpoint of speech adaptation. *Journal of Prosthetic Dentistry, 40,* 60–66.

Hanson, W., & Emanuel, F. W. (1979). Spectral noise and vocal roughness relationships in adults with laryngeal pathology. *Journal of Communication Disorders, 12,* 113–124.

Hardy, J. C., Netsell, R., Schweiger, J., & Morris, H. (1969). Management of velopharyngeal dysfunction of cerebral palsy. *Journal of Speech and Hearing Disorders, 34,* 123–137.

Henderson, D., & Steffel, V. L. (1981). *McCracken's removable partial prosthodontics* (6th ed., pp. 120–141, 168–175). St. Louis: Mosby.

Hixon, T. J. (1982). Speech breathing kinematics and mechanism inferences therefrom. In S. Grillner, B. Lindblom, J. Lubker, & A. Persson (Eds.), *Speech motor control* (pp. 75–93). Oxford: Pergamon Press.

Hixon, T. J., Goldman, M., & Mead, J. (1973). Kinematics of the chest wall during speech production: Volume displacements of the rib cage, abdomen, and lung. *Journal of Speech and Hearing Research, 16,* 78–115.

Hixon, T. J., Mead, J., & Goldman, M. (1976). Dynamics of the chest wall during speech production: Function of the thorax, rib cage, diaphragm, and abdomen. *Journal of Speech and Hearing Research, 19,* 297–356.

Hixon, T. J., & Putnam, A. H. B. (1983). Voice disorders in relation to respiratory kinematics. In W. H. Perkins, J. L. Northern, & D. R. Boone (Eds.), *Seminars in speech and language: Voice disorders in children and adults. Strategies of management* (Vol. 4, pp. 217–232). New York: Thieme-Stratton.

Hollien, H. (1976). Status report on instrumentation useful for craniofacial research. *Cleft Palate Journal, 13,* 138–155.

Hollien, H. (1977). The registers and ranges of the voice. In M. Cooper & M. H. Cooper (Eds.), *Approaches to vocal rehabilitation.* Springfield, IL: Thomas.

Horii, Y. (1982). Jitter and shimmer differences among sustained vowel phonations. *Journal of Speech and Hearing Research, 25,* 12–14.

Isshiki, N. (1964). Regulatory mechanism of voice intensity variation. *Journal of Speech and Hearing Research, 7,* 17–29.

Karnell, M. P., Ibuki, K., Morris, H. L., & Van Demark, D. R. (1983). Reliability of the nasopharyngeal fiberscope (NPF) for assessing velopharyngeal function: Analysis by judgment. *Cleft Palate Journal, 20,* 199–208.

Kelso, J. A. S., Tuller, B., & Harris, K. S. (1983). A "dynamic pattern" perspective on the control and coordination of movement. In P. MacNeilage (Ed.), *The production of speech* (pp. 137–174). New York: Springer-Verlag.

Kipfmueller, L. J., & Lang, B. R. (1972). Treating velopharyngeal inadequacies with a palatal lift prosthesis. *Journal of Prosthetic Dentistry, 27,* 63–72.

Kuehn, D. P. (1982). Assessment of resonance disorders. In N. J. Lass, L. V. McReynolds, J. L. Northern, & D. E. Yoder (Eds.), *Speech, language, and hearing: Vol. II. Pathologies of speech and language* (pp. 499–525). Philadelphia: Saunders.

Kuehn, D. P., & Moll, K. L. (1976). A cineradiographic study of VC and CV articulatory velocities. *Journal of Phonetics, 3,* 303–320.

Laine, T., Warren, D. W., Dalston, R. M., & Morr, K. E. (1988). Screening of velopharyngeal closure based on nasal airflow rate measurements. *Cleft Palate Journal, 25,* 220–225.

LaVelle, W. E., & Hardy, J. C. (1979). Palatal lift prosthesis for treatment of palatopharyngeal incompetence. *Journal of Prosthetic Dentistry, 42,* 308–315.

Lawson, W. A., & Bond, E. K. (1969). Speech and its relation to dentistry. *The Dental Practitioner, 19,* 150–156.

Leeper, H. A., & Graves, D. K. (1984). Consistency of laryngeal airway resistance in adult women. *Journal of Communication Disorders, 17,* 153–163.

Leeper, H. A., & Sills, P. S. (1986). Prosthetic and speech management of patients with velopharyngeal incompetence. *Human Communication Canada, 10,* 5–20.

Lloyd, R. S., Pruzansky, S., & Subtelny, J. D. (1957). Prosthetic rehabilitation of a cleft palate patient subsequent to multiple surgical and prosthetic failures. *Journal of Prosthetic Dentistry, 8,* 216–230.

Marshall, R. C., & Jones, R. N. (1971). Effects of a palatal lift prosthesis upon the speech intelligibility of a dysarthric patient. *Journal of Prosthetic Dentistry, 25,* 327–333.

Mason, R., & Simon, C. (1977). An orofacial examination checklist. *Language, Speech and Hearing Services in Schools, 8,* 155–164.

Matsuya, T., Miyazaki, T., & Yamaoka, M. (1974). Fiberscopic examination of velopharyngeal closure in normal individuals. *Cleft Palate Journal, 11,* 286–291.

Matsuya, T., Yamaoka, M., & Miyazaki, T. (1979). A fiberoptic study of velopharyngeal closure in patients with operated cleft palates. *Plastic and Reconstructive Surgery, 63,* 497–500.

Mazaheri, M. (1976). Indications and contraindications for prosthetic speech appliances in cleft palate. *Journal of Plastic and Reconstructive Surgery, 30,* 663–669.

Mazaheri, M., & Mazaheri, E. H. (1976). Prosthodontic aspects of palatal elevation and palato–pharyngeal stimulation. *Journal of Prosthetic Dentistry, 35,* 320–327.

Mazaheri, M., & Millard, R. T. (1965). Changes in nasal resonance related to differences in location and dimension of speech bulbs. *Cleft Palate Journal, 2,* 167–175.

McWilliams, B. J., & Bradley, D. P. (1964). A rating scale for evaluation of video tape recorded X-ray studies. *Cleft Palate Journal, 1,* 88–94.

McWilliams, B. J., Lavorato, A. S., & Bluestone, C. D. (1973). Vocal cord abnormalities in children with velopharyngeal valving problems. *Laryngoscope, 83,* 1745–1753.

Mead, J., Bouhuys, A., & Proctor, D. F. (1968). Mechanisms generating subglottic pressure. In A. Bouhuys (Ed.), Sound production in man [Special issue]. *Annals of the New York Academy of Sciences, 155,* pp. 177–181.

Minsley, G. E., Warren, D. W., & Hairfield, W. M. (1991). The effect of cleft palate speech and prostheses on the nasopharyngeal airway and breathing. *Journal of Prosthetic Dentistry, 65,* 122–126.

Miyazaki, T., Matsuya, T., & Yamaoka, M. (1975). Fiberscopic methods for assessment of velopharyngeal closure during various activities. *Cleft Palate Journal, 12,* 107–114.

Moller, K. T., & Starr, C. D. (1984). The effects of listening conditions on speech ratings obtained in a clinical setting. *Cleft Palate Journal, 21,* 65–69.

Molt, L. F. (1990). Use of the nasometer in palatal prosthesis configuration adjustments. *Nasometer application notes* (pp. 56–59). Pine Brook, NJ: Kay Elemetrics.

Moon, J. B., & Smith, W. L. (1987). Application of cine computed tomography to the assessment of velopharyngeal form and function. *Cleft Palate Journal, 24,* 240–243.

Morr, K. E., Warren, D. W., Dalston, R. M., & Smith, L. R. (1989). Screening of velopharyngeal inadequacy by differential pressure measurements. *Cleft Palate Journal, 26,* 42–45.

Muntz, H. R., D'Antonio, L. L., Gay, W. D., & Marsh, J. (1985, May). *The use of fiberoptic nasendoscopy for fitting palatal lift prostheses and the management of velopharyngeal dysfunction.* Paper presented at the 13th World Congress of Otorhinolaryngology, Miami Beach, FL.

Netsell, R. (1969). Subglottal and intraoral air pressure during intervocalic /t/ and /d/. *Phonetica, 20,* 68–73.

Netsell, R., & Daniel, B. (1979). Dysarthria in adults: Physiologic approach to rehabilitation. *Archives of Physical Medicine and Rehabilitation, 60,* 502–508.

Oral, K., Aramany, M. A., & McWilliams, B. J. (1979). Speech intelligibility with the buccal flange obturator. *Journal of Prosthetic Dentistry, 41,* 323–328.

Osberg, P. E., & Witzel, M. A. (1981). The physiologic basis for hypernasality during connected speech in cleft palate patients: A nasendoscopic study. *Journal of Plastic and Reconstructive Surgery, 67,* 1–5.

Palmer, J. (1974). Analysis of speech in prosthodontic practice. *Journal of Prosthetic Dentistry, 31,* 605–614.

Parel, S. M., Branemark, P-I., & Janson, T. (1986). Osseointegration in maxillofacial prosthetics. *Journal of Prosthetic Dentistry, 55,* 490–494.

Peterson, S. J. (1975). Nasal emission as a component of the misarticulation of sibilants and affricatives. *Journal of Speech and Hearing Disorders, 40,* 106–114.

Pigott, R. W. (1969). The nasendoscopic appearance of normal palatopharyngeal valve. *Journal of Plastic and Reconstructive Surgery, 43,* 19–24.

Reisberg, D. J., Gold, H. O., & Dorf, D. S. (1985). A technique for obturating palatal fistulas. *CLeft Palate Journal, 22,* 286–289.

Riski, J. E., Hoke, J. A., & Dolan, E. A. (1989). The role of pressure flow and endoscopic assessment in successful palatal obturator revision. *Cleft Palate Journal, 26,* 56–62.

Rosen, M. S., & Bzoch, K. R. (1958). The prosthetic speech appliance in rehabilitation of patients with cleft palate. *Journal of the American Dental Association, 57,* 203–210.

Rosenbek, J. C., & Netsell, R. (1984). Treating the dysarthrias. In J. C. Rosenbek (Ed.), *Seminars in speech and language: Current views of dysarthria.* New York: Thieme-Stratton.

Sato, Y., Sato, M., Yoshida, K., & Tsuru, H. (1987). Palatal lift prostheses for edentulous patients. *Journal of Prosthetic Dentistry, 57,* 204–208.

Schneider, E., & Shprintzen, R. (1980). A survey of speech pathologists: Current trends in the diagnosis and management of velopharyngeal insufficiency. *Cleft Palate Journal, 17,* 249–253.

Schneiderman, C. R., & Mann, M. (1978). Air flow and intelligibility of speech of normal speakers and speakers with a prosthodontically repaired cleft palate. *Journal of Prosthetic Dentistry, 39,* 193–199.

Seaver, E. J., Dalston, R. M., Leeper, H. A., & Adams, L. E. (1991). A study of nasometric values for normal nasal resonance. *Journal of Speech and Hearing Research, 28,* 715–721.

Sharry, J. J. (1981). Miscellaneous partial prosthodontics. In D. Henderson & V. L. Steffel (Eds.), *McCracken's removable partial prosthodontics.* St. Louis: Mosby.

Shaughnessy, A. L., Netsell, R., & Farrange, J. (1983). Treatment of a four-year-old with a palatal lift prosthesis. In W. R. Berry (Ed.), *Clinical dysarthria* (pp. 216–230). Austin, TX: PRO-ED.

Shelton, R. L., & Blank, J. L. (1984). Oronasal fistulas, intraoral air pressure, and nasal airflow during speech. *Cleft Palate Journal, 21,* 91–99.

Shelton, R. L., Lindquist, A. F., Arndt, W. B., Elbert, M. A., & Youngstrom, K. A. (1971). Effect of speech bulb reduction on movement of the posterior pharyngeal wall of the pharynx and posture of the tongue. *Cleft Palate Journal, 8,* 10–17.

Shelton, R. L., Lindquist, A. F., Chisum, L., Arndt, W. B., Youngstrom, K. A., & Stick, S. L. (1968). Effect of prosthetic speech bulb reduction on articulation. *Cleft Palate Journal, 5,* 195–204.

Shelton, R. L., Lindquist, A. F., Knox, A. W., Wright, V. L., Arndt, W. B., Elbert, M., & Youngstrom, K. A. (1971). The relationship between pharyngeal wall movements and exchangeable speech appliance sections. *Cleft Palate Journal, 8,* 145–158.

Shelton, R. L., & Lloyd, R. S. (1963). Prosthetic facilitation of palatopharyngeal closure. *Journal of Speech and Hearing Disorders, 28,* 55–66.

Shelton, R. L., & Trier, W. C. (1976). Issues involved in the evaluation of velopharyngeal closure. *Cleft Palate Journal, 13,* 127–137.

Shiere, F. R., Fox, A., & Perry, C. C. (1962, November). Removable partial prosthesis for the cleft palate patient. *Dental Clinics of North America,* 837–849.

Shprintzen, R., Lencione, R., McCall, G., & Skolnick, M. L. (1974). A three dimensional cinefluoroscopic analysis of velopharyngeal closure during speech and non-speech. *Cleft Palate Journal, 11,* 412–428.

Sills, P. S., & Leeper, H. A. (1984). *An investigation of changes in speech behaviour using a palatal lift prosthesis* (Final Report). Toronto: Ontario Ministry of Health.

Skolnick, M. L., & Cohn, E. R. (1989). *Videofluoroscopic studies of speech in patients with cleft palate.* New York: Springer-Verlag.

Smith, B. E., Fiala, K. J., & Guyette, T. W. (1989). Partitioning model nasal airway resistance into its nasal cavity and velopharyngeal components. *Cleft Palate Journal, 26,* 327–330.

Smitheran, J., & Hixon, T. J. (1981). A clinical method for estimating laryngeal airway resistance during vowel production. *Journal of Speech and Hearing Disorders, 46,* 138–146.

Starr, C. (1979). Dental and occlusal hazards to normal speech production. In K. R. Bzoch (Ed.), *Communicative disorders related to cleft lip and palate* (pp. 66–76). Boston: Little, Brown.

St. Louis, K. O., & Ruscello, D. M. (1981). *The Oral Speech Mechanism Screening Examination.* Baltimore: University Park Press.

Stringer, D. A., & Witzel, M. A. (1989). Comparison of multiview videofluoroscopy and nasopharyngoscopy in the assessment of velopharyngeal insufficiency. *Cleft Palate Journal, 26,* 88–90.

Subtelny, J. D., Sakuda, M., & Subtelny, J. D. (1966). Prosthetic treatment for palatopharyngeal incompetence: Research and clinical implications. *Cleft Palate Journal, 3,* 130–158.

Taub, S. (1966). The Taub oral panendoscope: A new technique. *Cleft Palate Journal, 3,* 328–346.

Templin, M. C., & Darley, F. L. (1969). *The Templin–Darley Tests of Articulation* (2nd ed.). Iowa City: University of Iowa Bureau of Educational Research and Service.

Van Demark, D. R. (1974). Assessment of articulation for children with cleft palate. *Cleft Palate Journal, 11,* 200–208.

Van Demark, D. R., Bzoch, K., Daly, D., Fletcher, S., McWilliams, B. J., Pannbacker, M., & Weinberg, B. (1985). Methods of assessing speech in relation to velopharyngeal function. *Cleft Palate Journal, 22,* 281–285.

Van Demark, D. R., Kuehn, D. R., & Tharp, R. F. (1975). Prediction of velopharyngeal competency. *Cleft Palate Journal, 12,* 5–11.

Van Demark, D. R., Morris, H., & Vandehaar, C. (1979). Patterns of articulation abilities in speakers with cleft palate. *Cleft Palate Journal, 16,* 230–239.

Warren, D. W. (1964). Velopharyngeal orifice size and upper pharyngeal pressure-flow patterns in normal speech. *Journal of Plastic and Reconstructive Surgery, 33,* 148–162.

Warren, D. W. (1975). The determination of velopharyngeal incompetence by aerodynamic and acoustic techniques. *Clinics in Plastic Surgery, 2,* 299–304.

Warren, D. W. (1982). Aerodynamics of speech. In N. J. Lass, L. V. McReynolds, J. L. Northern, & D. E. Yoder (Eds.), *Speech, language, and hearing: Vol. 1. Normal processes* (pp. 219–245). Philadelphia: Saunders.

Warren, D. W. (1986). Compensatory speech behaviors in cleft palate: A regulation/control phenomenon. *Cleft Palate Journal, 23,* 251–260.

Warren, D., Dalston, R., Trier, W., & Holder, M. (1985). A pressure-flow technique for quantifying temporal patterns of palatopharyngeal closure. *Cleft Palate Journal, 22,* 11–19.

Warren, D. W., & DuBois, A. B. (1964). A pressure-flow technique for measuring velopharyngeal orifice area during continuous speech. *Cleft Palate Journal, 1,* 52–71.

Weiss, C. E. (1971). Success of an obturator reduction program. *Cleft Palate Journal, 8,* 291–297.

Weiss, C. E., & Louis, H. (1972). Toward a more objective approach to obturator reduction. *Cleft Palate Journal, 9,* 157–160.

Williams, W. N. (1971). Applications of radiological measures. In K. R. Bzoch (Ed.), *Communicative disorders related to cleft lip and palate* (pp. 163–171). Boston: Little, Brown.

Wong, L. P., & Weiss, C. E. (1972). A clinical assessment of obturator-wearing cleft palate patients. *Journal of Prosthetic Dentistry, 27,* 632–639.

Wood, M. T., & Warren, D. W. (1971). Effect of cleft palate prosthesis on respiratory effort. *Journal of Prosthetic Dentistry, 26,* 213–218.

Zajac, D. J., & Linville, R. N. (1989). Voice perturbation of children with perceived nasality and hoarseness. *Cleft Palate Journal, 26,* 226–230.

CHAPTER 7

Otologic and Audiologic Concerns and Treatment

Rolf F. Ulvestad and Jane E. Carlstrom

Ulvestad and Carlstrom discuss the structure and function of the eustachian tube, the relation of middle ear pathology to dysfunction of the tube, and the manner in which a cleft palate may contribute to tube dysfunction. They stress the importance of early identification and treatment and the role of the otolaryngologist and the audiologist in the management of pathology and hearing loss.

1. *What are the two major functions of the eustachian tube, and how does a child's growth affect these functions?*

2. *Why might the presence of a cleft palate affect eustachian tube functions? How does surgical repair of the palate affect these functions?*

3. *How does information obtained from pure-tone hearing tests differ from that obtained from tympanometry?*

4. *Under what conditions are tympanostomy tubes considered to be useful in treating middle ear problems?*

5. *Why might children with cleft palate develop laryngeal problems?*

The otolaryngologist brings to the cleft palate team a surgical background with a foundation in anatomy, physiology, and pathophysiology of the auditory and vestibular systems, the upper aerodigestive tract, including the trachea, larynx, and pharynx, the oral cavity, and paranasal sinuses and nose. The ear, with its divisions into external, middle, and inner ear, and the eustachian or auditory tube connecting the middle ear and nasopharynx are intimately related to the structure and function of the nasopharynx and palatal mechanisms and are the focus of discussion in this chapter.

An otolaryngologist's training in these and other areas required by the specialty generally begins after medical school with 1 or 2 years of general surgical residency, where the resident benefits from learning about the fluid or electrolyte changes and pulmonary problems common to all surgical patients. For the following 3 or 4 years, the otolaryngologist focuses on the head and neck. The specialist learns medical and surgical techniques related to problems of hearing loss and hearing rehabilitation, as well as surgical treatments for benign and malignant tumors of the head and neck, including those of the larynx, pharynx, oral cavity, tongue, sinuses, salivary glands, and related areas. The otolaryngologist also learns facial plastic and reconstructive techniques used to correct defects caused by the removal of such tumors, or those caused by acute and delayed problems of facial trauma. In the latter group, fractures of the mandible, maxilla, and nose are common, resulting from motor vehicular accidents. Less common are fractures of the larynx, with potential loss of the normal airway and phonation necessary for speech, and fractures of the temporal bone that may result in damage to the middle and inner ear and secondary hearing loss. Nontraumatic functional and cosmetic deformities of the ears, nose, and other facial structures are frequent surgical problems that also are of concern to the otolaryngologist. As reflected in their training, otolaryngologists are expected to correctly manage and repair these types of injuries and conditions.

Following successful completion of residency in otolaryngology, a physician may be eligible to take an extensive certification examination and, if passed, become certified by the American Board of Otolaryngology. Some otolaryngologists choose to gain additional expertise in particular facets of the specialty, such as head and neck tumor surgery, otology, facial plastics, allergy or pediatric otolaryngology.

The patient with a cleft represents a challenge to the otolaryngologist, for the deformity affects many important structures and functions. When the patient is seen with representatives of multiple specialties in a comprehensive cleft palate or craniofacial deformities clinic, the specialists can share their insights with each other. The otolaryngologist and audiologist are the professionals on the team who have the greatest interest in the problems of the ear and hearing, which affect nearly all children with cleft palates. Although otitis media is the second most common illness of childhood, behind only a common cold, its frequency in the normal population is far less than in the cleft palate population. As with all disease treatment processes, treating ear disease requires an understanding of the etiology, of characteristic diagnostic tools and findings, and of appropriate treatment, as based on the pathophysiology. This chapter focuses on the etiology, diagnosis, and treatment of otitis media in the child with cleft palate.

ETIOLOGY OF AUDITORY TUBE DYSFUNCTION

Structure and Function of the Auditory Tube

Sound conduction from the environment to the brain, where it is perceived as meaningful speech, music, and so forth, is dependent in part on normal aeration or ventilation of the middle ear (Figure 7.1). Ventilation of the middle ear is only one function of the eustachian or auditory tube system. Via the auditory tube, pressure within the middle ear, or medial to the tympanic membrane, is equalized with ambient or atmospheric pressure, lateral to the tympanic membrane (Figure 7.2). A second function of the auditory tube is to provide an outlet from the middle

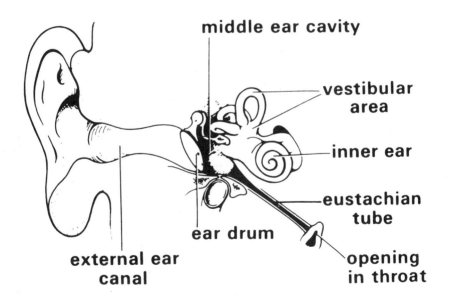

Figure 7.1 Anatomical features of the external, middle, and inner ear.

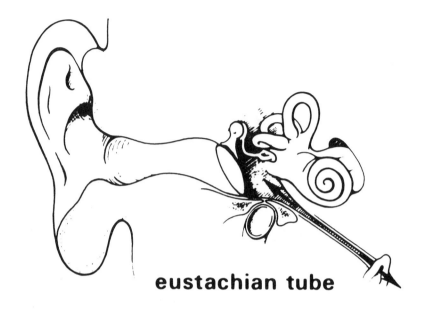

eustachian tube

Figure 7.2 The eustachian tube connects the middle ear cavity to the nasopharynx. Arrows indicate air movement through the tube.

ear for fluid and the by-products of middle ear inflammation (Figure 7.3). Dysfunction of the auditory tube is the etiological event common to nearly all middle ear disease, with several known or proposed factors leading to dysfunction of the tube mechanism.

The auditory tube changes its angle of inclination with age, and much has been written in the medical and lay literature about the different inclinations. The auditory tube lies in a sulcus (sulcus tubarius) on the base of the skull. The infant and young child's skull is relatively flat; as a result, the auditory tube lies in a relatively flat plane (Figure 7.4). The inferior anterior end of the tube that communicates with the nasopharynx is closely associated with bony structures of the posterior midface. As these structures grow downward and forward with age, the effect is to angulate the base of the skull; therefore, the auditory tube becomes more vertically oriented. The horizontal position of the tube in the infant and young child decreases the ability of the tensor veli palatini muscle to dilate the tube effectively (Figure 7.5). Because this is a muscle of the soft palate, it may be compromised by a cleft. Dilation is necessary to permit the passage of air into the middle ear for pressure equalization. The activity of these muscles in swallowing explains the common admonition for airplane passengers to chew gum

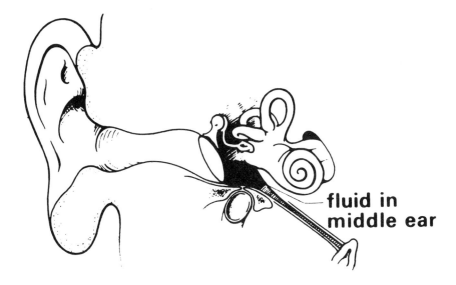

fluid in middle ear

Figure 7.3 The eustachian tube is the outlet for fluid and by-products. The black area indicates a collection of fluid in the middle ear.

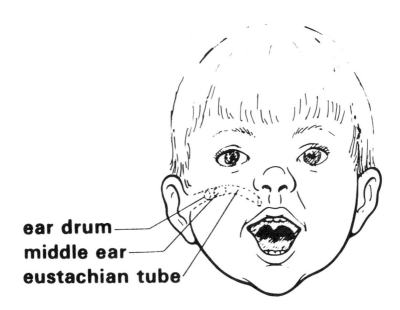

ear drum
middle ear
eustachian tube

Figure 7.4 Eustachian tube in a child. Note that the nasopharyngeal and middle ear openings are on a horizontal plane. In adults, the nasopharyngeal opening is lower than the middle ear opening.

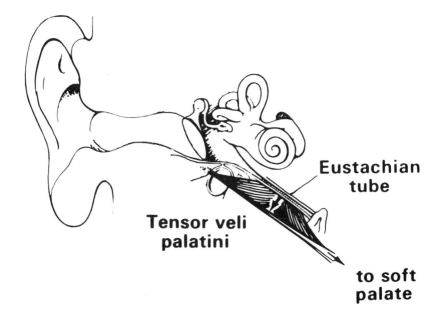

Figure 7.5 Tensor veli palatini muscle contraction (note arrow) dilates the eustachian tube and allows air pressure to be equal on both sides of the eardrum.

or swallow when pressure changes are encountered, as in take-off and landing. The pop or click one hears is the rapid passage of a bolus of air into the middle ear with partial equalization of pressure as the auditory tube is dilated by the swallowing mechanism.

The horizontal position of a child's tube also facilitates the retrograde passage of the nasopharyngeal bacteria into the middle ear. This disadvantage is further aggravated by the recumbent position. Saliva, milk, or formula also may pool in the auditory tube orifice while the child is in the recumbent position. This is one reason why parents are advised to avoid putting a child to bed with a bottle and to keep the child upright while feeding. Swallowing allows opening of the tube and permits passage of this contaminated culture media into the middle ear, with a resultant otitis. This problem is aggravated by the presence of an unrepaired cleft palate, permitting free flow into the nasopharynx. As children grow, the bottle gives way to the cup used in the upright position, the inclination of the skull base and auditory tube become more favorable, and the muscular dilators of the tube become more efficient. Theses factors contribute to the decrease in the frequency of otitis in normal children with increasing age.

In addition to tubal inclination, the morphology of the auditory tube may be a factor in tubal dysfunction. Bluestone (1971) suggested that the tube in persons with cleft palates may be "floppy" or hypercompliant. This excessive compliance may be due to the quality of the cartilage itself, muscular dysfunction, or other unrecognized factors. Rood and Stool (1981) have summarized other forces either shown or proposed to affect auditory tube function. These include muscular forces noted earlier, and factors related to tympanum–nasopharynx pressure, surface tension, mucociliary activity, middle ear muscle function, adenoid hypertrophy, muscle edema, and blockage of tubal lymphatics.

Palatal Muscle Factors

The relationship of the tensor palatini muscle group to the lateral wall of the auditory tube is influenced by the position of the hamulus and bony palate (Figure 7.6). Changes in the position of the pterygoid plate also influence angulation and the force vectors resulting from muscular contraction.

Tympanum–Nasopharyngeal Pressures

A hypercompliant auditory tube in a child with a cleft palate may be subject to collapse of the opening or lumen, from pressure differences on either side of the tube. The collapse of the lumen results in tubal obstruction. Also, increased positive nasopharyngeal pressure could force nasopharyngeal secretions through the lumen in a hypercompliant system. Although pressure differences between the nasopharynx and the middle ear exert an effect in a normal ear, the child with a cleft palate is likely to be more susceptible to these differences.

Surface Tension

A surface active agent that lowers the surface tension of fluid within the alveoli of the lung is well established. A similar substance or surfactant has been proposed in the mucous membrane of the auditory tube. Rood and Moyce (1980) demonstrated surface activity in washings from otologically normal human subjects, but specific data from the cleft population is lacking.

Mucociliary Activity

The mucosa lining the auditory tube and middle ear is typical of the respiratory tract, with a ciliated border on the cells of the lumen. The cilia beat in rhythmic waves toward the nasopharynx and, when functioning normally, serve to sweep mucus and debris from the middle ear and tube. When the mucosa is inflamed and edematous, the ciliary clear-

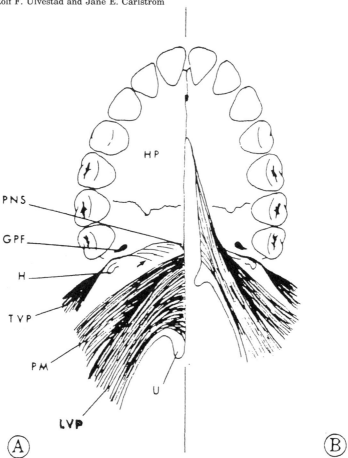

Figure 7.6 Diagram of normal (A) and cleft palate (B) muscles. HP = hard palate; PNS = posterior nasal spine; GPF = greater palatine foramen; H = hamulus; TVP = tensor veli palatini muscle; PM = palatopharyngeus muscle; LVP = levator palatini muscle; and U = uvulas muscle. (From "Anatomy and Physiology Related to Cleft Palate: Current Research and Clinical Implications" by W. Maue-Dickson and D. R. Dickson, 1980, *Plastic and Reconstructive Surgery, 65,* p. 87. Copyright 1980 by American Society of Plastic and Reconstructive Surgeons, Inc. Reprinted with permission.)

ing activity is less efficient and may cease altogether. Chronic inflammation also causes a decrease in the number of cilia-bearing cells and an increase in the number of mucus-producing cells in the middle ear. It is this transformation that contributes to the formation of the chronic mucoid or "glue" ear. In some conditions (e.g., in Kartagener's syndrome), the direction of the cilia beat is reversed; as may be expected, these individuals have a higher incidence of middle ear problems.

Middle Ear Muscles

On contraction, the tensor tympani, which is attached to the malleus, pulls the malleus and tympanic membrane medially. The tensor tympani and tensor palatini are part of the same muscle group, and all the muscles contract as a group. It has been postulated that contraction of the tensor tympani pulls the tympanic membrane medially, decreasing the volume of the middle ear and serving to pump mucus and debris from the middle ear and down the auditory tube toward the naso-pharynx. Specific information on the effects of this mechanism is not available; however, defects in the seal of this air space, such as a perforation or a tympanostomy tube, would negate the pump effect. As yet, this hypothesis remains unproven.

Adenoid Hypertrophy

Much attention has been given to the role of the adenoids and their contribution to velopharyngeal closure in the cleft palate population. Where palatal length is inadequate, the beneficial effect of the adenoid mass may be significant. However, adenoid tissue also may play a role in the incidence of otitis. Bluestone, Cantekin, and Berry (1982) noted that adenoid size alone may not predict auditory tube dysfunction, but that most children with large adenoids have obstruction to the flow of radio-opaque medium from the nasopharynx to the middle ear. Such flow would be against the normal flow and ciliary beating. The effect of the obstruction may be mixed, with total or near total obstruction leading to inadequate ventilation and the development of middle ear disease; this suggests that partial obstruction by lymphoid (and adenoid) tissues in the area of the nasopharynx and eustachian tube may be beneficial in the patient with cleft palate. If, as Bluestone et al. suggested, the auditory tube in the cleft population is hypercompliant, the adenoid mass may act to limit the retrograde flow of nasopharyngeal secretions, bacteria, and so on, into the middle ear and may decrease the incidence of middle ear infection. However, these relationships are not consistent and need further investigation. Because of the above concerns, adenoidectomy is rarely done in the patient with a cleft. If contemplated, its potential benefits should be compelling, and, in both cleft and noncleft patients, care must be taken to avoid injury to the tubal orifice during surgery. Postsurgical scarring may compromise a tube that otherwise might function satisfactorily.

The tonsils, which are lower in the pharynx, may influence palate function in some cases. Tonsil hypertrophy may have adverse effects, such as a vocal resonance distortion, difficulty swallowing solid food, airway obstruction, sleep apnea and corpulmonale, hearing failure, or a combination of these problems. In the patient with cleft palate, however, the tonsils may be a valuable source of tissue to obturate the posterior nasal airway and decrease nasal resonance. This must be considered when contemplating tonsillectomy (see Chapter 10).

Mucosal Edema

Obstruction of the auditory tube by edema of the mucosa may lead to middle ear pathology. Edema may result from infection, immunological response or allergies, or direct irritation. Parents and clinicians are well aware of the likelihood of otitis in some children following an upper respiratory infection or "runny nose." The same process that causes mucosal edema and leads to rhinorrhea may cause mucosal edema of the auditory tube, with resultant obstruction. The mucosal edema of allergic rhinitis likely extends into the auditory tube, where obstruction may result. Direct irritation of the mucosa by reflux of oral cavity fluids, such as milk or formula, may also lead to edema and tubal obstruction. A child with an unrepaired or nonobturated cleft, or one with velopharyngeal incompetence following surgical repair, is at higher risk for reflux, particularly if allowed to lie supine during feeding.

Blockage of Tubal Lymphatics

Rood and Stool (1981) noted that obstruction of the lymphatic system surrounding the auditory tube may lead to tubal dysfunction. The lymphatic system is a means of draining interstitial fluids (i.e., body fluid and tissue outside the arterial or venous system). The swelling associated with an allergic reaction is the result of interstitial fluid that must be cleared by lymphatics. Lymphatic obstruction may lead to an increase in interstitial fluid, which may compromise the auditory tube.

The factors discussed in the previous subsections all play a role in the etiology of tubal dysfunction in the general pediatric population. Some, such as muscle abnormalities, increased tubal compliance, or mucosal edema, have greater significance in the cleft population. The next section of this chapter deals with the pathology that develops once tubal dysfunction, whatever its cause, is present.

MIDDLE EAR PATHOLOGY RESULTING FROM AUDITORY TUBE DYSFUNCTION

The middle ear normally contains 4 to 9 ml of air, which is absorbed through the mucosa at a rate of 1 ml per day (Curtis & Clemis, 1979). The auditory tube must allow a sufficient flow of air to replace that loss, or negative pressure will develop in the middle ear. Normal tubal function allows middle ear pressure to remain at, or near, atmospheric pressure, despite a steady absorption of air from the middle ear. The normal tube can also equalize the much more rapid changes in atmospheric pressure that are encountered in air travel or elevator riding in tall buildings.

If negative pressure or a relative vacuum of sufficient degree persists in the middle ear, the result is a middle ear effusion as the body forms a middle ear liquid, or "fluid ear," to fill the void. Middle ear effusion is extremely common in people with cleft palate or cleft lip and palate (Paradise, Bluestone, & Felden, 1969), but no more common in people with cleft lip only than in the normal population. It is the abnormality of the palate function and morphology that leads to the tubal dysfunction responsible for the effusion.

The middle ear mucosa changes rapidly with tubal dysfunction and may influence both the type and the amount of the effusion. Curtis and Clemis (1979) found that after complete obstruction of the tube, the mucosa undergoes metaplastic changes, with the appearance of mucus-secreting cells, 25 hours after total obstruction. After 60 hours, there is extensive change to mucus-producing cells. Middle ear effusions have differing characteristics, due in part to the mechanism of their formation. A *transudate* is a thin fluid with high water content and a low level of cells, protein, and solid material, whereas an *exudate* has relatively low water level and higher levels of protein, solid materials, and cells. White blood cells yield a purulent or puslike character to the exudate. Hemorrhage will result in a bloody effusion, most commonly after an acute pressure trauma, such as on an airplane flight or during a rapid descent in an automobile through a mountain pass. A secretory effusion is generally mucoid. Most effusions fail to fall into a single category, but have a combination of characteristics. Senturia (1970), in an often-quoted article, suggested that the mucopurulent and mucoid effusions are characteristics of middle ear mucosal inflammation, whereas the serous and purulent types may be representative of an acute process.

Aspiration of nasopharyngeal secretions, with normal bacterial contamination, into the middle ear by a relative vacuum may result in acute otitis media. Acute otitis media with effusion is usually bacterial in origin, whereas chronic otitis media may be due to high negative middle ear pressure alone. Again, the division is rarely clear-cut in clinical practice, as chronic effusions may be repeatedly subject to acute bacterial contamination. Tubal inflation–deflation studies by Bluestone (1978; Bluestone, Cantekin, Berry, & Paradise, 1975) show that patients with unrepaired cleft palates are unable to equalize applied negative pressure by swallowing. Auditory tube dysfunction leading to high negative middle ear pressure may be considered the primary cause of the nearly universal occurrence of middle ear disease in that population.

Following repair of the cleft palate, the frequency of the middle ear effusion is reduced due to several factors. Age alone will improve the tubal angle of inclination, the degree of tubal cartilage support, and the dilator muscle vectors, as discussed earlier. The surgical technique also influences the frequency of otitis. Morgan, Dellon, and Hopper (1983) reported that a palatoplasty with a retrodisplacement of the levator palatini muscle results in decreased frequency of conductive hearing loss, presumably because of a decrease in frequencies of middle ear effusions, when compared with palatoplasty procedures that do not incorporate levator retrodisplacement. However, even with surgical correction of the palate, the incidence of otitis in the cleft population exceeds that in the noncleft population, and careful monitoring of middle ear function is essential.

DIAGNOSIS

Medical Evaluation

Monitoring of middle ear function and the diagnosis of pathology is essential to minimizing the educational and social sequelae of middle ear disease and hearing loss. Educating parents to recognize the signs and symptoms of ear disease is important. Possible signs or symptoms of acute ear disease in children include decreased response to auditory stimuli, pulling or rubbing the ears, fever, irritability, and diarrhea.

The physician's assessment of the middle ear begins with otoscopy, either with a standard office otoscope or the operating microscope (Figure 7.7). The appearance of the tympanic membrane and the middle ear, which can be seen through the membrane, provides extremely valuable information about the status of the middle ear and auditory tube function. Most otolaryngologists have available the binocular operating room microscope. With binocular vision, increased magnification, and superior light transmission, the operating microscope can be invaluable in providing greater detail of structures and functions in problem ears. In addition, pneumatic otoscopy provides important information about the movement of the tympanic membrane. With experience, one can differentiate between normal mobility and the decreased mobility due to middle ear effusion (Figure 7.8).

Audiologic Evaluation

In addition to otoscopy, audiologic evaluation is an integral part of the assessment plan. Although the incidence of sensorineural hearing loss in children with cleft palates is similar to that in the general population, the middle ear disorders that are almost universally experienced

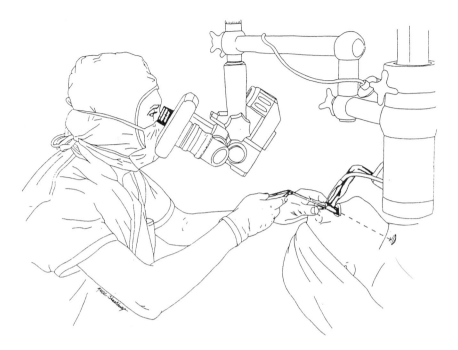

Figure 7.7 Binocular operating room microscope. (From *Surgical Care of Voice Disorders* (p. 34) by W. J. Gould and V. Lawrence, 1984, New York: Springer-Verlag. Copyright 1984 by Springer-Verlag. Reprinted with permission.)

by children with cleft palates frequently cause fluctuating conductive hearing loss. The audiologist's contribution to the diagnostic process includes providing information about the nature and degree of any hearing loss and about the effects of the hearing loss on communication.

The importance of early and periodic audiologic evaluation for children with cleft palates cannot be overemphasized. These children are at risk for communication problems related to the speech mechanism. Due to the presence of more obvious speech mechanism problems, the invisible handicap of a mild hearing loss is easily overlooked as a contributing factor to delays in speech and language development. Early diagnosis and remediation of hearing impairment is important to the child's speech and language development. Even children with very mild hearing losses may be more susceptible to communication and psychoeducational problems (Bess, 1985). The Joint Committee on Infant Hearing (1982) identified anatomic malformations involving the head or neck, including cleft palate, as one of seven high-risk factors for hearing loss in infants. The committee recommended that infants who are at risk should have hearing tests by 3 months of age, but no later than 6 months.

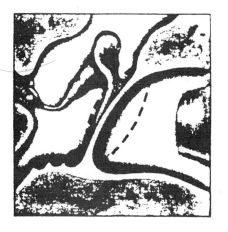

Normal

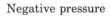

Negative pressure

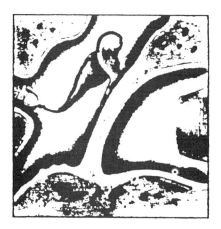

Thickened membrane

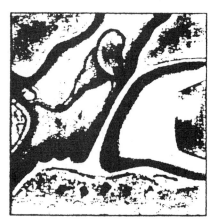

Fluid in middle ear

Figure 7.8   During pneumatic otoscopy, a slight positive or negative pressure causes a
normal eardrum to move easily. When there is negative pressure in the middle
ear, the tympanic membrane becomes retracted and does not move well when
positive pressure is applied. When the membrane is thickened, mobility is
decreased in response to positive and negative pressures. Mobility is severely
limited when fluid is present in the middle ear. (From "Pneumatic Otoscopy:
Getting the Most out of the Ear Exam" by R. H. Schwartz, 1983, *Journal
of Respiratory Diseases, 4*(5), p. 85. Copyright 1983 by Cliggott Publishing
Co. Reprinted with permission.)

Although children of any age may be evaluated, the audiologic assessment protocol will vary with the child's age and level of function. The audiometric test techniques most commonly used to obtain information about the hearing status of the individual with a cleft palate include acoustic immitance testing; behavioral tests of hearing, including pure-tone and speech audiometric testing; and auditory brainstem response measures.

Acoustic immitance.   Because of the high incidence of otitis media in children with cleft palates, *tympanometry* is an essential part of the audiological evaluation. Tympanometric test results indicate nothing about the child's hearing status, but are good predictors of middle ear disease.

To produce a tympanogram, an airtight seal is obtained by placing a probe tip in the ear canal. The probe contains three tubes that are connected to (a) a pressure pump to vary the air pressure in the ear canal from +200 to −400 daPa, (b) a sound source that generates a constant low-frequency probe tone, and (c) a microphone that measures the level of the reflected sound in the ear canal (Figure 7.9). The tympanogram plots the eardrum's mobility, measured by the change in the sound pressure level in the ear canal, as that pressure is changed.

Tympanometry provides a measure of the mobility of the eardrum and gives information about middle ear pressure. Results are described by the height and location of the tympanogram's admittance or compliance peak. A very high admittance peak is characteristic of a flaccid

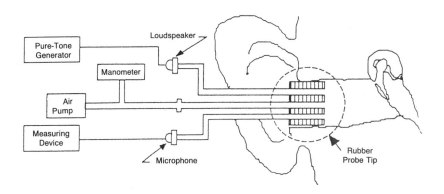

Figure 7.9 Components of an acoustic immitance instrument (tympanometer). (From *Audiology: The Fundamentals* (p. 201) by F. H. Bess and L. E. Humes, 1990, Baltimore: Williams and Wilkins. Copyright 1990 by Williams and Wilkins. Reprinted with permission.)

tympanic membrane or, more rarely, a disarticulation of the middle ear bones (Figure 7.10e). A very low peak admittance reflects a stiff system (Figure 7.10d). The location of the pressure peak for a normal middle ear is between +50 and −100 daPa (Figure 7.10a). A negative peak pressure outside this range is characteristic of eustachian tube malfunction (Figure 7.10b). If the tympanogram is flat, the result may indicate the presence of fluid behind the eardrum, the presence of an eardrum perforation, or occlusion of the ear canal by cerumen (Figure 7.10c). Most acoustic immitance instruments allow the audiologist to differentiate among these causes for flat tympanograms by giving an estimate of equivalent ear canal volume. A flat tympanogram with an abnormally large equivalent volume suggests the presence of a perforated eardrum or functioning ventilation tube. An ear filled with cerumen will show an abnormally low equivalent volume.

Tympanograms may be obtained on children of any age; however, results for infants under 4 months of age may be difficult to interpret by the rules used to define normal and abnormal adult tympanograms. Results of tympanometry for some neonates show what appear to be normal pressure peaks in the presence of middle ear fluid, but flat tympanograms in neonates may be interpreted as abnormal. By the time children reach the age of 4 months, their tympanograms look similar to those of adults (Margolis & Shanks, 1985).

In addition to tympanometry, two other acoustic immitance measures—a test of eustachian tube function and acoustic reflex testing—may be included in the assessment protocol. In an ear with negative middle ear pressure or an eardrum perforation, the test of eustachian tube function looks for a change in middle ear pressure with a swallow or a change in pressure in the ear canal. The opening of the eustachian tube is reflected in change in pressure toward normal, 0 daPa.

Acoustic reflex thresholds for pure tones and noise may be used to detect sensorineural hearing loss in the presence of normal middle ear function. Unfortunately, acoustic reflex testing may be of limited value in a patient with a fluid-filled middle ear or an eardrum that is not intact, conditions that are common to a high proportion of children with cleft palates. Acoustic reflex thresholds are also difficult to determine if the child is moving, crying, or talking.

Audiometric brainstem response testing. Audiometric brainstem response (ABR) audiometry is generally used to measure hearing in children for whom behavioral thresholds for tones or speech cannot be obtained because of the child's level of development or cooperation. In most cases, the child is placed under sedation, electrodes are attached to the skin with conducting paste, and a series of clicks or tone bursts is presented through earphones. The test provides information about the integrity of the peripheral auditory system by measuring the elec-

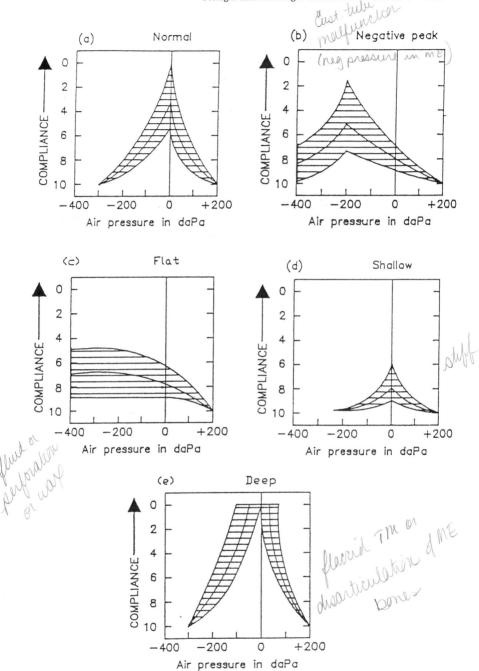

Figure 7.10 Normal and abnormal tympanograms. (From *Audiology: The Fundamentals* (p. 104) by F. H. Bess and L. E. Humes, 1990, Baltimore: Williams and Wilkins. Copyright 1990 by Williams and Wilkins. Reprinted with permission.)

trical response to sound presented to each ear. If the responses obtained to stimuli presented via air conduction suggest the presence of a hearing loss, testing may be carried out using a signal transmitted through the bone conduction vibrator to help determine the nature of the hearing loss.

The information obtained via ABR testing gives information about the child's hearing without demanding a voluntary response to sound. Because the signal is presented through earphones, each ear can be tested independently, allowing detection of a unilateral hearing loss. The stimuli most commonly used for ABR evaluation primarily reflect the status of hearing in the higher frequency range. Test results may miss a low-frequency or very mild hearing loss. The ABR is useful for those children for whom behavioral threshold measures are difficult to obtain or interpret, but it should not be used in lieu of the audiogram. As soon as possible, behavioral threshold testing should be accomplished.

Behavioral tests of hearing.   Testing the hearing of infants and young children requires modification of the stimuli to be presented and the acceptable response, depending on the age and cognitive level of the child being tested. A variety of testing techniques must be used creatively to generate audiograms for young children.

For infants from birth to about 6 months of age, the audiologic evaluation is likely to include *behavioral observation audiometry*. For this type of test, the infant is placed in an infant seat or on a parent's lap in the calibrated spot in the sound booth, and warble tones, speech, or noises are presented through speakers. Changes in the child's behavior following presentation of the sound stimuli are then noted by one or more examiners. These changes may include reflexive responses to sound, eye blinks, a startle response, changes in sucking patterns, quieting, arousal, and rudimentary localization responses. Because infants are likely to habituate to the test stimuli after a few presentations, the audiologist must base estimates of hearing on limited information. The infant's activity state at the time of the evaluation affects the probability that a response will occur, as well as the type and quality of the response.

Behavioral observation audiometry is used to rule out severe hearing losses, but is less reliable for determining mild to moderate hearing losses. The responses noted should be labeled minimal response levels rather than hearing thresholds, because even infants with normal hearing may not respond to the test stimuli until they are well above the threshold of hearing. The auditory behavior index for infants shown in Table 7.1 (from Northern & Downs, 1984) describes the expected auditory responses for children with normal hearing as a function of developmental age.

By the time the child reaches the age of 6 months, *visual reinforcement audiometry* (VRA) or *conditioned orienting response* (COR) testing

TABLE 7.1

Auditory Behavior Index for Infants Stimulus and Level of Response

Age	Noisemakers (Approx. SPL)	Warbled Pure Tones (dB HL)	Speech (dB HL)	Expected Response	Startle to Speech (dB HL)
0–6 weeks	50–70 dB	78 dB	40–60 dB	Eye widening, eye blink, stirring or arousal from sleep, startle	65 dB
6 weeks– 4 months	50–60 dB	70 dB	47 dB	Eye widening, eye shift, eye blink, quieting; beginning rudimentary head turn by 4 months	65 dB
4–7 months	40–50 dB	51 dB	21 dB	Head turn on lateral plane toward sound; listening attitude	65 dB
7–9 months	30–40 dB	45 dB	15 dB	Direct localization of sounds to side, indirectly below ear level	65 dB
9–13 months	25–35 dB	38 dB	8 dB	Direct localization of sounds to side, directly below ear level, indirectly above ear level	65 dB
13–16 months	25–30 dB	32 dB	5 dB	Direct localization of sound on side, above, and below	65 dB
16–21 months	25 dB	25 dB	5 dB	Direct localization of sound on side, above, and below	65 dB
21–24 months	25 dB	26 dB	3 dB	Direct localization of sound on side, above, and below	65 dB

Note. Decibel (dB) is a unit of intensity referenced to hearing loss (HL) or sound pressure level (SPL). From *Hearing in Children* (p. 145) by J. L. Northern and M. P. Downs, 1991, 4th ed., Baltimore: Williams and Wilkins. Copyright 1991 by Williams and Wilkins. Reprinted with permission.

techniques are used to increase the number of responses elicited by reinforcing the naturally occurring head turn localization response. A typical sound field arrangement for COR audiometry is diagramed in Figure 7.11. The test stimuli (warble tones, narrow band noise, or speech) are presented through the loudspeakers. As the child turns to seek the source of the sound, a visual reinforcer (usually a lighted or moving toy) is activated. Once the child has learned to associate the sound with the interesting visual event, the audiologist decreases the

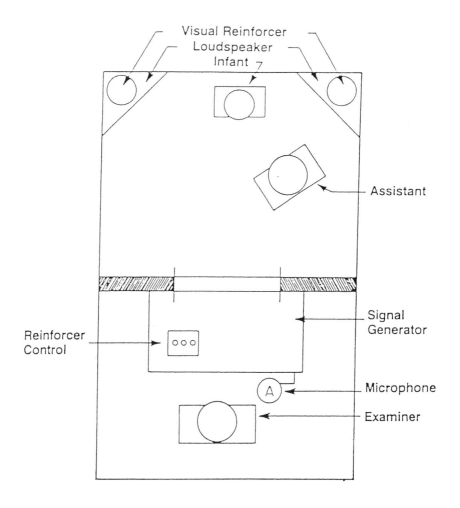

Figure 7.11   Diagram of a sound field setup for conditioned orienting response audiom-
etry. (From "Tests of Hearing—The Infant" by W. R. Hodgson, in *Hearing Disorders in Children* (p. 201) by F. N. Martin (Ed.), 1987, Austin, TX: PRO-ED. Copyright 1987 by PRO-ED, Inc. Reprinted with permission.)

stimulus intensity and begins the search for minimal response levels. The accuracy of the estimate of hearing threshold increases with the child's developmental level. The results of sound field audiometry give an estimate of hearing thresholds for the better ear, but may miss a unilateral hearing loss. If the child will tolerate earphone placement, VRA can be used to obtain results for each ear.

Visual reinforcement testing techniques are useful until the child outgrows interest in the reinforcer. After the child is 2 to 2½ years old, *conditioned play audiometry* is the test technique most frequently used by the pediatric audiologist. The child is conditioned to respond by performing a repetitive task (e.g., putting a block in a container, a peg in a hole, a ring on a stick, or a piece in a puzzle) each time the tone is heard. The game, usually accompanied by social reinforcement for correct responses, serves as a motivation device to extend the number of responses that can be obtained during the evaluation. Play audiometry may be used with warble tone or speech stimuli presented through the loudspeakers or with pure tones or speech presented via earphones or bone conduction vibrator. Most children can be trained to respond by raising their hands when the tone is heard by the time they are 4 years old.

Although the hearing loss caused by otitis media is generally conductive in nature, it is important to remember that some children with cleft palates may have a sensorineural hearing loss. Bone conduction thresholds give information about the nature of the hearing loss. The presence and size of an air–bone gap helps to classify the loss as conductive, sensorineural, or mixed.

Thresholds for hearing speech are useful in confirming the pure-tone test results. Toddlers and infants are expected to respond to speech at lower levels that to pure tones (Table 7.1), whereas speech thresholds for older children and adults should agree closely with their thresholds for pure tones. *Speech awareness thresholds* are obtained in the same manner as thresholds for pure tones. When the child is able to identify body parts, clothing items, or pictures of familiar objects, *speech reception thresholds* can be measured using a point-to-the-picture or point-to-the-object response. Older children with intelligible speech are tested in the same manner as adults, by being asked to repeat the target words.

Tests of speech recognition are performed at levels above threshold and provide information about the hearing impaired child's ability to understand speech. A variety of speech recognition (discrimination) tests have been developed for use with young children. Some require the child to repeat the words; others require the child to point to a picture of the word. The test selected must include words within the child's vocabulary. Word lists presented at low or normal conversational levels can give information about how difficult it is for the child to understand speech in a quiet listening environment and help demonstrate the effects of the hearing loss to the parents.

Nature and Implications of Hearing Loss

The hearing loss due to otitis media is conductive in nature and may range from 0 decibels (dB) to about 55 dB hearing loss (HL). A typical audiogram for a child with middle ear disease shows a flat mild hearing loss of about 25 dB HL (Dobie & Berlin, 1979). Middle ear fluid may affect one or both ears or may cause a fluctuating hearing loss. A child with a fluctuating conductive hearing loss receives inconsistent speech information and may completely miss some of the less intense speech sounds. Although there is some disagreement concerning the effects of a slight or mild hearing loss on child development, numerous studies of children with a history of recurrent otitis media suggest that these children are at risk for early delays in speech and language development and for later academic problems. The extent of the long-term effects of an early mild hearing loss is difficult to predict for an individual child. Davis (1986) and Matkin (1986) suggested that the frequency of episodes of otitis media, the length of time the hearing is impaired, and the degree of hearing loss interact with environmental variables and child characteristics to influence the development of communication skills.

Audiologic Follow-Up and Monitoring

Children with middle ear problems require frequent audiologic monitoring. Hearing evaluation and tympanometry should be repeated following completion of each medical treatment for otitis media. Monitoring should be done every 3 to 6 months until hearing is judged to be stable, and thereafter on an annual basis.

The audiologist provides parents and teachers with information about the nature of the child's hearing problems and with suggestions for reducing the communication problems caused by the hearing loss. For children with recurrent conductive hearing loss, development of communication skills and academic progress need careful monitoring by teachers and speech–language pathologists.

If results of the hearing evaluation reveal a sensorineural hearing loss or if a conductive hearing loss is not cleared through medical treatment, the use of amplification may be recommended. The audiologist must work closely with the otolaryngologist to make certain that occluding the child's ear with an earmold will not aggravate middle ear problems. Venting the earmold or using alternative methods of coupling the hearing aid to the child's ear (e.g., use of a bone conduction hearing aid or nonoccluding earphones with an FM amplification system) may need to be considered. Although hearing aids can benefit the child with a mild hearing loss, it is often difficult to persuade the parent or the child to try amplification. To the parent, the child may appear to have a problem with attention or "selective hearing" rather than a hearing problem. Demonstrating need for a hearing aid is a challenge for the audiologist.

Simply fitting a child with hearing aids is not enough. Close consistent monitoring of hearing aid function and use is essential. Studies of hearing aids worn by children in the schools indicate that approximately 50% are not functioning appropriately at any given time (Ross, 1977). A malfunctioning hearing aid serves as an expensive ear plug in an already impaired ear. Parents or school personnel should perform daily visual and listening checks of the child's hearing aids. The aids also should be evaluated by the audiologist every 3 to 6 months for the preschool and elementary child and at least annually for older children.

MEDICAL TREATMENT

Although the incidence of middle ear disease in cleft palate patients is very high, the hearing loss and damage to middle ear structures from chronic effusions, inflammation, and negative pressure are largely preventable. To ensure prevention, the child with a cleft palate must be followed otologically and audiologically on a frequent basis (every 6 months or less). As previously discussed, the greater incidence of effusions is due primarily to structural abnormalities associated with the cleft, but is also subject to the same factors causing effusions in the noncleft population (e.g., allergy, upper respiratory infection, and adenoid hypertrophy). Because the basis of the problem is largely structural, the treatment is largely surgical. Nonetheless, nearly all patients deserve a trial of conservative medical therapy.

Antibiotics are the mainstay of medical treatment for middle ear disease, in addition to time alone. Antibiotic therapy has been shown to speed the resolution of middle ear effusions, whereas decongestants or decongestant–antihistamine medications (typical cold medicines) have not. A 7- to 10-day course of corticosteroid therapy may resolve the effusion if the auditory tube dysfunction is due to swelling from allergic rhinitis (i.e., hay fever). If, after 90 days and one or more courses of medication, the middle ear effusion persists, then tympanostomy tube insertion needs to be considered.

Myringotomy and Tympanostomy Tube Insertion

When the goal is to provide optimal ventilation through the auditory tube, to ensure equal middle ear and atmospheric pressure, a simple reliable surgical procedure on the auditory tube remains elusive. Ventilation via the tympanic membrane, with myringotomy and tympan-ostomy tube (ventilation or PE tube) insertion, is the most common surgical procedure. The myringotomy enables the surgeon to suction the effusion from the middle ear. The PE tube, or grommet, prevents the rapid healing of the tympanic membrane and permits ventilation of the middle ear. This is a brief outpatient procedure with minimal risk. The otolaryngologist can choose from a variety of tube designs. The debate, if one exists, is usually not whether the tubes are to be placed, but when is the optimal time. Paradise (1976) and Bernstein (1978) opt for routine insertion of tubes in the patient with cleft palate, whereas others wait until hearing loss or pathological changes in the tympanic membrane develop. It should be emphasized to parents that, although tympanostomy tubes provide ventilation necessary to the middle ear, they do not correct the underlying anatomical pathology. Therefore, when the tube is extruded by the tympanic membrane and the perfora-tion is healed, the entire process of negative pressure formation, the resultant effusions, and hearing loss may begin again. The tympanic membrane is constantly replacing itself and, as it does, it gradually extrudes the tube, which then migrates laterally along with the wax and dead skin cells. (This migration is the natural cleaning mechanism of the ear and is often disrupted by the use of cotton swabs to clean the ear.)

The growth rate of the tympanic membrane is unrelated to the matu-ration of the auditory tube, and tympanostomy tubes frequently need to be replaced as they are extruded, if middle ear problems reoccur. Some tube designs have large inner flanges to resist extrusion and may re-main in place several years, as opposed to 18 months for a "standard" tube. A higher rate of residual perforation may be quite acceptable in a patient when a longer than average history of middle ear problems is anticipated (e.g., in the patient with a cleft palate). Although there are inevitable differences among physicians about the use and timing of tympanostomy tubes, Buckingham (1970) summarized the issue well with the statement, "It is far easier to ventilate the middle ear to pre-vent the formation of a reversible, chronic, adhesive otitis media or cholesteatoma than to wait until development of such conditions and to try and correct them surgically" (p. 40).

Simple Mastoidectomy

The mastoid bone, honeycombed with air cells and communicating with the middle ear, is a potential site of an infection, upon extension of an acute otitis media. Prior to the era of antibiotics, acute mastoiditis was fairly common, and the treatment was exoneration of the air cells via a surgical approach from behind the external ear. Acute mastoiditis is less frequent now, and the cortical, or simple, mastoidectomy is less often used.

Tympanoplasty, With or Without Mastoidectomy

A frequent sequelae of chronic otitis media, in both the cleft and the noncleft populations, is damage to the ossicular chain, tympanic membrane, and mastoid air cells. Correction at this point is usually beyond ventilation via tubes, and surgical intervention is typically indicated. The principle of this surgical procedure is to remove damaged air cells from the mastoid, reconstruct the ossicular chain to provide the best possible sound conduction, repair damage to the tympanic membrane, and provide adequate middle ear ventilation. Again, it is hoped that with careful observation and attention to the early development of ear problems, and the use of tympanostomy tubes in the cleft population, procedures such as tympanoplasty and mastoidectomy can be avoided.

NASAL PROBLEMS

In the cleft palate or craniofacial team approach, concerns for disruptions of the nasal anatomy and function as a result of the cleft palate and its management are shared by the plastic or pediatric surgeon, the speech pathologist, and the otolaryngologist. (The management of these deformities is covered in Chapter 3.) The normal nose serves to warm, filter, and humidify inspired air, and the nose of the patient with a cleft palate should ideally provide the same functions after repair. In actuality, the failure of the palate to merge often leaves the nasal septum markedly deviated to one side (usually to the side of the cleft). This deviation often persists even after the initial repair of the palate and produces nasal airway obstruction (Warren, Hairfield, & Dalston, 1990). This septal deformity, the loss of cartilage support, collapse of the nasal ala, and narrowing of the anterior nares, are common problems in the cleft population. Perhaps for too long, nasal function has been a neglected area; however, there is now evidence that increasing attention is being given to its importance. For example, the wide line pharyngeal flap used to remediate speech production may significantly compromise nasal patency. The creation of an adequate nasal airway via correction of septal deformity and external nasal deformities, as well as pharyngeal flap design and modification, must be coordinated with facial growth, development of dentition, orthodontic treatment, and the continued assessment and concerns for speech. Again, the value of the interdisciplinary team approach is readily apparent.

LARYNGEAL PROBLEMS

Although much attention is paid to the quality of speech produced by a patient with a cleft palate, it is the vocal folds of the larynx that produce the sound that is later modified by the effects of the cleft palate. No evidence suggests that laryngeal problems will be inherent due to the cleft lip and palate. However, laryngeal problems may develop due to laryngeal compensations in which speakers engage as they try to deal with their velopharyngeal inadequacy. McWilliams, Lavorato, and Bluestone (1973) reported a high incidence of vocal nodules in people with cleft palates, which they feel may be due to compensatory speech habits.

Laryngeal problems are found in a cross-section of the population, and the otolaryngologist is responsible for the diagnosis as well as the medical and surgical treatment of them. Indirect laryngoscopy, or examination of the larynx in the clinical setting, traditionally involves the use of a head mirror and a laryngeal mirror. The latter is placed against the soft palate and angled so as to visualize the larynx inferiorly. The laryngeal mirror gives the best clarity for viewing the larynx, but its use requires practice, and few non-otolaryngologists are able to use it successfully. The fiberoptic laryngoscope/pharyngoscope (Figure 7.12) is somewhat easier to use and, although the optical quality is not as good as a mirror, it can be of great value. It provides the opportunity to examine areas not otherwise accessible. This scope can be used to visualize the motion of the velum and the lateral pharyngeal wall during phonation, and to obtain an excellent view of the posterior nares and nasopharynx that might otherwise be impossible, particularly in a child who has had pharyngeal flap surgery. When used with a videorecorder, this instrument provides a record that can be used for further study and can be compared with other recordings.

SUMMARY

The problems created by the presence of a cleft lip and palate are diverse an challenging. Those problems facing the otolaryngologist—providing optimal nasal function and appearance, striving to ensure healing that enhances a child's receptive language and facilitates expressive language skills, and helping to maintain normal laryngeal voice production despite palatal abnormalities—are at the center of successful cleft palate management. At the same time, each of these concerns of the otolaryngologist overlaps those of adjoining or related specialties. The audiologist and otolaryngologist work together to prevent or remediate hearing problems in the child with a cleft palate. The importance of the interdisciplinary team approach cannot be overstated.

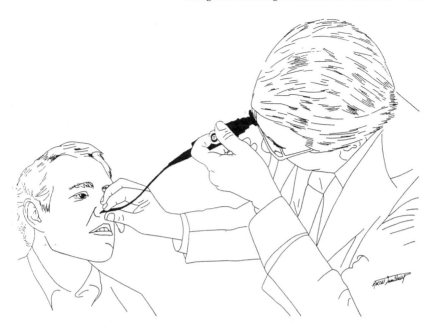

Figure 7.12 Flexible naso/pharyngo/laryngoscope. (From *Surgical Care of Voice Disorders* (p. 32) by W. J. Gould and V. Lawrence, 1984, New York: Springer-Verlag. Copyright 1984 by Springer-Verlag. Reprinted with permission.)

REFERENCES

Bernstein, L. (1978). Maxillofacial clefts. In B. Jazbi (Ed.), *Advances in Oto-rhino-laryngology. Pediatric Otorhinolaryngology.* Basel: S. Karger.

Bess, F. H. (1985). The minimally hearing-impaired child. *Ear and Hearing, 6,* 43–47.

Bess, F. H., & Humes, L. E. (1990). *Audiology: The fundamentals.* Baltimore: Williams and Wilkins.

Bluestone, C. D. (1971). Eustachian tube obstruction in the infant with cleft palate. *Annals of Otology, Rhinology and Laryngology, 80*(Suppl. 2), 1–30.

Bluestone, C. D. (1978). Eustachian tube function and allergy in otitis media. *Pediatrics, 61,* 753–760.

Bluestone, C. D., Cantekin, E. I., & Berry, Q. C. (1982). Symposium in prophylaxis and treatment of middle ear effusion. *IV Physiology of the Eustachian Tube in the Pathogenesis and Management of Middle Ear Effusion. Laryngoscope,* 1654–1670.

Bluestone, C. D., Cantekin, E. I., Berry, Q. C., & Paradise, J. L. (1975). Eustachian tube ventilatory function in relation to cleft palate. *Laryngoscope, 82,* 333–338.

Buckingham, R. A. (1970). Changes in the tympanic membrane with eustachian tube malfunction. *Otolaryngology Clinics of North American, 3,* 15–44.

Curtis, A., & Clemis, J. (1979). Middle ear effusion: Part I. Pathophysiology. *Journal of Continuing Education in Otorhinolaryngology and Allergy, 41,* 13–25.

Davis, J. M. (1986). Remediation of hearing, speech, and language deficits resulting from otitis media. In J. F. Kavanagh (Ed.), *Otitis media and child development* (pp. 182–191). Parkton, MD: York Press.

Dobie, R., & Berlin, C. (1979). The influence of otitis media on hearing and development. *Annals of Otology, Rhinology and Laryngology, 88*(Suppl. 60), 54–63.

Gould, W. J., & Lawrence, V. (1984). *Care of voice disorders.* New York: Springer-Verlag.

Hodgson, W. R. (1987). Tests of hearing—The infant. In F. N. Martin (Ed.), *Hearing disorders in children* (pp. 185–216). Austin, TX: PRO-ED.

Joint Committee on Infant Hearing. (1982). Position statement. *ASHA, 24,* 1017–1018.

Margolis, R. H., & Shanks, J. E. (1985). Tympanometry. In J. Katz (Ed.), *Handbook of clinical audiology* (3rd ed., pp. 438–475). Baltimore: Williams and Wilkins.

Matkin, N. D. (1986). The role of hearing in language development. In J. F. Kavanagh (Ed.), *Otitis media and child development* (pp. 3–11). Parkton, MD: York Press.

Maue-Dickson, W., & Dickson, D. R. (1980, January). Anatomy and physiology related to cleft palate: Current research and clinical implications. *Plastic and Reconstructive Surgery, 65,* 83–90.

McWilliams, B. J., Lavorato, A. S., & Bluestone, C. D. (1973). Vocal cord abnormalities in children with velopharyngeal valving problems. *Laryngoscope, 83*(11), 1745–1753.

Morgan, R. F., Dellon, A. L., & Hopper, J. E. (1983). Effects of levator retrodisplacement on conductive hearing loss in the cleft palate patient. *Annals of Plastic Surgery, 10,* 306–308.

Northern, J. L., & Downs, M. P. (1991). *Hearing in children.* Baltimore: Williams and Wilkins.

Paradise, J. L. (1976). Management of middle ear effusion in infants with cleft palate. *Annals of Otology, Rhinology and Laryngology, 85*(Supp. 2, Pt. 2), 285–288.

Paradise, J. L., Bluestone, C. D., & Felden, H. (1969). The universality of otitis media in 50 infants with cleft palate. *Pediatrics, 44,* 35–42.

Rood, S. R., & Moyce, A. (1980). *The identification of a surface agent within the adult human eustachian tube.* Paper presented at the annual meeting of the American Speech–Language–Hearing Association, Houston.

Rood, S. R., & Stool, S. E. (1981). Cleft palate related otopathologic disease. *Otolaryngology Clinics of North America, 14,* 865–884.

Ross, M. (1977). A review of studies on the incidence of hearing aid malfunctions. In F. B. Withrow (Ed.), *The condition of hearing aids worn by children in a public school program* (HEW Publication No. OE 77-05002). Washington, DC: U.S. Government Printing Office.

Schwartz, R. H. (1983). Pneumatic otoscopy: Getting the most out of the ear exam. *Journal of Respiratory Diseases, 4*(5), 82–92.

Senturia, B. (1970). Classification of middle ear effusion. *Annals of Otology, Rhinology, and Laryngology, 798,* 358–370.

Warren, D., Hairfield, W., & Dalston, E. (1990). The relationship between nasal airway size and nasal–oral breathing in cleft lip and palate. *Cleft Palate Journal, 27,* 46–50.

CHAPTER 8

Early Phonological Development and the Child with Cleft Palate

Patricia A. Broen and Karlind T. Moller

> *Broen and Moller describe a process by which children acquire the sound system of their language. They review several models of phonological development that have been described in the literature and argue that these models do not, for the most part, adequately account for some of the unique speech productions seen frequently in children with cleft palate. They conclude that all children are active learners attempting to sound like others and that several levels of speech need to be considered if speech–language pathologists are to understand the acquisition of phonological skills by any child. The authors review how speech characteristics of speakers with cleft palate have previously been described and discuss the impact of structural problems, such as frequent middle ear problems, faulty velopharyngeal closure, and dental hazards, on production of normal speech.*
>
> 1. *Broen and Moller make the point that previously proposed models of phonological development fail to adequately account for the maladaptive pattern frequently seen in children with cleft palate. Do you agree? Does it seem reasonable to think of a glottal stop as a "creative" way to sound like others?*
> 2. *How does Broen and Moller's statement "The accuracy of the speech is constrained by the child's perception of what is to be produced and the child's physical ability to produce what is perceived" apply to the child with cleft palate?*

3. *What are the two contrasting error patterns typically described in speakers with cleft palate? Why is one considered more undesirable than the other?*
4. *What can we conclude from studies of children who are acquiring their first 50 words? What can we conclude from studying 30-month-old children or from studying children undergoing pharyngeal flap surgery? What additional studies are needed?*

Speech–language pathologists have known for a long time that children with cleft palate sometimes develop unusual patterns of articulation, patterns that are not seen in other children and that cannot be accounted for in a simple way by the differences in their speech mechanisms. Also, some children with cleft palate develop these "maladaptive" or "back" patterns of articulation, whereas other children who appear to have similar structural mechanisms do not. Following surgical intervention (e.g., primary palatal repair), changes in articulation are often slow to occur, even though the speech mechanism may be capable of functioning adequately; that is, patterns of misarticulation observed prior to surgery may persist, and speech–language pathologists do not always understand why.

This chapter describes a process by which children, including the child with cleft palate, might acquire the sound system of their language. Within this model of speech production, the errors of the child with cleft palate are seen as the more or less natural outcome of the interaction between a child who learns language normally and a non-normal speech mechanism. The speech production errors of children with cleft palate are considered within a model of phonological development that views the child as an active, creative language learner. Menn (1983) commented that "We have evolved a notion of the young child as a creature of some intelligence who is trying to solve a problem: the problem of sounding like her companions when communicating with them" (p. 3). This is the perspective that is developed in this chapter. The young child is described as an active problem solver who is attempting to produce speech that sounds like the speech he or she hears. For any child, this means that he or she must hear a sample of speech, recognize those aspects of the sample that are important, and reproduce them. Even the young child with normal oral structures lacks the motor control (and perhaps the insight) to produce accurate, well-articulated speech at first. Normal children adopt strategies to accommodate to the discrepancy between the speech they hear and their ability to produce speech, but as they become more skillful and more insightful, the match between their speech and the speech of others becomes better.

For some children with cleft palate, learning to sound like their companions is particularly difficult because the equipment with which they attempt to produce speech is faulty. The child with cleft palate has the normal ineptitude found in any young child *plus* the inability to separate the oral and nasal cavities, the likelihood that the speech heard will be distorted or attenuated by an intermittent hearing loss, and the possibility that the speech produced may be distorted by dental hazards. Thus, the acquisition of normal sounding speech is difficult.

In this chapter, we examine what strategies normal children appear to use in learning their phonological system, what is the nature of the cleft palate child's problems, and how these problems might affect phonological learning. We also examine the speech patterns of several young children with cleft palate and relate those patterns to possible strategies for phonological learning. First, however, we examine some'older models of phonological learning.

PHONOLOGICAL ACQUISITION

The Autonomic Model

Any description of a child's speech production assumes some model of the sound system and some model of the learning process. In the past, speech–language pathologists have used a model that assumed that children learned a set of individual sounds, one at a time, and that the learning of one sound was relatively unrelated to the learning of other sounds (Spriestersbach, Darley, & Rouse, 1956; Templin, 1957) or to the learning of language in general. This reflects what has been described as a taxonomic or autonomic model of phonology (Hyman, 1975). Within this model, the child was seen as learning the correct production of each phoneme. It was assumed that some sounds were easier to learn than others, and thus were mastered first. More difficult sounds were learned later. This model was reflected in testing procedures that examined individual sounds, with little attention to the phonemic context in which they occurred, or to the phonetic content of the errors themselves. Errors might be described as "omissions," "distortions," or "substitutions," but the specific nature of the substitution or distortion was not of primary interest. Within this model, speech–language pathologists sought the order and age of acquisition of various sounds so that they could assess the productions of children, to identify those children who were sufficiently delayed in their acquisition to require some sort of intervention.

Within such a model, the behavior of the child with a cleft palate was a puzzle. Although it was generally the case that little attention was paid to the specific errors that children made, the errors made by children with cleft palate were so unusual that they seemed to require some kind of explanation. Children with cleft palate used glottal stops, pharyngeal fricatives, nasal fricatives, and other "maladaptive" approximations that seldom occurred in the speech of other children (Bzoch, 1965; Sherman, Spriestersbach, & Noll, 1959; Trost, 1981). The children persisted in using these patterns in the face of attempts to teach more accurate articulation, and even after successful reconstructive surgery (Morris, 1979). These patterns were described as learned patterns of articulation, where "learned" had a negative connotation.

Features, Rules, and Processes

More recently, other linguistic models were applied to phonological acquisition in normal children, and speech–language pathologists attempted to adapt these models to the description and treatment of children with speech production problems. Normal children were described as learning a set of distinctive features or distinctive feature contrasts (Jakobson, 1968; McReynolds & Huston, 1971; Menyuk, 1968), as learning a set of phonological rules that relate the child's output to the adult model (Compton, 1970; Dinnsen, 1984; Ingram, 1974a, 1974b; Smith, 1973), or as learning to suppress natural phonological processes that act together to simplify speech (Ingram, 1976; Shriberg & Kwiatkowski, 1980; Stampe, 1969). Although the underlying theoretical positions differed, all of these approaches did several things that the autonomic-based models failed to do: They described the phonological context in which the errors occurred, the phonetic nature of the error, and both the context and the error in terms of features or natural classes rather than individual phonemes. For example, a child who substituted [p] for /b/, [t] for /d/, [k] for /g/, [f] for /v/, [s] for /z/, and [tʃ] for /dʒ/ at the ends of words would be described, within a distinctive feature model, as lacking a word-final voicing *contrast*. The same child might be described as having a *rule* that devoices word-final obstruents (stops, fricatives, and affricates) or as exhibiting a word-final devoicing *process*.

Distinctive features.   Each of these models or approaches made a different assumption about the nature of the child's learning and about what is learned. Jakobson (1968) proposed that the child learns a set of *phonemic contrasts* (or distinctive feature oppositions). His account of phonological acquisition in children was intended more as a demonstration of the power of a particular model of adult phonology than as an account of the acquisition process, but his account of phonological acquisition was accepted with little question for a number of years.

As detailed descriptions of phonological acquisition in individual children were compared with the predictions made by Jakobson (Leopold, 1953; Moskowitz, 1970; Smith, 1973; Velten, 1943), it became clear that a strict interpretation of his proposed order of acquisition for feature contrasts was not supported by the data. Each time a child's speech was examined, the order and the plan of acquisition were modified until his proposal could no longer be made consistent with all of the data. Each child was different. No single order of acquisition of phonemic contrasts was consistent across all children. Although there were general trends, there were always exceptions. It also became apparent that any adequate account of phonological learning would have to describe more than the acquisition of phonemes or distinctive feature contrasts. In addition to changes that affect the production of individual sounds, children made modifications in their speech that appeared to function primarily to simplify or modify the structure of syllables. For example, a child might delete final consonants or omit approximants and fricatives from consonant clusters or intrude a vowel between the consonants in consonant clusters. All of these changes acted to simplify the syllable structure of the speech the child produced so that words tended to be produced with consonant–vowel (CV) syllables. Even adding a diminutive suffix (e.g., "dog" becoming "doggy") served to replace a CVC syllable structure with a CVCV structure, and might represent a kind of simplification.

The speech that children produce can differ from the adult model in other ways not predicted by Jakobson. Children are often observed to do a kind of distance assimilation, not common in adult speech, in which the place of articulation of one consonant in a word assimilates to the place of articulation of another, nonadjacent consonant. For example, "dog" might become [gɔg], with the /d/ assimilating to the place of articulation of the final /g/. This might occur even though /d/ is produced correctly in "daddy" and "down." Some children prefer a particular sound, replacing all word-initial obstruents, for example, with /d/ (Broen & Jons, 1979) or all word-final fricatives with /tʃ/ (Becker & Broen, 1972). None of these patterns would be predicted by a Jakobson-type distinctive feature model of phonological acquisition.

Phonological rules. Phonological rules are devices for representing the regularities that occur in speech. In the child phonology literature, they have usually been used to describe the relationship between the child's production and the adult model. The standard form for such phonological rules is as follows:

Some phoneme or natural class of phonemes in the adult model	→	changes in a particular way in the child's speech	in some phonetic environment

For example, the following rule could be written to describe the speech of the child mentioned earlier who devoiced word-final obstruents:

$$[+\text{obstruent}] \rightarrow [-\text{voice}] /\text{\_\_\_\_\_}\#$$

That is, phonemes that are [+obstruent] in the adult model will also be [−voice] in the child's speech when they occur at the end of a word.

Some child phonologists write rules simply to capture regularity observed in the relationship between the child's productions and the adult model; others interpret the rule as a representation of the process the child goes through in translating some underlying representation of the adult target to the child's output form (Dinnsen, 1984). Only in the latter case is a claim made about the child's knowledge of the process by which the child creates speech. Phonological rules, in this latter case, are descriptions of the structure of the child's language and only indirectly of the relationship between the child's productions and the adult model. (See Dinnsen, 1984, for a more complete account.)

In the child with a cleft palate, there are two possible sources for the observed differences between the child's speech and the adult model. Differences can be the direct result of structural differences, such as the child's inability to separate the oral and nasal cavities. For example, nasal resonance associated with vowels and weak or inaudible obstruent consonants would appear to be the direct result of the coupling of the oral and nasal cavities. They are the kinds of changes that occur when velopharyngeal incompetence occurs in an otherwise normal adult (Isshiki, Honjow, & Morimoto, 1968). Differences may also reflect the child's active creative attempt to match the adult model with a speech mechanism that is inadequate for the task. The use of glottal stops for oral stops or frictionalized nasal air for oral fricatives may reflect attempts by the child with cleft palate and inadequate velopharyngeal closure to match at least some aspects of the ambient model. In treating the child, it may be necessary to separate these two sources of error, but phonological rules can be used to describe the systematicity or lawfulness in either case. We return to these issues later.

Phonological processes.   Stampe (1969) argued that a child begins with a set of *innate phonological processes* and that the child's task is to learn to suppress or modify only those processes that are inconsistent with the language the child is learning. Like Jakobson, Stampe was primarily interested in explaining some aspects of adult phonology, and he used child phonology as a tool. In doing so, he made a significant contribution, not necessarily because he was right or because he accounted for all of the variability in the data, but because he directed attention to some aspects of speech that had previously been ignored and because he provided some new ways of interpreting the production patterns that were observed in children's speech. The initial interpretation of Stampe's work for individuals interested in the clinical application of a phonological process model was done by Ingram (1976). Many of the labels now used for phonological processes were created by Ingram. Since that time, several proposals have been made for the analysis of misarticulated speech within a phonological process model (Hodson & Paden, 1981; Ingram, 1981; Shriberg & Kwiatkowski, 1980; Weiner, 1979), and at least one paper (Lynch, Fox, & Brookshire, 1983) examined the speech of two children with repaired clefts within such a model.

The concept of the phonological process is very attractive to speech–language pathologists because it provides (a) a way to identify and label error patterns, (b) a causal explanation of sorts for those error patterns, and (c) a rationale for therapy at something other than the single-phoneme level. However, even Stampe's model did not account for all of the patterns of speech observed in young normal children. Taken in its strictest form, Stampe's proposal predicts that all children follow similar, but not necessarily identical, paths to mastery and that their progress is orderly. It also predicts that a single set of phonological processes is common to all children. At least three findings are inconsistent with these predictions: The units of learning differ from one child to another, progress toward mastery is not always orderly, and children learning the same language exhibit different error patterns.

Not only does no single order of acquisition hold across all children, but some children start learning at the word level or at the phrase level (Peters, 1977), whereas others begin with sounds. Some children avoid words they are unable to produce (Ferguson & Farwell, 1975), whereas other children are content to use a single sequence of sounds for many different words (Priestly, 1977). There seems to be no single path from first word to adultlike speech, but rather many different paths.

The concept that children make increasingly fine distinctions as they move toward mastery of the sound system is attractive and logical, but it does not seem to be true. Children are sometimes able to produce words quite accurately at a young age, only to lose that ability as they become older. These are the "progressive idioms" that Ingram (1976) described. The classic example is the word "pretty" in the speech of Leopold's (1947) daughter Hildegard. Ferguson and Farwell (1975) describe the sequence of productions from [prɪti] when the child was 10 months old to [bɪdi] at 22 months. This kind of regressive change has been observed in other children as well (Smith, 1973).

Children make creative errors. The error pattern that occurs when one child is unable to produce a class of sounds may differ from the error pattern that occurs when another child is unable to produce the same class of sounds. For example, when children are unable to produce fricative consonants, most children substitute stops, but some substitute glides. Some children substitute alveolar consonants for velars, but others substitute velars for alveolars. Children often "prefer" a particular sound, or class of sounds, and substitute that for other similar sounds. For one child, the preferred sound may be labial; for another, the preferred class may be nasals (Ingram, 1979). Some children actually add to the production of a phoneme, producing what appears to be a more complex sound (Fey & Gandour, 1982).

In summary, the errors observed in normal children as they are learning the phonological system of their language do not appear to be the residue from processes that have not yet been suppressed or modified, or to be the result of a lack of feature contrasts. Although some error patterns can be described in this way, others clearly cannot. Often the error patterns observed in children can be described by phonological rules; that is, the child's speech pattern is predictable, and it is possible to make some general statement about the nature of the error pattern and to use a phonological rule to describe that pattern. This statement may be useful, but it is not an explanation. It is merely a form of description.

A Model of Phonological Learning

Menn (1983) and Studdert-Kennedy (1983, 1987) proposed that what is needed is an account of phonological acquisition in which the child is an active, creative participant, using the motor skills and the perceptual knowledge currently available to produce some approximation of the adult speech forms. Within such a model, the child's task is to learn to produce the complex series of motor gestures that will result in speech that "sounds like" the speech that the child hears. The child accomplishes this by a series of successive approximations, gradually producing speech that is more like the adult model. Different children match different parts of the model, and some children wander into cul-de-sacs that do not lead directly to adultlike speech.

This account has several parts. First, the child's intent is to produce meaningful speech, and the child's attention is on the meaning, not on the form. Second, the child must learn the motor gesture or sequence of motor gestures that correspond to a particular acoustic event, and putting these gestures together is a major part of the problem. Third, the child eventually produces speech that has the fine detail of the speech that is heard, not merely the phonemic contrasts; that is, the child eventually learns to produce the fine phonetic detail of what is heard, even though all of the detail is not required for communication. The child hearing a New England dialect will learn the phonetic detail of that dialect, whereas the child hearing a Midwestern dialect will reproduce that.

Learning can and does occur at several levels. The child may at times learn to produce whole words or phrases that are phonemically unanalyzed. Hildegard's (Leopold, 1947) early production of "pretty" probably reflects this kind of learning. The child will also eventually learn to produce the syllable structures that occur in the target language, although CV and VC syllables appear to be easier to produce than syllables that contain a sequence of two or more consonants with no intervening vowel. A sequence of syllables with the same or similar consonants (i.e., reduplication) is usually produced before syllable sequences that contain different consonants. Some of the differences between the young child's speech and the adult model will reflect the degree to which the child has mastered the complex syllable structures that occur in the language.

Children also learn at a distinctive feature level. They often demonstrate that they can produce some features of a class of sounds before others. The child in our previous example, who substituted voiceless sounds for voiced sounds in word-final positions, substituted a stop or fricative with correct place of articulation. Only the voicing of the child's production was incorrect. The child who substitutes alveolar consonants for velar consonants will generally substitute [t] for /k/, [d] for /g/, and [n] for /ŋ/, maintaining manner, voicing, and nasality, while changing place of articulation. These kinds of errors may be described as distinctive feature errors or as phonological process errors. In either case, an accurate description of the error recognizes that many, but not all, of the features of the child's production match the target. Children may use both auditory and visual information in attempting to reproduce speech. For example, very young children can recognize the visual representation of the speech they hear (Kuhl & Meltzoff, 1982), and, whereas children with normal vision learn to produce highly visible phonemes (e.g., /m/) very early, children who are blind do not (Mills, 1983).

The learning process is "cognitive" in that children are actively experimenting to match the visual and acoustic attributes of speech, and different children discover different approximations to the target language. At any time, a child may appear to use one or more of the following "strategies" in producing speech: avoiding words that cannot be produced or favoring sounds or sound sequences that have been mastered; modifying some features of a class of sounds while producing other features more accurately; using phonological rules that conspire to simplify the syllable structure of the words (e.g., deleting consonants from consonant clusters); assimilating the place of articulation or voicing or manner of one phoneme in a word to that of another phoneme; or reordering the place of articulation of sequential phonemes. All of these changes take place while the child is attempting to communicate through speech.

Thus, if we are to understand the speech productions of normal young children (or children with cleft palate), we may have to look at speech at several levels. In some instances, we need to look at whole words. In other instances, regularities are apparent at the level of the syllable, phoneme, or feature. The accuracy of the speech is constrained by the child's perception of what is to be produced and the child's physical ability to produce what is perceived. The same constraints hold for the child with cleft palate: The speech that this child produces is the result of the child's perception of the structure of the target language and the child's ability to produce the sequences of motor gestures required to reproduce that structure. Like other children, children with cleft palate explore their capability to produce speech, and different children arrive at different solutions to the speech production task as they are learning. No normal child can produce accurate speech without a period of learning. The child with a cleft palate is no different, except that the solutions arrived at by this child may be different because what the child can produce may be restricted by inadequate velopharyngeal closure and dental hazards, and what the child hears may be distorted by a conductive hearing loss.

THE CHILD WITH CLEFT PALATE

Children with cleft palate are essentially normal children who will be expected to follow normal paths in learning to produce speech. However, children with cleft palate may differ from children without clefts in that their velopharyngeal mechanisms may not be adequate for normal speech production, they may not hear as well some of the time, and their dental situation may present hazards along the way. In the following sections, we describe briefly the speech characteristics that have been observed in children with cleft palate and the possible contribution of hearing and oral–pharyngeal differences to their speech, and attempt to account for phonological learning in children with cleft palate.

Speech Characteristics

Most studies describe the speech of older children and adults with cleft palate within a taxonomic phonological model (Bzoch, 1979; Fletcher, 1978; McWilliams, Morris, & Shelton, 1984; Moll, 1968; Morris, 1968; Wells, 1971; Westlake & Rutherford, 1966). The majority of the studies describe production only as correct or incorrect and either list the frequency with which individual sounds are in error or compare the number of errors made by children with cleft palate with normative data. The focus is often on the relationships among articulatory performance and variables such as type of cleft (Byrne, Shelton, & Diedrich, 1961; Bzoch, 1956, 1965; Counihan, 1956; Spriestersbach, Moll, & Morris, 1961), surgical procedures used to close the palate (Byrne et al., 1961; Spriestersbach & Powers, 1959), physiological and anatomical factors (Spriestersbach & Powers, 1959; Starr, 1956; Subtelny, Koepp-Baker, & Subtelny, 1961; Van Demark & Van Demark, 1967), and age of testing (Bzoch, 1965; Counihan, 1956; Morris, 1962; Olson, 1965; Starr, 1956). The following represents a summary of the findings of those studies:

- At all ages, children with cleft palate as a group scored below the mean on articulation tests, but there was wide variation within the group, and many children developed normal articulation.
- Speech sounds requiring intraoral pressure (i.e., stops, fricatives, and affricates or [−sonorant] phonemes) were most frequently in error, and nasal consonants and semivowels were least affected. Among the [−sonorant] consonants, fricatives and affricates, particularly /s/ and /z/, were misarticulated more often than stops.
- No particular place of articulation was more vulnerable than others; compensatory patterns of articulation were noted for all places of articulation.
- Within an individual, there was often inconsistency in the presence or absence of an error and in the nature of the error.
- The more complex the utterance, the greater the likelihood of articulation errors.
- The less adequate the velopharyngeal and dental structures, the greater the inconsistency and the greater the influence of phonetic complexity.
- Inappropriate compensatory articulation and audible nasal air emission occurred frequently in speakers with cleft palate.

In addition to these rather general descriptions, two contrasting error patterns have been described as occurring in individuals with cleft palate (McWilliams et al., 1984; Morley, 1970). In one case, place and manner of articulation were reasonably accurate, but speech was accompanied by nasal emission and [−sonorant] consonants were weak. The other pattern involved what Bzoch (1979) has called "gross substitutions" (e.g., glottal stops, pharyngeal fricatives, and nasal fricatives) for other consonants. Trost (1981) added to these descriptions midpalatal and pharyngeal stops, linguavelar nasal fricatives, and simultaneously produced oral and glottal stops. Both of these patterns of articulation were associated with velopharyngeal inadequacy; however, the latter pattern, referred to variously as the "maladaptive," "compensatory," or "posterior" pattern, was less desirable in that it frequently interfered with assessment of velopharyngeal potential and was difficult to modify once habituated.

Hearing

All children with cleft palate are at risk for middle ear effusion and associated conductive hearing loss (see Chapter 7). The effects of mild conductive hearing loss on phonological acquisition in normal children are not fully understood, but evidence indicates that children with recurrent middle ear problems are slower to acquire speech production skills. In addition, some attributes of the speech of individuals with cleft palate are also observed in the speech of individuals with hearing losses. For example, glottal stops have been reported in the babbling of hearing impaired infants (Oller & Eilers, 1988) and in the speech of young children with histories of middle ear disease (Shriberg & Smith, 1983). Intermittent nasality is also a characteristic of the speech of hearing impaired individuals.

Oral Structures

Inadequate velopharyngeal closure remains the primary structural problem in persons with cleft palate. The child with an unrepaired cleft palate and frequently the child who has undergone initial palatal repair are unable to separate the oral cavity from the nasal cavity. Palatal fistulae following initial repair and delayed hard palate closure (primary veloplasty) present similar problems in that they prevent a complete separation of the oral and nasal cavities. The child may also have to contend with dental hazards, including missing or malposed teeth in the area of an alveolar cleft and anterior–posterior and transverse arch discrepancies. The dental problems are dealt with in a more comprehensive way in Chapters 4 through 6 on oral surgery, orthodontics, and prosthodontics. In this chapter, the primary interest centers on the possible effects of velopharyngeal differences on speech.

Inadequate velopharyngeal closure in speakers who have acquired normal speech skills results in hypernasal resonance distortion, distortion of [−sonorant] consonants by nasal air emission, or substitutions of nasal for non-nasal sounds (Bernthal & Beukelman, 1977; Isshiki et al., 1968). Patients who become adventitiously velopharyngeally incompetent following surgical resection of the soft palate or portions of the maxilla demonstrate these characteristics. This pattern of speech production resembles one of the patterns observed in children and adults with cleft palate, but not the other. The use of places of articulation that differ markedly from the target sound (e.g., glottal stops for oral stops or nasal fricatives for oral fricatives) does not occur in individuals who learn to speak with a normal speech mechanism and subsequently become velopharyngeally incompetent. These patterns occur only in individuals who learn to speak with an inadequate velopharyngeal mechanism.

The Problem

Phonological learning in children with cleft palate has been a puzzle because the children do not seem to behave like other children. Often their productions do not seem to be reasonable approximations to the speech to which they are exposed. They make errors that cannot be accounted for in a simple way by the differences in their speech mechanisms. For example, lack of velopharyngeal closure does not "cause" glottal stops or pharyngeal fricatives. In addition, given the same or similar structural problems, children demonstrate very different phonological patterns. However, it is probably the case that, like the errors of other children, the errors of the child with cleft palate reflect a creative attempt to match the adult model rather than a simple inability to reproduce certain aspects of the speech signal or inaccurate learning. Also, like normal children, some children with cleft palate probably begin to learn speech at a phrase level, some at a word level, and others at a phoneme level. The following section describes the speech of several children with cleft palate. The children represent different points in the speech development process and different degrees of cleft involvement.

EXAMPLES FROM THE SPEECH OF CHILDREN WITH CLEFT PALATE

This section examines the speech of young children with cleft palate from several perspectives, including the nature of syllables and whole words produced by very young children, the manner class substitutions that occur in older preschool children, and the patterns of change that occur with structural modification. The examples come from studies of (a) children who are acquiring their first 50 words, (b) 30-month-old children, and (c) children undergoing pharyngeal flap surgery. These are interesting and important time intervals in that they represent (a) the very beginnings of meaningful speech, (b) a period when children are actively and rapidly acquiring a phonological system, and (c) a time when there is a substantial change in the velopharyngeal mechanism.

Early Vocabulary

Children typically begin to use meaningful speech sometime during their second year. The transition from babbling to speech is generally gradual, with the child's babbling or nonmeaningful vocalizations becoming more speechlike (Oller, 1986) and the child's early speech having many of the characteristics of babbling (Locke, 1983). For example, as in babbling, early words often include reduplication, and the child uses primarily oral stops, nasals, and glides.

This section examines the first 20 words produced by two children with cleft palate (Table 8.1), both of whom exhibited velopharyngeal problems at the time the samples were obtained. The samples come from a larger study of the first 50 words produced by a group of normal children and a group of children with cleft palate (Estrem, 1984; Estrem & Broen, 1989). Both children described here had complete clefts of the

TABLE 8.1
The First 20 Words Produced by Two Children
with Clefts of the Hard and Soft Palate

Child 1		Child 2	
Gloss	Transcription	Gloss	Transcription
light	n:a:	bye	əaɪ:
bye	bā:	thank you	hā:kʊ
mommy	ma:mi	hi	gaɪ
banana	ɲæɲə	Katy	ʕeɪʕɪ:
mine	ma:	hot	hɔtˈ
here	hi:	sock on	ɔkā
hi	həaɪ:	Ben	bɛ̃
milk	mæ:	block	mɔʔ
hair	he	cup	bəʔ
more	m:ə	eye	aɪ
owie	awɪ	good	gʊ̧
no	no	ball	ba̧
water	wa:wa	cracker	æʔə
toe	do	doggie	gɔ̧gi̧
hello	aow	kitty	gəʔgi̧
ear	aɪ	horsie	ho:ʔgi̧
egg	ɛʔ	papa	ba̧ba̧
what	əʔ	dolly	gəʔgi̧
horsie	naʔɪ	good girl	gʊgə̧
ball	ma	what	wə̃

Other selected examples from the first 50 words:

wheel	wi	night night	gaɪga̧
yellow	jɛwə	coffee	gəgɪ̧
round	wāʔ	glasses	gə̧
read	wi:	Jaques	ʔgəʔgə̧
dog	dɔʔ	banana	ɲæɲə
whale	we:ow	chicken	ɲæɲə

Note. From "A Comparison of the Speech Patterns and Word Choices of Very Young Children With and Without Cleft Palates" by T. Estrem, 1984, unpublished master's thesis, University of Minnesota, Minneapolis.

hard and soft palates with primary palatal surgery at about 18 months. Child 1 began to talk at 22 months, 4 months after surgery, whereas Child 2 began to talk at 16.5 months, 1.5 months before surgery. The children were assumed to have inadequate velopharyngeal closure because Child 1 was recommended for pharyngeal flap surgery by a multidisciplinary team and Child 2 had an unrepaired palate at the time this speech sample was taken. However, the two children approached the task of producing speech in different ways, as reflected in the phonetic characteristics of the words they attempted to produce, in their strategies for producing the words, and in the frequency of accurate productions.

In many respects, the productions of both children were similar to the productions one would expect from any young child. For example, final consonants were generally absent in both samples (Table 8.1). Very young normal children often have been observed to produce open syllables, that is, syllables that contain no final consonants, as these young cleft palate speakers did. With the exception of the voiceless glide /h/, all word-initial consonants were voiced and, in two-syllable words, the consonant of the first syllable was usually repeated in the second syllable. Again, these phonological patterns—word-initial consonant voicing and reduplication—are characteristic of the speech of normally developing children.

These two samples also exhibit phonological patterns that have been described as characteristic of the speech of children with cleft palate. Both children sometimes used glottal stops where the target word had an oral stop, and Child 2 also produced glottal stops preceding some velar stops. Child 2 produced one word with pharyngeal fricatives (i.e., "Katy" was pronounced as [ʕeɪʕiː]). Child 2 appeared to "prefer" velar stops, particularly [g].[1] This phoneme was produced posterior to the usual place of articulation for [g] and may have been produced by elevating the velum with the tongue body, although no direct evidence indicated that this was the case.

Child 1 appeared to fit Ferguson and Farwell's (1975) description of children who used words that contain sounds they were able to produce. About 75% of the target words in his sample began with phonemes that were [+sonorant], that is, with nasals, glides, and vowels. These sounds would be expected to be easier because they do not require the increased intraoral air pressure that [−sonorant] sounds (i.e., stops, fricatives, affricates) require. Child 1's vocabulary was modified in another way. The words he attempted were single-syllable words about 75% of the time. This combination of single-syllable words and word-initial phonemes that he produced with some accuracy made Child 1's speech fairly intelligible in spite of his structural problems. Later, as his vocabulary increased, his speech became less accurate.

Child 2, on the other hand, selected words that contained sounds that she was unable to produce. A large proportion of the words she attempted began with oral stops, fricatives, and consonant clusters. Only 5 of the first 20 words began with [+sonorant] consonants. As might be expected, her productions were not very accurate. In addition, about 50% of the words she tried to produce were multisyllabic words. Her 14th word was doggie [gɔgi]. From that point on, she produced a number of words as [gVgV] or some variation of this pattern. Later in the sample she produced some [ŋVŋV] words that seem to represent a similar or related pattern. It appeared that she adopted a particular pattern of sounds or a "template" (Priestly, 1977) and used that template for a number of different multisyllabic words.

These samples illustrate a number of things. First, children with cleft palate learn to talk in much the same way that normal children do; they use CV syllables, use voiced word-initial consonants, and demonstrate reduplication. They may even use a template or preferred sound pattern for many words, as some normal children do. However, they also differ from normal children and from each other. Some phonological characteristics that have been attributed to speakers with cleft palate may be present from the time they begin to talk. These two children differed in the kinds of words they attempted and in their strategies for producing those words (Table 8.1), but they both provide evidence that their early speech is influenced by their cleft palates. Child 1 could be described as taking a conservative approach to talking. He did not begin to talk until he was almost 2 years old. At that time, he chose single-syllable words most of the time (70%) and words that began with nasals and approximants (70%), sounds that would be expected to be easier for a child with inadequate velopharyngeal closure. His production of the word-initial consonant was accurate 60% of the time.

Child 2, on the other hand, was more adventuresome. She began to talk with an open palate, 45% of her first 20 words were either two syllables or two words, and 75% began with oral stops or fricatives. These are the sounds that are expected to be difficult for a child with inadequate velopharyngeal closure. Her word-initial consonant productions were accurate only 30% of the time. Like normal children, Child 2 used reduplicated syllables, and she adopted a template and used it for several words. However, unlike normal children, she used backed velar stops, and produced pharyngeal fricatives and glottal stops in her first words.

The very early speech of children with cleft palate may provide insights into the source of some of their compensatory production patterns and, although some aspects of phonological acquisition are similar to those observed in normal children, differences can be identified early.

30-Month-Old Children

Most studies of the production of speech sounds in children with cleft palate begin with children who are 3 or 4 years old (Dorf & Curtin, 1982; O'Gara & Logemann, 1988). Despite some notable exceptions (Prather, Hedrick, & Kern, 1975; Stoel-Gammon & Cooper, 1984), the same is generally true for studies of normal children. However, the third year is an active time for phonological learning, and this may be a critical year for the child with cleft palate. Speech patterns established during this time may either lay a strong foundation for accurate speech or start the child with cleft palate down a path that leads to undesirable articulatory patterns.

This section considers data from a study of three groups of 30-month-old children: (a) those with cleft palate who required improved velopharyngeal closure (Group 1), (b) those with cleft palate who did not require improved velopharyngeal closure (Group 2), and (c) an age-matched group of normal children (Group 3) (Broen, Felsenfeld, & Kittelson-Bacon, 1986). Five children were in each group. The children were chosen, retrospectively, from a larger longitudinal study of speech development in children with cleft palate. They were chosen because they had either age-appropriate speech or pharyngeal flap surgery by the time they were 5 years old; that is, by age 5, a decision had been made regarding the adequacy of their velopharyngeal mechanism. The study examined the production of word-initial [−sonorant] consonants (i.e., stops, fricatives, and affricates) by these children when they were 30 months old. Both imitated and spontaneous speech samples were obtained. The production of word-initial consonants by the three groups was compared in several ways. The data reported here come from the imitative speech sample, but conclusions based on the spontaneous speech sample were similar even though not all phonemes were represented in the spontaneous sample.

Group 1 children averaged 36.2 errors in 45 productions of [−sonorant] consonants, Group 2 children averaged 20.8 errors, and Group 3 children averaged 13.2 errors (Table 8.2). The performance of Group 1 children was statistically significantly different from that of Group 2 and that of Group 3 children, but Groups 2 and 3 were not different from each other. Overall, children who required secondary management of the velopharyngeal mechanism tended to make more errors than other children in the production of stops, fricatives, and affricates.

Some of the children's errors involved inappropriate use of the voicing feature: Sounds that should have been voiced were voiceless, or sounds that should have been voiceless were voiced. Group 1 children averaged 24.4 such voicing errors, Group 2 children 10.1, and Group 3 children 1.2. The performance of Group 1 children differed significantly

TABLE 8.2

A Comparison of 45 Productions of Word-Initial [−Sonorant] Consonants
Produced by Children with Cleft Palate Who Required Secondary Palatal
Surgery (Group 1), Children with Cleft Palate Who Did Not Require
Secondary Palatal Surgery (Group 2), and Normal Children (Group 3)

	Group		
Error Type	1	2	3
Overall errors	36.2	20.8	13.2
Voicing errors	24.4	10.1	1.2
Place errors	16.4	13.7	9.2
[+Sonorant] substitutions	22.8	2.0	0.2

Note. The table presents the mean number of errors that fall into each category.

from that of Group 3, but the performance of children in Group 2 did
not differ from that of Groups 1 and 3. Place errors were more evenly
distributed. Although Group 1 children made more place errors (16.4)
than children in Groups 2 (13.7) and 3 (9.2), none of the differences among
the groups was significant for place of articulation.

The most striking difference among the groups was in the frequency
with which [+sonorant] consonants were substituted for [−sonorant] consonants. An average of 22.8 of the 45 [−sonorant] consonants in the
sample were produced by Group 1 children as [+sonorant] consonants.
Group 2 children averaged only 2.0 such errors, and Group 3 children
only 0.2. That is, the children who ultimately required improvement
of velopharyngeal closure tended to substitute nasals, glides,[2] and vowels
for stops, fricatives, and affricates. This type of error was rarely made
by the children with cleft palate who acquired normal speech and was
almost never made by the normal group.

Even though many of the errors made by Group 1 children could
be described as involving a particular feature change (i.e., [+sonorant]
consonants for [−sonorant] consonants), the children in this group did
not sound like one another. Each child appeared to preserve some aspects
of the target sounds and to sacrifice others, but they made different
choices. For example, one child tended to produce nasal stops for [+voice]
oral consonants and [h] for [−voice] consonants, preserving the voicing
contrast, but sacrificing place of articulation among the voiceless sounds.
Another child produced nasals or voiced glides for [−sonorant] consonants, neutralizing the voicing contrast, but often preserving place

of articulation. These kinds of tradeoffs were necessary if the child was to produce audible speech that approximated the target language. In this study, there were children who used two or three different consonants as substitutions for a single phoneme, reflecting the "inconsistency" that has been described in previous studies. This was true in both the imitative and the spontaneous samples.

The child described in the error matrix shown in Figure 8.1 substituted nasals and glides for obstruent consonants. She had some tendency to produce nasals for [+voice] consonants and to produce glides, primarily [h], for [−voice] consonants. Most of the non-nasal productions were transcribed as "nasalized" (see the lower portion of the matrix). This child might be described as inconsistent in that there were often two or three different productions for a single phoneme, but even when there was variation, the error productions were almost always [+sonorant].

Regardless of the particular substitutions or the manner of obtaining the sample, all of the Group 1 children could be described as frequently substituting [+sonorant] consonants for [−sonorant] consonants or as substituting consonants that required less intraoral pressure for those that required more. Some of the error patterns preserved voicing, some preserved place of articulation, and some preserved the oral–nasal contrast. They all allowed the child to produce audible speech with a less than perfect mechanism. Some of these patterns led in a relatively effortless way to accurate speech once velopharyngeal closure was improved; others did not.

Several observations can be made from this study. The children with cleft palate, even those who acquired age-appropriate speech with no intervention beyond primary palatal surgery, tended to be slower than the children without clefts to acquire accurate speech production skills. The children with cleft palate and inadequate velopharyngeal closure tended to substitute [+sonorant] consonants for [−sonorant] consonants. However, this describes both desirable and undesirable compensatory patterns of articulation. These patterns of articulation were apparent when the children were 2½ years old, long before the children would be expected to have adultlike speech.

Pharyngeal Flap Surgery

Children with cleft palate sometimes undergo procedures that result in substantial changes in their oral–pharyngeal structures and that have a significant effect on their ability to produce speech. Pharyngeal flap surgery (as described in Chapter 3) is one such procedure. The primary rationale for this procedure is to improve speech, but correct speech sound production does not necessarily occur immediately after surgery.

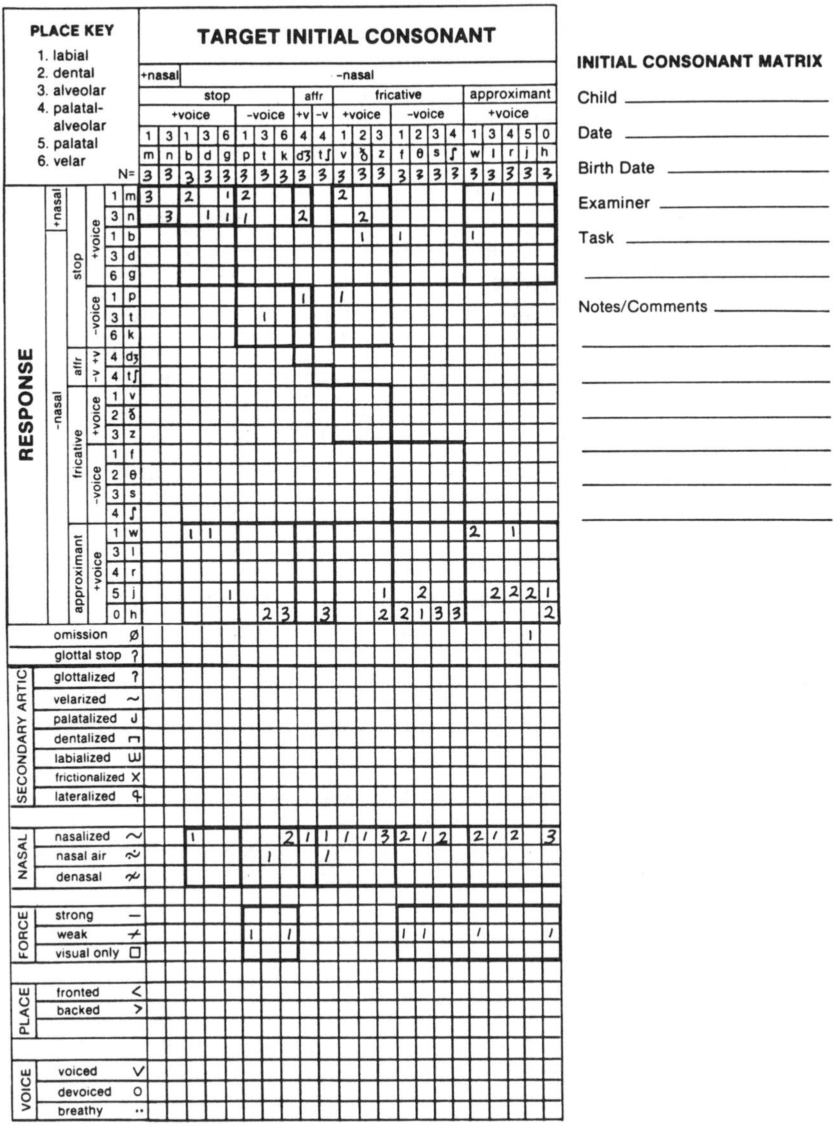

PLACE KEY
1. labial
2. dental
3. alveolar
4. palatal-alveolar
5. palatal
6. velar

TARGET INITIAL CONSONANT

INITIAL CONSONANT MATRIX

Child _____

Date _____

Birth Date _____

Examiner _____

Task _____

_____

Notes/Comments _____

_____

_____

_____

_____

_____

Figure 8.1   Error matrix for a Group 1 child with cleft palate.

It is not uncommon for articulation patterns observed prior to surgery to continue for a period of time. This may seem puzzling, because most children are hyponasal following surgery; however, given the model of phonological learning that we have been considering, one would not expect the change to be immediate. If the child has learned to accommodate to inadequate velopharyngeal closure in a certain manner, the child must learn new speech production patterns following surgery. The change may not be as simple as learning to coordinate velopharyngeal port constriction with other aspects of speech production. To deal appropriately with the child who has had such surgery requires an understanding of the rate of change and the nature of the changes that occur following surgery. At this time, these data are limited.

This section describes the course of change in the speech production of two children following pharyngeal flap surgery (Letcher, Broen, & Moller, 1986). The descriptions are based on samples of word-initial consonant production that were obtained from the children just prior to surgery, 1 month after surgery, and at about 3-month intervals until each child's speech was considered age appropriate. The relationship between the child's productions and the adult model is described in terms of a set of phonological rules that reflect that relationship. The rules are not intended to represent the *process* by which the child produces speech.

Bob. Bob had a unilateral complete cleft of the lip and palate. His palate was repaired at 17 months, and the pharyngeal flap was performed at 43 months. The rules in Table 8.3 describe his production of word-initial consonants prior to pharyngeal flap surgery and at intervals following surgery. Prior to surgery, Bob produced almost all voiced stops, fricatives, and affricates as nasal stops (Rule 1). Place of articulation was preserved in that labial consonants were produced as [m] and nonlabial consonants as [n]. Voiceless stops (Rule 2) were generally produced correctly as voiceless stops, and about half of the time they were accompanied by audible nasal air emission (NAE). Voiceless fricatives (Rule 3) were correct with NAE about half of the time and produced as [h] about half of the time.

One month after surgery, correct productions were no longer accompanied by audible nasal air, but productions that were not correct prior to surgery were often incorrect. For example, voiced [−sonorant] consonants (both stops and fricatives) were still produced as nasals about 29% of the time, but were always produced as stops. Voiceless fricatives were still produced as [h] about one-third of the time. Three months after surgery, these rules no longer characterized Bob's speech. However, he was still making errors (Figure 8.2), and at least some of his errors appeared to be related to his strategies for producing speech prior to surgery.

Prior to surgery, Bob's voiceless stops and voiceless fricatives were correct at least some of the time and distinct from each other. Voiceless stops were generally stops, and voiceless fricatives were either fricatives or [h]. However, both voiced stops and voiced fricatives (and the

TABLE 8.3
Frequency of Occurrence of Three Phonological Rules in Bob's Speech
Prior to and Following Pharyngeal Flap Surgery

		Session		
Rule		Prior to Surgery	1 Month	3 Months
1. +voice −sonorant → stop +nasal		21/23 (91%)	6/21 (29%)	0/21 (0%)
2. −voice −continuant → [+NAE][1]		5/10 (50%)	0/9 (0%)	
3a. +voice fricatives → [h]		6/13 (46%)	4/12 (33%)	0/12 (0%)
3b. +voice fricatives → [+NAE]		6/13 (46%)	0/12 (0%)	

NAE = nasal air emission.

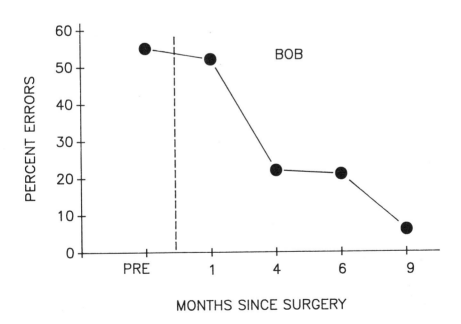

Figure 8.2 The percentage of consonants produced incorrectly by Bob prior to surgery
and 1, 4, 6, and 9 months after surgery.

voiced affricate) were produced as nasal stops. No productive distinction was made between voiced stops and fricatives. Voiced fricatives were still produced as voiced stops (but not nasal) more than 50% of the time 6 months after surgery. This error pattern, labeled "stopping," has been observed in both young normal children and phonologically delayed children. By 9 months postsurgery, Bob produced voiced fricatives correctly. The errors remaining in Bob's speech 9 months after surgery were age appropriate within class shifts in place of articulation (e.g., [f] for /θ/ and [w] for /l/).

In summary, Bob accommodated to his inability to achieve velopharyngeal closure in two ways. Either he produced the appropriate sound and allowed the audible NAE to occur (not really an accommodation), or he substituted a sound, which he was able to produce, that matched some of the features of the target sounds. For the [−voice] fricatives, he substituted the voiceless glide [h]; for the [+voice] stops and fricatives, he substituted a nasal stop with approximately the same place of articulation. Following surgery, productions that were correct but accompanied by NAE, became correct; productions that had been modified in some way took longer to change; and at least some of the errors that persisted at 6 months after surgery seemed to reflect his collapsing of the stop–fricative contrast in the voiced sounds prior to surgery.

Carol. Carol also had a unilateral complete cleft lip and palate. Her palate was repaired at 17 months, and the pharyngeal flap was performed at 33 months. The rules in Table 8.4 characterize Carol's word-initial consonant production prior to surgery and at intervals following surgery. Prior to surgery, Carol substituted glottal stops for velar stops (Rule 1) and glottalized other stops (Rule 2) (i.e., she produced a simultaneous glottal and oral stop for nonvelar oral stops). Affricates were produced in the same way, with both oral and glottal stopping. Both voiced and voiceless fricatives were generally produced as voiceless fricatives accompanied by NAE (Rule 3). Therefore, she preserved the voicing contrast and the oral–nasal contrast by glottalizing oral stops. She preserved the stop–fricative distinction (but not the voicing distinction among the fricatives) by producing fricatives as voiceless fricatives accompanied by NAE.

One month after surgery, velar stops were still produced as glottal stops. Glottalized productions of other stops still occurred, but were less frequent. By 7 months postsurgery, this glottal stop pattern had almost disappeared. The other error that appeared to be related to velopharyngeal incompetence was the presence of audible NAE during the production of fricatives and affricates. Unlike Bob, audible NAE did not disappear from Carol's speech immediately after surgery. No change had occurred in the frequency of NAE 1 month after surgery, and

TABLE 8.4

Frequency of Occurrence of Phonological Rules in Carol's Speech
Prior to and Following Pharyngeal Flap Surgery

		Session			
Rule		Prior to Surgery	1 Month	4 Months	7 Months
1. −nasal velar → glottal stop stop		5/6 (83%)	2/6 (33%)	2/6 (33%)	0/6 (0%)
2. −nasal −velar → glottalized stop		7/12 (58%)	3/12 (25%)	1/13 (8%)	1/12 (8%)
3. fricatives → +NAE −voice		15/21 (71%)	15/22 (68%)	7/21 (33%)	2/21 (9%)

NAE = nasal air emission.

4 months later one-third of her fricatives were still accompanied by NAE. It seemed clear that during this time Carol was actively using audible fricationalized nasal air as a feature of fricative production. It might be more accurate to call her productions nasal fricatives, except that there was usually an oral component also. Following surgery, it was difficult for Carol to produce the fricationalized nasal air, particularly simultaneous with the oral fricative. It required visible effort on her part. In Bob's speech, the audible NAE seemed to be a passive product of velopharyngeal incompetence, but in Carol, it was an active addition to her fricative productions that probably made fricatives more audible, just as the glottalization of oral stops made them more audible and distinct from nasal stops. Another way to phrase this is that Carol appeared to add a feature (glottalization) to the production of oral stops and a feature (fricationalized NAE) to the production of fricatives. These were not the "passive" result of velopharyngeal incompetence, but active, creative attempts to produce audible speech that matched the ambient model.

Seven months after surgery, Carol produced very few errors in word-initial consonants (Figure 8.3), and most of her errors seemed to be related to her strategies for dealing with velopharyngeal inadequacy. Place of articulation and voicing were never significant problems for her, and these aspects were correct 7 months after surgery.

These two children dealt with the problems associated with producing speech with an inadequate velopharyngeal mechanism in two differ-

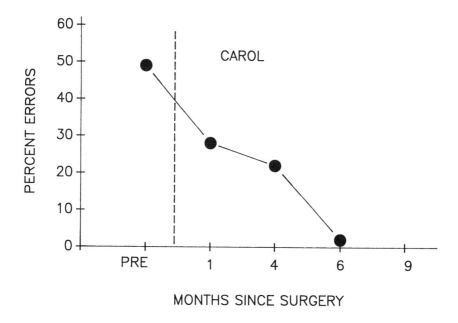

Figure 8.3 The percentage of consonants produced incorrectly by Carol prior to surgery and 1, 4, and 6 months after surgery.

ent ways. Each preserved some phonemic contrasts while merging or not preserving others. Audible nasal air emission was present in the speech of both children prior to surgery, but seemed to function differently in the two children. In one case (Bob), the changes that occurred following surgery suggest that the NAE was simply a by-product of poor velopharyngeal closure, whereas in the other case (Carol), NAE appeared to be a productive feature of fricative consonants that had to be "unlearned" following surgery.

Summary.   These examples are not meant to provide normative information or definitive descriptions of how children with cleft palate speak. They are intended as examples of ways of looking at the speech of children with cleft palate and of ways in which children with cleft palate are similar to and different from normal children. If normal children are active and creative as they learn to produce speech, so are children with cleft palate, but their creativity may lead them in different directions. Although children with cleft palate may sound different from normal children, the processes by which they attempt to produce speech may be very similar.

NOTES

1. [ɡ̞] represents a backed velar stop.
2. Following Chomsky and Halle (1968), [h] and [ʔ] were considered glides.

ACKNOWLEDGMENTS

The preparation of this chapter and the research reported here were supported in part by the Center for Research in Learning, Perception, and Cognition and the National Institute of Child Health and Human Development grant HD-07-151; in part by Social and Behavioral Sciences research grant 12-90 from the March of Dimes Birth Defects Foundation; and in part by a grant from the Ralph B. Kersten Research Fund. We also wish to thank both the University of Minnesota Cleft Palate Maxillofacial Clinic and the Minnesota Services for Children with Handicaps for their help.

REFERENCES

Becker, M., & Broen, P. (1972). A therapy program based on a distinctive feature analysis of misarticulation: A case study. *Journal of the Minnesota Speech and Hearing Association, 11,* 85–94.

Bernthal, J. E., & Beukelman, W. R. (1977). The effect of changes in velopharyngeal orifice area on vowel intensity. *Cleft Palate Journal, 14,* 63–77.

Broen, P. A., Felsenfeld, S., & Kittelson-Bacon, C. (1986). Predicting from the phonological patterns observed in children with cleft palate. In *Proceedings of the 11th University of Wisconsin Symposium on Research in Child Language Disorders.* Madison: University of Wisconsin.

Broen, P. A., & Jons, S. M. (1979). The perception and production of speech by a misarticulating child. In H. L. Pick, Jr., H. W. Stevenson, A. Steinschneider, J. E. Singer, & H. Leibowitz (Eds.), *Psychology: From practice to theory.* New York: Plenum.

Byrne, M. C., Shelton, R. L., & Diedrich, W. M. (1961). Articulatory skill, physical management, and classification of children with cleft palates. *Journal of Speech and Hearing Disorders, 26,* 326–333.

Bzoch, K. R. (1956). *An investigation of the speech of pre-school cleft palate children.* Unpublished doctoral dissertation, Northwestern University, Evanston, IL.

Bzoch, K. R. (1965). Articulation proficiency and error patterns of preschool cleft palate and normal children. *Cleft Palate Journal, 2,* 340–349.

Bzoch, K. R. (1979). Measurement and assessment of categorical aspects of cleft palate speech. In K. R. Bzoch (Ed.), *Communicative disorders related to cleft lip and palate.* Boston: Little Brown.

Chomsky, N., & Halle, M. (1968). *Sound patterns of English.* New York: Harper and Row.

Compton, A. J. (1970). Generative studies of children's phonological disorders. *Journal of Speech and Hearing Disorders, 35,* 315–339.

Counihan, D. T. (1956). *A clinical study of the speech efficiency and structural adequacy of operated adolescent and adult cleft palate persons.* Unpublished doctoral dissertation, Northwestern University, Evanston, IL.

Dinnsen, D. A. (1984). Methods and empirical issues in analyzing functional misarticulation. In M. Elbert, D. A. Dinnsen, & G. Weismer (Eds.), *Phonological theory and the misarticulating child* (ASHA Monograph No. 22). Rockville, MD: American Speech–Language–Hearing Association.

Dorf, D. S., & Curtin, J. W. (1982). Early cleft palate repair and speech outcome. *Plastic and Reconstructive Surgery, 70,* 74–79.

Estrem, T. (1984). *A comparison of the speech patterns and word choices of very young children with and without cleft palates.* Unpublished master's thesis, University of Minnesota, Minneapolis.

Estrem, T., & Broen, P. A. (1989). Early speech productions of children with cleft palate. *Journal of Speech and Hearing Research, 32,* 12–23.

Ferguson, C. A., & Farwell, C. B. (1975). Words and sounds in early language acquisition: English initial consonants in the first fifty words. *Language, 51,* 419–439.

Fey, M., & Gandour, J. (1982). Rule discovery in early phonology acquisition. *Journal of Child Language, 9,* 71–82.

Fletcher, S. G. (1978). *Diagnosing speech disorders from cleft palate.* New York: Grune and Stratton.

Hodson, B. W., & Paden, E. P. (1981). Phonological processes which characterize unintelligible and intelligible speech in early childhood. *Journal of Speech and Hearing Disorders, 46,* 369–373.

Hyman, L. (1975). *Phonology: Theory and analysis.* New York: Holt.

Ingram, D. (1974a). Fronting in child phonology. *Journal of Child Language, 1,* 233–241.

Ingram, D. (1974b). Phonological rules in young children. *Journal of Child Language, 1,* 49–64.

Ingram, D. (1976). *Phonological disability in children.* New York: Elsevier.

Ingram, D. (1979). Phonological patterns in the speech of young children. In P. Fletcher & M. Garman (Eds.), *Language acquisition.* Cambridge: Cambridge University Press.

Ingram, D. (1981). *Procedures for the phonological analysis of children's language.* Baltimore: University Park Press.

Isshiki, M. D., Honjow, I., & Morimoto, M. (1968). Effects of velopharyngeal incompetence upon speech. *Cleft Palate Journal, 5,* 297–310.

Jakobson, R. (1968). *Child language, aphasia, and phonological universals.* The Hauge: Mouton.

Kuhl, P., & Meltzoff, A. N. (1982). The bimodal perception of speech in infancy. *Science, 218,* 1138–1141.

Leopold, W. F. (1947). *Speech development of a bilingual child: A linguist's record. Vol. 2. Sound-learning in the first two years.* Evanston, IL: Northwestern University.

Leopold, W. F. (1953). Patterning in children's language learning. *Language Learning, 5,* 1–14.

Letcher, L. M., Broen, P. A., & Moller, K. T. (1986). *A longitudinal study: Phonological changes associated with pharyngeal flap surgery.* Paper presented at the annual meeting of the American Speech–Language–Hearing Association, Detroit.

Locke, J. L. (1983). *Phonological acquisition and change.* New York: Academic Press.

Lynch, J. I., Fox, D. R., & Brookshire, B. L. (1983). Phonological proficiency of two cleft palate toddlers with school-age follow-up. *Journal of Speech and Hearing Disorders, 48,* 274–285.

McReynolds, L. V., & Huston, K. (1971). A distinctive feature analysis of children's misarticulations. *Journal of Speech and Hearing Disorders, 36,* 155–166.

McWilliams, B. J., Morris, H. L., & Shelton, R. L. (1984). *Cleft palate speech.* St. Louis: Mosby.

Menn, L. (1983). Development of articulatory, phonetic, and phonological capabilities. In B. Butterworth (Ed.), *Language production: Volume 2. Development, writing, and other language processes.* New York: Academic Press.

Menyuk, P. (1968). The role of distinctive features in children's acquisition of phonology. *Journal of Speech and Hearing Research, 11,* 138–146.

Mills, A. (1983). The acquisition of speech sounds in the visually-handicapped child. In A. E. Mills (Ed.), *Language acquisition in the blind child: Normal and deficient.* London: Croom Helm.

Moll, K. L. (1968). Speech characteristics of individuals with cleft lip and palate. In D. C. Spriestersbach & D. Sherman (Eds.), *Cleft palate and communication.* New York: Academic Press.

Morley, M. E. (1970). *Cleft palate and speech* (7th ed.). Baltimore: Williams and Wilkins.

Morris, H. L. (1962). Communication skills of children with cleft lips and palates. *Journal of Speech and Hearing Research, 5,* 79–90.

Morris, H. L. (1968). Etiological bases for speech problems. In D. C. Spriestersbach & D. Sherman (Eds.), *Cleft palate and communication.* New York: Academic Press.

Morris, H. L. (1979). Evaluation of abnormal articulation patterns. In K. R. Bzoch (Ed.), *Communicative disorders related to cleft lip and palate.* Boston: Little Brown.

Moskowitz, A. (1970). The two-year stage in the acquisition of English phonology. *Language, 46,* 426–441.

O'Gara, M. M., & Logemann, J. A. (1988). Phonetic analysis of the speech development of babies with cleft palate. *Cleft Palate Journal, 25,* 122–134.

Oller, D. K. (1986). Metaphonology and infant vocalizations. In F. Lindblom & R. Zetterstrom (Eds.), *Precursors of early speech.* Basinstoke, Hamshire: Macmillan.

Oller, D. K., & Eilers, R. E. (1988). The role of audition in infant babbling. *Child Development, 59,* 441–449.

Olson, D. A. (1965). *A descriptive study of the speech development of a group of infants with unoperated cleft palates.* Unpublished doctoral dissertation, Northwestern University, Evanston, IL.

Peters, A. M. (1977). Language learning strategies. *Language, 53,* 560–573.

Prather, E. M., Hedrick, D. L., & Kern, C. A. (1975). Articulation development in children aged two to four years. *Journal of Speech and Hearing Disorders, 40,* 179–191.

Priestly, T. M. S. (1977). One idiosyncratic strategy in the acquisition of phonology. *Journal of Child Language, 4,* 45–66.

Sherman, D., Spriestersbach, D. C., & Noll, J. D. (1959). Glottal stops in the speech of children with cleft palates. *Journal of Speech and Hearing Disorders, 24,* 37–42.

Shriberg, L. D., & Kwiatkowski, J. (1980). *Natural process analysis.* New York: Wiley.

Shriberg, L. D., & Smith, A. J. (1983). Phonological correlates of middle-ear involvement in speech-delayed children: A methodological note. *Journal of Speech and Hearing Research, 26,* 293–297.

Smith, N. V. (1973). *The acquisition of phonology.* Cambridge: Cambridge University Press.

Spriestersbach, D. C., Darley, F. L., & Rouse, V. (1956). Articulation of a group of children with cleft lips and palates. *Journal of Speech and Hearing Disorders, 21,* 436–445.

Spriestersbach, D. C., Moll, K. L., & Morris, H. L. (1961). Subject classification and articulation of speakers with cleft palates. *Journal of Speech and Hearing Research, 4,* 362–372.

Spriestersbach, D. C., & Powers, G. R. (1959). Nasality in isolated vowels and connected speech of children with cleft palates. *Journal of Speech and Hearing Research, 2,* 40–45.

Stampe, D. (1969). The acquisition of phonetic representation.*Papers from the 5th Regional Meeting of the Chicago Linguistic Society* (pp. 443–454). Chicago: Chicago Linguistic Society.

Starr, C. (1956). *A study of some of the characteristics of the speech and speech mechanisms of a group of cleft palate children.* Unpublished doctoral dissertation, Northwestern University, Evanston, IL.

Stoel-Gammon, C., & Cooper, J. (1984). Patterns of early lexical and phonological development. *Journal of Child Language, 11,* 247–271.

Studdert-Kennedy, M. (1983). On learning to speak. *Human Neurobiology, 2,* 191–195.

Studdert-Kennedy, M. (1987). The phoneme as a perceptuomotor structure. In A. Allport, D. Mackay, W. Printz, & E. Scheerer (Eds.), *Language perception and production* (pp. 67–84). New York: Academic Press.

Subtelny, J., Koepp-Baker, H., & Subtelny, J. D. (1961). Palatal function and cleft palate speech. *Journal of Speech and Hearing Disorders, 26,* 213–224.

Templin, M. C. (1957). *Certain language skills in children* (Institute of Child Welfare Monograph Series 26). Minneapolis: University of Minnesota Press.

Trost, J. E. (1981). Articulatory additions to the classical description of the speech of persons with cleft palate. *Cleft Palate Journal, 18,* 193–203.

Van Demark, D. R., & Van Demark, A. H. (1967). Misarticulation of cleft palate children achieving velopharyngeal closure and children with functional speech problems. *Cleft Palate Journal, 4,* 31–37.

Velten, H. V. (1943). The growth of phonemic and lexical patterns in infant language. *Language, 19,* 440–444.

Weiner, F. F. (1979). *Phonological process analysis.* Austin, TX: PRO-ED.

Wells, C. F. (1971). *Cleft palate and its associated speech disorders.* New York: McGraw-Hill.

Westlake, H., & Rutherford, D. (1966). *Cleft palate.* Englewood Cliffs, NJ: Prentice-Hall.

CHAPTER 9

Evaluation of Velopharyngeal Function

Jerald B. Moon

> *Moon provides a comprehensive review and analysis of procedures used to evaluate velopharyngeal function. He stresses the importance of listeners' judgments of the presence of hypernasality in determining the presence of velopharyngeal incompetence, and discusses advantages and disadvantages in the use of kinematic, acoustic, and airflow measurements in confirming listeners' judgments and providing further information on the nature of velopharyngeal function.*

1. *What are the limitations of visual intraoral examinations in assessing velopharyngeal function?*
2. *What observations can be made from videofluoroscopy that provides frontal views of velopharyngeal function? Why are clinicians interested in these observations?*
3. *What observations of velopharyngeal function can be made from nasally inserted endoscopes? What does Moon consider to be the main disadvantage to the use of endoscopes?*
4. *How does the Nasometer use sound pressure measurements to derive the measure of nasalance?*
5. *How can measurements of air pressure and airflow be used to determine the size of the orifice that exists when velopharyngeal closure is incompetent?*

All speech clinicians involved with persons with cleft palate regularly face the challenge of evaluating a velopharyngeal (VP) mechanism to determine how it works, or why it does not work as it should. The results of VP evaluation are also important to surgical and dental colleagues serving on interdisciplinary teams because these specialists are frequently called upon to treat a VP mechanism that does not function appropriately for speech. In this chapter, I present some of the instruments that the diagnostician may use for VP evaluations.

Before I continue, however, some discussion regarding terminology used to describe VP function is warranted. Terms such as *inadequacy, incompetence,* and *insufficiency* appear in literature references and clinic reports. As alluded to by Loney and Bloem (1987), application of these different terms in a redundant or contradictory manner hinders discussion of the problem, especially in the context of a multidisciplinary team. Loney and Bloem recommended that insufficiency be used to refer to any malformation resulting in imperfect closure. This term would encompass the terms incompetence and inadequacy. Folkins (1988) correctly pointed out that use of the term *perfect* may cause some significant problems of interpretation. Is "perfect" closure a prerequisite to normally perceived speech? The term incompetence was suggested by Loney and Bloem (1987) to describe a deficit in neuromuscular functioning, whereas they proposed inadequacy as a descriptor of imperfect VP closure caused by a deficit of tissue.

Although it may be true that VP disorders are routed in anatomical (structural) and/or neuromuscular (movement) deficits, Folkins (1988) argued that we do not yet possess the quantitative ability, or the theoretical need, to separate speakers on the basis of neuromuscular versus structural deficits. Incompetent is defined in the dictionary as "lacking the qualities needed for effective action" and "inadequate to or unsuitable for a particular purpose" (*Webster's Seventh New Collegiate Dictionary,* 1965). This definition implies not causation, but simply that an end result cannot be attained. The end result in this case is speech that is perceived to be within normal limits. Therefore, the term incompetent is applied throughout this chapter to refer to abnormal function of the VP mechanism.

Evaluation of any mechanism must be based on knowledge of normal form and function; that is, the diagnostician must know the anatomy of the normal VP mechanism (form), and must understand the physiological events associated with normal VP movement (function). A number of excellent descriptions of VP anatomy appear in the literature, and the reader is referred to reviews by Dickson (1975), Kuehn (1979), Lubker (1975), and McWilliams, Morris, and Shelton (1984). For purposes of orientation, a schematic diagram of the head showing the VP region in relation to other craniofacial structures and cavities is pre-

sented in Figure 9.1. The physiological events associated with VP closing and opening gestures during speech (i.e., function) are complex. It
is beyond the scope of this chapter to discuss the physiology of VP function in detail; however, because this discussion of instrumental analysis of the velopharynx is predicated on a basic understanding of the
physiological events associated with normal VP movement, a brief
review of those events is presented here.

Kinematics

Normal VP closure is thought to consist of a velar and a pharyngeal
movement component (Skolnick, McCall, & Barnes, 1973). The velar
component includes elevation and posterior elongation or stretching
of the velum. Numerous investigators (Mourino & Weinberg, 1975;
Neiman & Simpson, 1975; Simpson & Chin, 1981; Simpson & Colton,
1980) have documented the fact that, during closure, the velum is elon-
gated relative to rest. According to Skolnick et al. (1973), the pharyngeal component includes all movements of the nasopharyngeal walls.
No distinction is made between lateral and posterior pharyngeal wall
movement, and the nasopharyngeal walls are thought to move as a
single functional unit. It is generally accepted, however, that mesial
movement of the lateral pharyngeal walls constitutes a most significant aspect of the "nasopharyngeal" component (Iglesias, Kuehn, &
Morris, 1980). The relative contribution of the velum and lateral pharyngeal walls to closure has been studied by Croft, Shprintzen, and Rakoff
(1981), Skolnick (1975), and Zwitman, Sonderman, and Ward (1974), who
described a number of patterns, ranging from exclusive velar movement
to exclusive lateral pharyngeal wall movement.

Acoustics

Acoustic events associated with VP function involve the movement of
vibrational energy through the vocal tract. During normal speech production, VP closure serves to impede the transmission of sound energy
into and through the nasal cavity. The sound resonator, in this case,
comprises the pharyngeal and oral cavity. Differing oral cavity shapes
that result from articulator movements give rise to different acoustic
filters. The passage of acoustic energy through these filters produces
complex sounds with different spectral "shapes" that are perceived as
different oral speech sounds (Daniloff, Schuckers, & Feth, 1980; Peterson
& Barney, 1952). In some instances (e.g., nasal consonants /m/, /n/, /ŋ/),
the VP mechanism offers minimal impedance to sound transmission
relative to a much greater oral impedance. Here, the nasal tract contributes to sound resonation and the oral cavity outlet is closed. Energy
in the nasal airway is dissipated in two principal ways: While the

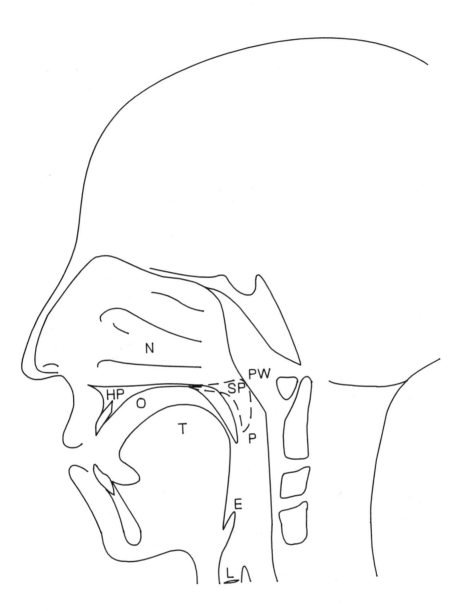

Figure 9.1 Sagittal schematic view of the head showing structures of the oral and pharyngeal region in relation to other craniofacial structures. Soft palate (SP) shown
at rest (solid line) and during /s/ production (dotted line). N = nasal cavity;
O = oral cavity; P = oropharynx; HP = hard palate; PW = posterior pharyngeal wall; E = epiglottis; L = larynx; T = tongue.

primary output is an acoustic signal at the nares, some energy can also be expected to vibrate the nasal mucosa and cartilage and the overlying bones. This vibration is easily demonstrated by placing a finger on the nasal bone while humming.

Aerodynamics

Perhaps the most basic physiological event associated with normal speech production is the movement of a pressurized air stream through the vocal tract. The aerodynamics of speech production has been studied extensively (Stathopoulos & Weismer, 1985; Thompson & Hixon, 1979; Warren, 1979, 1982). Simply stated, normal oral articulation involves no (or at least very little) nasal airflow and a large pressure drop across the VP orifice. The result is an infinite (or at least very large) VP aerodynamic resistance and the ability to develop oral airflows and air pressures of sufficient magnitude to produce appropriately resonated speech output. Conversely, normal nasal resonance involves airflow through the nasal cavity. Lowering of the velum to allow for the passage of air results in a much lower pressure drop across the VP port and much lower VP resistance. The magnitude of these parameters depends, among other things, on the amount of VP opening present.

Instrumental Evaluation

The many approaches to instrumental evaluation of the VP mechanism vary from fairly simplistic in concept and design to highly sophisticated. VP evaluation is usually done because someone perceives that an individual's speech deviates from normal. It is widely accepted that the ear is the first and primary diagnostic tool:

> If the individual's speech is "normal" sounding during conversational speech, then there is no need to do any further testing—except for research purposes ... The most valid measure of adequate functioning is the sound produced while talking. When conversational speech deviates from normal, our task is to determine why. (Bensen, 1977, p. 46)

Ultimately, by simply listening, a speech clinician judges a person's speech to be within normal limits or suspects a potential VP problem that warrants, as termed by McWilliams et al. (1984), a definitive assessment.

Simply described, the VP mechanism is a valve that must open and close during a variety of speech and nonspeech tasks. Given that a patient is suspected of speaking with a dysfunctional system, the clinician should evaluate the structure of the VP mechanism, and its ability to move appropriately during speech. The structure of the mechanism is best evaluated by comparing it with normal. Study of the motion (kinematics) of the mechanism can be accomplished in a number of ways. One can simply watch the mechanism move, or one can evaluate the consequences of VP movement. For example, acoustic and aerodynamic events in the vocal tract are known to be intimately related to movements of VP structures. In defining VP inadequacy, Schwartz (1975) referred to "an opening between the nasopharynx and the oropharynx during speech of sufficient magnitude to produce a condition of acoustic coupling between nose and mouth great enough for trained listeners to perceive a quality called hypernasality," and to "an opening between oral and nasopharynx great enough to allow an escape of air from the nose during the production of high intraoral air pressure consonants and to thereby create a condition known as nasal emission" (p. 305).

Lubker and Moll (1965) referred to those evaluative approaches that allow the diagnostician to make direct observations of the articulatory structures as "direct techniques," and those approaches that provide data that may be used to make inferences regarding VP movement as "indirect techniques." Evaluative techniques may be grouped further into primary measures (measures of structure and movement per se) and secondary measures (acoustics and aerodynamics); that is, *primary* measures are those that allow for evaluation of the *structure* and *kinematics of the VP mechanism,* whereas *secondary* measures are those that involve an evaluation of the *consequences of VP function* on other speech physiological parameters. These groupings are illustrated in Table 9.1.

TABLE 9.1

Evaluative Techniques Used to Assess Velopharyngeal Form and Function

	Direct	Indirect
Primary measures	Lateral still radiography Frontal still radiography Motion picture radiography Ultrasound Endoscopy Magnetic resonance imaging Unaided eye visual exam	Phototransducer Electromyography Movement transduction
Secondary measures Acoustics		Listener judgment Sound spectrography Sound pressure Accelerometry
Aerodynamics		Air pressure Airflow

This categorization is not meant to suggest that primary measures are more important than secondary measures. The distinction is offered simply to differentiate between the types of data that might be collected that provide information about the VP mechanism and its function. This information should contribute to the clinical decision regarding what the speaker can and cannot do velopharyngeally to produce acceptable speech.

DIRECT PRIMARY MEASURES

Direct primary measures used to evaluate the structure and movement abilities of the VP mechanism include visual intraoral examination, a number of radiographic procedures, magnetic resonance imaging, ultrasound, and endoscopy.

Visual Intraoral Examination

It seems intuitively obvious to begin an evaluation of the VP mechanism by looking in the mouth (Figure 9.2). In fact, 88% of the speech pathologists surveyed by Schneider and Shprintzen (1980) utilized intra-

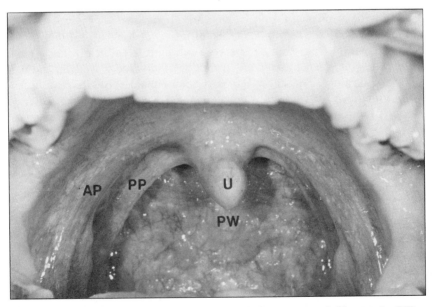

Figure 9.2 Intraoral view of the oral cavity and pharynx at rest. U = uvula; PW = posterior pharyngeal wall; AP = anterior faucial pillar; PP = posterior faucial pillar.

oral examination in assessing VP function. Intraoral examination should be targeted toward an inspection of the lips, teeth, tongue position and function, tonsils, hard palate, soft palate, uvula, and pharyngeal walls (Hirschberg, 1986; McWilliams et al., 1984). Various questions should be considered: How do these structures function during speech? Are there any observable fistulae in the hard or soft palate? Is there notching of the uvula that would indicate a submucous cleft of the palate? Does the velum move on phonation? What is the extent of movement? Does it move symmetrically? Does the length of the velum appear normal? Is there pharyngeal wall movement on phonation?

Neither researchers nor clinicians uniformly agree on the utility of the unaided visual examination of the oral cavity. Yules and Chase (1971) suggested that one should view the mechanism to estimate

> length of soft palate, soft palate thickness, palate closure, quickness of motion, amplitude of motion, depth of nasopharynx, presence or absence of Passavant's ridge, presence or absence of an adenoidal mass, movement of posterior and lateral pharynx, characteristics of the hard palate, . . . , presence or absence of fistulas. (p. 454)

Hirschberg (1986) advocated estimation of the thickness, length, and mobility of the soft palate; the condition of the lateral and posterior pharyngeal walls; and the extent of any VP gap.

Others support the view that, although the intraoral examination can provide some useful information and should not be ignored, it should be much more limited in scope. Evaluation of length and mobility of the soft palate from this perspective can be misleading (Pigott, 1980). The posterior pharyngeal wall cannot be visualized well from the front of the oral cavity. The soft palate may show considerable movement from this view, but still not contact a recessed posterior pharyngeal wall. McWilliams et al. (1984) suggested a number of aspects of VP form and function that cannot be assessed reliably on visual exam. These include

> the adequacy of velar length, palatal elevation, movement of lateral and posterior pharyngeal walls, VP valving, occult submucous cleft palate wherein the levator muscles insert into the hard palate instead of forming a muscle sling for velar elevation . . . , [and] malformation of the musculus uvulae. (p. 287)

Using lateral-view cinefluorography as the referent, Eisenbach and Williams (1984) evaluated the accuracy of statements made on the basis of unaided visual examination of the VP mechanism. Statements regarding velar length, depth of nasopharynx, VP closure, and velar mobility were compared with objective data obtained from cinefluorographic films. Rates of agreement ranged from 52% (velar mobility) to 71% (VP closure). The overall rate of agreement was only 60%. Not surprisingly, the data supported the view that more objective assessments of VP form and function should be utilized.

Lateral Still Radiography

Lateral-view still or cephalometric radiography represents one of the oldest instrumental approaches to the evaluation and study of the VP mechanism. One of the earlier applications of this technique for the study of speech was reported by Hixon (1949), who used lateral-view still radiograms to assess the structure of the VP mechanism and surrounding tissues.

The technique of lateral-view still radiography involves positioning the patient between the X-ray tube and a sheet of X-ray film (Figure 9.3). The head is immobilized with rubber pads to ensure that the head is not tilted to one side. This also maintains each patient's head at a constant distance from the film, allowing for a constant magnification factor. Accurate measurements of the size of various structures can then be made from the exposed and developed film. High-speed electrons are emitted from the X-ray tube. They pass into the body part in their path, and are selectively absorbed by the tissue. The amount of absorption

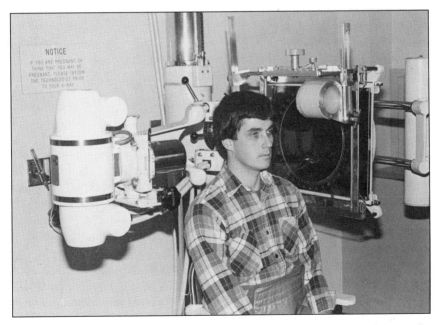

Figure 9.3 Positioning of the patient for lateral still radiograph. X-ray tube is on the left. Film holder is on the right.

depends on, among other things, the density of the tissue. Those electrons not absorbed pass through to the X-ray film, where the degree of exposure at any given point varies with the magnitude of electrons hitting it. The result is a radiograph or X-ray (Figure 9.4).

Because this approach involves a picture taken at one instant in time, the speech tasks that may be employed are somewhat limited. Typically, radiographs are taken at rest, during a sustained /s/, and perhaps during prolongation of a vowel. In some instances, a barium solution is injected either nasally or orally to coat the surfaces of the velum and pharyngeal walls (Cohn, Rood, McWilliams, Skolnick, & Abdelmalek, 1981). Because barium is a radiopaque material, it allows for better visualization of the margins of the velum and pharyngeal walls. The radiation exposure level for a single lateral still radiograph of the VP mechanism is about 0.01 to 0.02 roentgens.

Interpretation of lateral-view still radiographs may be subjective or objective. Van Demark, Kuehn, and Tharp (1975) developed a subjective X-ray rating scheme in an attempt to standardize interpretation of lateral radiograph images. They used the scale, in one instance, to predict the need for secondary management of the soft palate. On the

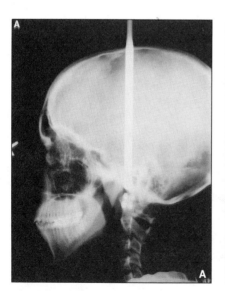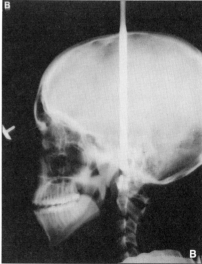

Figure 9.4 Lateral still radiographs taken at rest (A) and during production of /s/ (B). Vertical white bars are ear rods used for head immobilization. Elevation of the soft palate to contact the posterior pharyngeal wall may be seen during /s/ production.

basis of X-ray ratings alone, eventual outcome (i.e., pharyngeal flap required vs. not required) was correctly predicted in 92% of their patients.

The relationship between the presence of adenoid tissue and the ability to achieve VP closure in cleft palate is well documented. Subjective interpretation of lateral-view still radiographs was used by Mason and Warren (1980) to predict possible VP closure problems following adenoid size reduction. They suggested, however, that lateral-view still radiographs should not be used routinely for this purpose. Objective measurements taken from lateral-view still radiographs also have been used to document relationships among VP structures as a function of factors such as growth (Subtelny, 1957; Subtelny & Koepp-Baker, 1956) and surgical alteration.

Lateral-view still X-rays were once a mainstay of the evaluation process at some centers. An obvious advantage of this approach is that it allows for direct observation of the VP mechanism. One can readily assess structural features such as palatal length and adenoid pad presence. One can also assess relationships among structures. The procedure is relatively simple to complete, reliable, and provides quantifiable data. However, these positive aspects are outweighed by the liabilities of the approach. It is important to stress that the VP mechanism is a three-dimensional structure. Movements occur during opening and closing in both the sagittal (lateral) and frontal planes. By contrast, lateral X-rays are only two dimensional. Only structural features lying in the sagittal plane (anterior–posterior and superior–inferior) are represented. A second major disadvantage is that data collected is static in nature; that is, the radiograph depicts events occurring at one instant in time. The two common tasks (rest vs. prolonged [s]) yield information only on the extremes of movement. Events happening in between are not captured.

Proponents of the technique argue that velar "activity" seen on lateral-view still X-ray is an accurate indicator of velar activity actually occurring during ongoing speech. For example, Bzoch (1968) concluded that closure, or lack thereof, during repetitive consonant–vowel (CV) syllables as seen on lateral still radiographs was a valid predictor of VP integrity during connected speech. Similarly, Lubker and Morris (1968) stated that an estimate of the extent of VP opening can be reliably obtained from lateral still pictures taken during production of /s/. However, Shelton, Brooks, and Youngstrom (1964) argued that VP function as assessed during prolongation of an isolated phoneme is not indicative of functional status during speech. Williams and Eisenbach (1981) compared decisions regarding the functional status of the VP mechanism made from lateral still radiographs with those made from motion picture radiographs (to be discussed later). Inaccurate evaluation "of the competency or incompetency of the VP sphincter as viewed during the production of the sustained vowel /i/ would have occurred on 27% of the cases and 30% of the cases during the production of the CV syllable /pi/" (p. 49). The point is further illustrated by Stringer and Witzel (1989), who found that for assessing adequacy of closure, the lateral view alone produced a large number of false positives. Finally, the exposure to ionizing radiation must also be considered a disadvantage of this approach and, in fact, of all the radiographic approaches to be discussed in this section.

Despite its disadvantages, lateral-view still radiography continues to be part of the diagnostic battery in many clinics and centers. In Schneider and Shprintzen's (1980) survey, 50% of the speech pathologists who responded utilized lateral still radiographs in evaluation of VP function. Perhaps as a sign of growing apprehension toward lateral-view still radiography, only 10% of the respondents to Pannbacker et al.'s (1984) survey used the technique.

Frontal Still Radiography

The frontal view would seem useful in the evaluation of VP function because it should permit visualization of the lateral pharyngeal walls. An inherent problem with this view, however, is that the area of interest is hidden behind the bony facial structures. Kuehn and Dolan (1975) attempted to circumvent this problem using a technique that blurs structures outside the target area. Tomographic systems consist of three basic elements: an X-ray source, an object to be X-rayed, and recording material (e.g., film). Production of the tomographic effect involves moving any two of these elements synchronously in relation to the third element. As with other radiographic techniques, the patient is positioned between the X-ray source and the film. The technique differs from traditional approaches in that the X-ray source and film can be moved in opposite directions through an arc in the transverse plane (horizontal). Using information gathered from a lateral still radiograph, the equipment is adjusted such that the focal plane of the image is centered on the point of interest (Figure 9.5). By moving the film and X-ray tube while the film is being exposed, images of structures in front of and behind the target area (in this case the VP mechanism) are blurred while the image of the area of interest is clearly delineated. The tomogram is obtained simultaneously with a second lateral still radiograph while the patient prolongs a vowel sound. Kuehn and Dolan asserted that this technique permits measurement of the degree and level of lateral pharyngeal wall movement in relation to the velum and posterior pharyngeal wall. The result is, in essence, a static three-dimensional

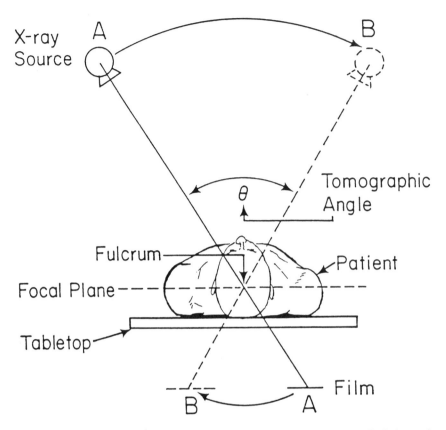

Figure 9.5 Example of a tomographic system. (From "A Tomographic Technique of Assessing Lateral Pharyngeal Wall Displacement" by D. Kuehn and K. Dolan, 1975, *Cleft Palate Journal, 12,* p. 202. Copyright 1975 by American Cleft Palate–Craniofacial Association. Reprinted with permission.)

representation of the VP mechanism (Iglesias et al., 1980). Radiation dosage was reported to be approximately 2 roentgens.

This technique has not been used extensively in research applications and is not used, to my knowledge, clinically. Frontal tomography represents an improvement on lateral still radiography and frontal still radiography in that (a) one can evaluate the magnitude and level of lateral pharyngeal wall movement in relation to other oral and oropharyngeal structures, and (b) the masking of the mechanism by overlying bony structures is removed. However, it suffers from the same liability as the lateral still radiograph in that it provides only a static view of a dynamic mechanism. Also, the radiation dosage is considerably higher.

Motion Picture Radiography/Videofluoroscopy

Recognizing the limitations of still radiographs regarding generalization from a static view to performance in connected speech, Carrell (1952) introduced lateral-view motion picture radiography to the study of VP function. In contrast to the lateral still technique, cineradiography allowed for the visualization of VP structures in motion.

The procedures involved in obtaining motion picture radiographs are not significantly different from those discussed for still radiographs. The patient is seated between the X-ray tube and the film at right angles to the path of the X-ray beam with the head stabilized to prevent image blurring movements. Instead of a sheet of photographic film, an intensifying screen and motion picture camera are used. Electrons hitting the intensifying screen cause it to emit light, which is then filmed by the movie camera. The intensity of light emitted at any point on the screen is a function of the number of electrons hitting the screen, which in turn varies with the density of the body part being traversed. With this technique, the speech sample is not limited to prolonged vowels or sibilants, but can include syllables, and sentences or connected speech.

Cineradiography (also referred to as cinefluoroscopy) has a rather extensive history of use in both clinical and research applications. Images may be rated with respect to extent of VP closure (McWilliams-Neely & Bradley, 1964) or measured to determine structural relationships in the pharyngeal cavity during speech (Moll, 1960, 1964). The technique has been employed in research studies to evaluate the mechanism of VP closure (Warren & Hofmann, 1961), articulatory movements (Wada, Yasumoto, Ikeoka, Fujika, & Yoshinaga, 1970), results of pharyngeal flap surgery (Harrington, 1970; Subtelny, McCormack, Subtelny, & Cichoke, 1960), velar movement (Kuehn & Moll, 1976; Lubker, 1968; Seaver & Kuehn, 1980; Shaw, Folkins, & Kuehn, 1980), and relationships between perceived nasality and VP movement (Karnell, Folkins, & Morris, 1985).

With advances in technology, the motion picture camera was replaced by video recording systems (McWilliams & Girdany, 1964). Video systems have some distinct advantages over cine systems. A much lower radiation dosage level is required for video systems than for cine or movie film systems. Video systems provide the ability to replay and evaluate the recorded exam immediately. Because cine systems use motion picture film, a developing process is involved. There are also, however, some inherent disadvantages involved with video recording systems. The standard camera speed of a cine unit is 24 frames per second, or 42 milliseconds per frame. Although this may be sufficient for clinical purposes (Shelton, Brooks, Youngstrom, Diedrich, & Brooks, 1963), it does not allow for precise documentation of articulatory movements that occur within a shorter time frame (Shelton & Trier, 1976). However, use of a high-speed cine camera allows for film speeds in excess of 100 frames per second (10 milliseconds per frame). Video systems do not have this capability. Standard video recorders function at a rate analogous to 30 cine frames per second. Although this is slightly faster than the standard cine speed, video systems do not possess the capability to operate at higher speeds.

Recognizing the inability of lateral-view projections to provide information regarding movement in the frontal plane, Skolnick (1969, 1970) introduced the concept of multiview videofluoroscopy. This approach is designed to assess VP function using three separate views (sagittal or lateral, frontal, base) projecting three anatomic planes (sagittal, coronal, transverse). The lateral view permits visualization of anterior–posterior velar movement and structural relationships between the soft palate and posterior pharyngeal wall. The frontal view permits visualization of lateral pharyngeal wall movement and vertical positioning of VP structures. The base view permits visualization of the sphincteric component of VP movement (Skolnick, 1970). Patient positioning for these three views is illustrated in Figure 9.6. For the frontal view, the patient is positioned facing the X-ray tube. For a base view, the subject lies prone on the fluoroscopy table with the head and shoulders elevated (sphinx position). The three views are filmed consecutively, but when interpreted, provide a composite three-dimensional "picture" of VP structure and function.

Although it is generally accepted that the lateral and frontal views can provide valuable diagnostic information, usefulness of the base view has been criticized (Shelton & Trier, 1976). Positioning for the basal view requires considerable hyperextension of the neck. Shelton and Trier cautioned that the closure phenomenon revealed on a base view may differ from that revealed on either a lateral or a frontal view. Williams and Eisenbach (1981) supported this view and proposed the use of only the lateral and frontal views. Omission of the base view negates the ability to directly observe the sphincteric component of closure; however, combined use of lateral and frontal views still allows for a three-dimension representation of the mechanism. In addition, Stringer and Witzel (1989) assessed the appropriateness of the Towne view (a cross-sectional view of VP function), concluding that it compared well with nasal endoscopic views of the velopharynx.

Multiview videofluoroscopy overcomes many of the disadvantages associated with the lateral-view still radiograph approach. It offers a view of the VP mechanism in motion during connected speech. It depicts,

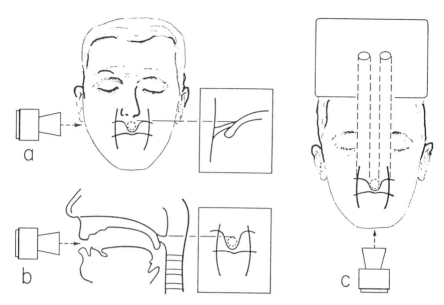

Figure 9.6 Radiographic positioning of patient for (a) lateral, (b) frontal, and (c) base views of the velopharyngeal mechanism. The patient depicted here has a pharyngeal flap. (From "Velopharyngeal Competence and Incompetence Following Pharyngeal Flap Surgery: Videofluoroscopic Study in Multiple Projections" by M. L. Skolnick and G. McCall, 1972, *Cleft Palate Journal, 9*, p. 2. Copyright 1972 by American Cleft Palate–Craniofacial Association. Reprinted with permission.)

through interpretation of multiple images, the VP mechanism in three dimensions. Multiple viewing techniques, be they two or three view, are not without liabilities, however. Because the multiple views are obtained consecutively, the patient is exposed to radiation two or three times. In addition, one must assume that the VP mechanism performs the same way each time. Despite these drawbacks, McWilliams et al. (1981) judged multiview videofluoroscopy to be a highly desirable tool. They compared videofluoroscopic data with data collected using manometry and pressure–flow techniques, using perceptual judgments of speech as the standard. Videofluoroscopic findings were "less variable and reflected what was heard in the speech pattern more often than did any of the other measures. In addition, videofluoroscopy provided a visual image of the mechanism that was not available from the other devices" (p. 7). Given the desirability of a three-dimensional interpretation, some might consider it surprising that this technique does not enjoy more widespread use. Whereas 72% of those surveyed by Schneider and Shprintzen (1980) used lateral-view cine- or videofluorography, only 24%

employed multiview techniques. Thirty-six percent of the respondents to the Pannbacker et al. (1984) survey reported using lateral views (still or video), whereas only 3% reported using multiview techniques.

Computed Tomography (CT Scan)

Computed tomography involves the mathematical, computer-assisted reconstruction of a "slice" of anatomy. The input to the mathematical reconstruction process is a series of X-ray transmission measurements made in a number of directions around the patient, but all located in the tomographic plane or "slice" of interest (Trefler, 1985). Conventional computed tomography produces images that reflect the varying attenuation of X-ray electrons by body tissue of various densities. Sensitive X-ray detectors are mounted in a gantry opposite the X-ray tube and measure the X-ray beam at different points after it has been transmitted through the body. A typical scan requires 2 to 4 seconds to complete. The patient is required to lay supine on a horizontal table with the head between the X-ray tube above and the detector bank below. The obtained image is a view of the target structure in the transverse plane. In the case of the VP mechanism, this would be somewhat analogous to the basal view.

Honjo, Mitoma, Ushiro, and Kawano (1984) have used computed tomography in the evaluation of VP closure. They reported that by using CT scans obtained at rest and during prolongation of a sound, "the dominant component of movement and its grade can be clearly visualized" (p. 624). Honjo et al. also suggested that these scans may be obtained on children if they can phonate a vowel for more than 3 seconds and if the level of VP closure can be determined.

Prior determination of the level of VP closure is a critical aspect of this technique. The slice width used by Honjo et al. (1984) was 3 mm. The examiner would have to be quite sure that the "slice" was positioned at both the proper angle and the proper height to capture the plane of maximal VP movement during an attempt at closure. The radiation dosage associated with the CT scan varies from 0.5 to 3 roentgens, considerably more than the lateral or frontal still radiograph.

The conventional CT scan produces only a static image from a sustained speech sound. Advances in CT imaging technology have led to the development of motion picture of cine-computed tomography. The cine-CT scanner is designed such that scan time has been reduced from 2 to 4 seconds to .65 seconds (Moon & Smith, 1987). Additional improvements allow for the scanning of multiple slices simultaneously. The patient to be evaluated is positioned in a fashion similar to that described for conventional CT scans. Prior to the actual scan, a localization scan, consisting of an exposure at each desired level, is obtained to ensure correct positioning. Series of CT scans are then obtained at each level. Each scan represents a single frame of the cine CT "movie," which may be viewed on a video monitor. Radiation dosage is 0.1 roentgen per scan.

The 650-millisecond scan rate does not allow for an accurate depiction of movement during ongoing speech. The speech task used by Moon and Smith (1987) in their description of this technique was an alternation of (a) inhalation through the nose, and (b) a short prolongation of /s/. This task was thought to allow an evaluation of the extremes of movement and possibly some visualization of movement between the extremes. Sample scans from a normal speaker are shown in Figure 9.7. The results of their investigation led Moon and Smith to suggest that

> cine CT technology may have some potential usefulness in the documentation of VP form and function. In its present state of development, it allows for visualization of all sides of the velopharynx at different tomographic levels. It also allows, to some degree, visualization of the motion of VP walls during phonatory and non-phonatory events. (p. 230)

Moon and Smith also commented on a number of liabilities of this system as used for VP function analysis: reduced resolution (as expressed by slice thickness of 8 mm), scan rate, radiation exposure level, possible effects of gravity on the VP mechanism when the patient is supine, and inability to combine simultaneously collected slices to obtain a three-dimensional composite image.

Magnetic Resonance Imaging

Magnetic resonance imaging (MRI) is based on principles involving magnetic properties of human tissue. Hydrogen nuclei (protons) reside in tissue having some water content. Protons act like spinning magnets that are all aligned when placed in a strong magnetic field, such as that provided by the MRI unit. In response to bombardment with radio-frequency pulses, alignment of the protons becomes perturbed. As they return to equilibrium, they give up energy in the form of radio waves that may be detected with a receiver (Vannier, 1984). These radio signals are decoded and displayed in the form of tomographic images. Contrast between tissues is achieved by using different sequences and timing of radio-frequency pulses (Dunn & Ehrhardt, 1984).

For an MRI image of the VP mechanism, the patient lies supine on a horizontal table, with the head placed inside the radio-frequency coils of the MRI unit. The head must be stabilized to minimize movement. Each image takes approximately 3 to 4 minutes.

To date, only one study demonstrating the application of this technology to speech production has appeared in the literature. Baer, Gore, Boyce, and Nye (1987) employed an MRI unit to obtain pharyngeal

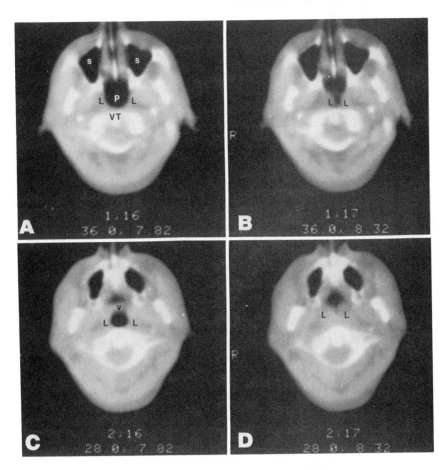

Figure 9.7 Cine computer tomography scans obtained from a normal adult male: A and B are scans obtained at Level 1; C and D are simultaneous scans at a level 8 mm lower. V = velum; L = lateral pharyngeal wall; VT = vertebra; S = sinus; P = pharynx. The velar prominance (V) is seen in C as the velum is elevated during /s/ production. (From "Application of Cine Computed Tomography to the Assessment of Velopharyngeal Form and Function" by J. Moon and W. Smith, 1987, *Cleft Palate Journal, 24,* p. 230. Copyright 1987 by American Cleft Palate–Craniofacial Association. Reprinted with permission.)

dimensions of speakers producing sustained vowels. The technology has not yet been applied to evaluation of the VP mechanism.

Magnetic resonance imaging is a potentially attractive approach to the evaluation of the VP mechanism because it does not involve radiation or other known biologic hazards. In addition, it provides better resolution than radiography (Dunn & Ehrhardt, 1984). However, its major disadvantage explains why the technique has not been applied to studying movement of VP structures: The collection of an image requires much more time than is feasible for the analysis of movement. Nonetheless, Baer et al. (1987) demonstrated the capability of using MRI technology to produce static images. With advances in technology, MRI will undoubtedly receive a great deal of attention as an alternative to radiographic imaging of the VP mechanism.

Ultrasound

The importance of lateral pharyngeal wall movement to the separation of the oral and nasal cavities and the inability of some instrumental techniques to allow visualization of that movement have been discussed earlier. Ultrasound has been investigated as a tool that might provide that information. When ultrasonic pulses are radiated into body tissue, acoustic echoes or reflections occur at boundaries between nonhomogeneous material (Ryan & Hawkins, 1976). This is especially true when the pulses meet a volume of air.

To assess lateral pharyngeal wall movement, a transducer is placed on the skin below the earlobe, and behind the ramus of the mandible (Parush & Ostry, 1986). The transducer employs a crystal that converts electrical signals into acoustic (ultrasound) pulses, which are in turn radiated through the neck skin into the body. Reflected pulses are received by the transducer and reconverted into electrical signals for display or recording. Transducers vary in the number of crystals used. Whereas some employ only a single crystal, others, such as the device used by Hawkins and Swisher (1978), employ 64 ultrasound crystals physically arranged linearly. The primary advantage of the multiple ultrasound source system is that it allows visualization of the vertical length of the pharynx, as opposed to a single point on the lateral pharyngeal wall (Hawkins & Swisher, 1978; Ryan & Hawkins, 1976).

The correct orientation of the transducer against the skin is somewhat of an art. Parush and Ostry (1986) described a typical protocol for orienting the transducer. The patient may be asked initially to swallow, a gesture involving large lateral pharyngeal wall excursions. Once the lateral pharyngeal wall is located, the patient may be asked to produce utterances with nasal and obstruent consonants while the transducer is manipulated to produce maximal output changes. Using multiple crystal transducers, Hawkins and Swisher (1978) were able to locate the lateral pharyngeal wall in less than 1 minute. By comparison, Ryan and Hawkins (1976) required several minutes to an hour to locate the lateral pharyngeal wall using a single-crystal transducer.

Images of lateral pharyngeal wall movement obtained using a single-crystal transducer appear basically as a moving dot on an oscilloscope screen. Inferior and superior deflections of the dot represent medial and lateral movement of the lateral pharyngeal wall (Figure 9.8). Images obtained using the multiple-crystal approach appear more like a video image. Hawkins and Swisher (1978) reported the quality of these images to vary considerably. Eighty percent of their images were judged to be average or poor in quality.

Although it is a nonradiographic technique, ultrasound has not become a popular tool in the analysis and evaluation of VP function. Kelsey, Minifie, and Hixon (1969) reviewed the use of this technology in monitoring speech production and concluded that it could be a useful diagnostic tool. However, there are no published reports of its use with velopharyngeally incompetent patients. Perhaps this is because only lateral pharyngeal wall activity may be viewed, and on only one side at a time. The technical difficulties involved with obtaining consistently useful, interpretable images may also limit its use.

Endoscopy

The endoscope is an optical instrument that allows for the illumination and visualization of internal body structures not easily visualized by the unaided eye. Light from an external light source is passed through the scope via either fiberoptic fibers or a series of lenses to illuminate

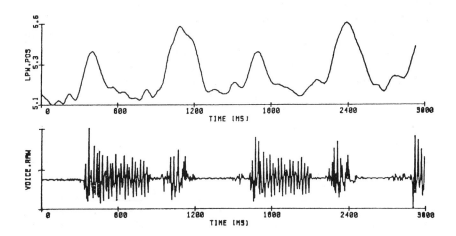

Figure 9.8 Medial movements of the lateral pharyngeal walls (upper trace) and the corresponding speech waveform (lower trace) during repetitions of the word "Sanka" as observed using a single-crystal ultrasound system. The units on the ordinate of the upper record correspond to the distance between the transducer and the lateral pharyngeal wall. (From "Superior Lateral Pharyngeal Wall Movements in Speech" by A. Parush and D. Ostry, 1986, *Journal of the Acoustical Society of America, 80,* p. 75. Copyright 1986 by Acoustical Society of America. Reprinted with permission.)

the area of interest. The image travels through a lens and more fiberoptic fibers to an eyepiece, which may be attached to a still or video camera for recording. Application of endoscopy to the assessment of VP form and function falls into a number of categorizations. In broad terms, these are oral versus nasal endoscopy and flexible versus rigid endoscopy.

One of the earliest reports of oral endoscopy of the VP mechanism was by Taub (1966). His "panendoscope" light source is a high-intensity incandescent lamp fastened adjacent to the lens. Because the lamp generates considerable heat, a tongue blade attachment is required to avoid burning the patient. The scope is passed along the upper surface of the tongue until the VP area comes into view. If the presence of the scope induces a gag reflex, a topical anesthesia is applied. Once the scope is inserted, the patient produces speech sounds while the examiner views the VP mechanism through the eyepiece, or records it on videotape (Willis & Stutz, 1972).

Although advances in endoscope technology have eliminated concerns about heat-radiating light sources, the technique of oral endoscopy enjoys limited use for a number of other reasons. Karnell and Morris (1985) suggested that the oral perspective may underestimate lateral pharyngeal wall movements in some patients. Insertion of a rigid endoscope into the oral cavity obstructs articulator movement and essentially limits the speech sample to low vowels and bilabial consonants. Also, oral insertion of an endoscope may be quite difficult, if not impossible, in patients with a gag reflex, and especially in children. Karnell and Morris did, however, point out that oral endoscopy and nasal endoscopy led to identification of identical valving patterns in 60% of their cases. Furthermore, they perceived that oral endoscopy resulted in more identifications of Passavant's ridge (anterior movement of the posterior pharyngeal wall) than did nasal endoscopy.

By far the more popular of the two options is nasal endoscopy. This technique involves the insertion of either a flexible or a rigid endoscope (Figure 9.9) through either the left or right nasal passage to view the VP mechanism from above. The rigid endoscope has gained popularity in Great Britain, primarily due to the work of Pigott and colleagues (Gilbert & Pigott, 1982; Pigott, 1980; Pigott & Makepeace, 1982). In contrast, the end-viewing flexible scope seems to be the instrument of choice in North America. Because of its superior optical characteristics, the rigid scope produces a sharper image than the flexible scope (Pigott, 1980); however, the flexible scope is typically easier to insert (Pigott & Makepeace, 1982).

Pigott (1980) provided an excellent review of the factors that should be taken into account when conducting endoscopy. These include the exam room and equipment, anesthesia, patient selection, scope insertion, and recording. The majority of endoscopic examinations of the VP

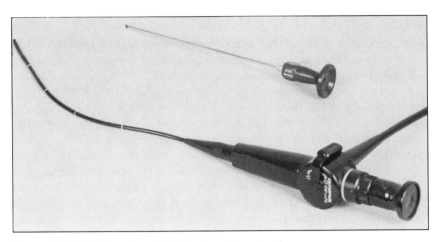

Figure 9.9 Rigid (upper) and flexible (lower) nasal endoscopes.

mechanism are likely to be conducted on children. As stated by Pigott, it is difficult to anticipate which children will tolerate the technique, and which will not. With the trend toward completing corrective surgery at earlier ages, there is growing demand to conduct nasal endoscopy on pre–school age children. The notion of allowing someone to pass a tube through the nose is undoubtedly terrifying to some children. It may be necessary to conduct a desensitization program and not even attempt to insert the scope fully until a second or third visit (M. Karnell, personal communication, 1987). The need to have a cooperative patient is of paramount importance. Little useful information will be obtained from viewing the VP mechanism of a child crying or sobbing uncontrollably who refuses to talk with the scope in place.

Many individuals will not tolerate passage of a 3- to 4-mm endoscope through the nose without some type of topical anesthesia. Endoscopes measuring less than 2 mm in diameter have recently become commercially available. Insertion of these endoscopes without anesthesia may be more feasible. It is important to have the patient blow his or her nose to remove any mucous buildup from the nasal passage. The more patent side of the nose can be determined by blocking each side independently and having the patient sniff. Cocaine, lidocaine, and ponticaine are examples of topical anesthetic agents that might be used if needed. A number of approaches can be used to apply the anesthesia. Some clinicians simply spray it in using an atomizer; others soak a cotton swab or gauze strip in the anesthesia and pass it through the passage along the intended course of the endoscope. The atomizer approach is thought to be simpler and less traumatic by its proponents; however, it results in anesthetization of tissue areas that would not require it. Regardless of which approach is used, application of anesthesia is a medical procedure and should be completed in the presence of a physician.

Assuming that the patient is willing to accept the scope and has been anesthetized (if needed), the insertion path of the scope is another consideration. One of two paths is typically chosen. The easier path is a lower one, along the floor of the nose underneath the inferior turbinate; however, the VP isthmus is then viewed rather obliquely, and a true representation of its function may be difficult to visualize. The optimal path lies just under the middle turbinate, through the middle meatus. By following this path, the viewing end of the fiberscope sits higher in the nasopharynx and can be deflected to look down on the VP mechanism from a more optimal angle (Figure 9.10). Once the scope is positioned, the patient can be instructed to complete any number of speech and nonspeech tasks. The speech sample used varies widely from clinician to clinician. Most samples include prolongations of vowels and fricatives, repetitions of high-pressure consonants (e.g., /pa/), sentences loaded with oral consonants, and words and sentences with oral and nasal consonants together (e.g., "hamper," "pimi").

A number of aspects of VP function may be evaluated using nasal endoscopy. These include the presence or absence of an adenoid pad and its contribution to closure, the extent of velar movement, the size of the VP port, and the contribution of lateral wall movement to closure. One can also look for evidence of bubbling mucous during speech attempts as indicative of incomplete VP closure. One must realize, however, that

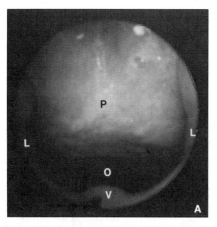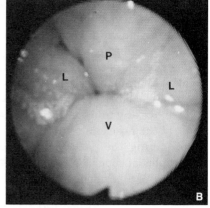

Figure 9.10 View of velopharyngeal region at rest (A) and during production of /s/ (B) using a flexible endoscope. P = posterior pharyngeal wall; L = lateral pharyngeal walls; V = velum; O = VP orifice.

the interpretation of data collected using endoscopy is largely subjective in nature. The orientation of the endoscope, its distance from the VP isthmus, and the distortion inherent in the endoscope image itself are possible sources of error in interpretation. In addition, the viewer must also be considered a source of error.

Relatively few attempts have been made to quantify or standardize endoscopic evaluations. Croft, Shprintzen, Daniller, and Lewin (1978) attempted to quantify the size of the VP orifice by inserting catheters of known diameter into the area of VP closure through the airway opposite the endoscope. They compared the diameter of the orifice as viewed through the scope with the known diameter of the catheter, also as viewed through the scope. They then calculated the area of the orifice. Ibuki, Karnell, and Morris (1983) made measurements of velar movement, size of the VP orifice, and extent of lateral pharyngeal wall movement from photographs taken through the endoscope during the subjects' production of sustained vowels or fricatives. They concluded that "a trace-and-measure procedure can be used on NPF [nasal endoscope] still photographs that gives reliable data" (p. 103). However, measurements of movement of the lateral pharyngeal wall opposite the side of insertion were not reliable. The conclusions reached by Ibuki et al. were criticized by Shprintzen (1983), who pointed out that a side-viewing endoscope (an endoscope with the lens oriented at 90 degrees, which is rarely used clinically) was used in place of an end-viewing endoscope (one with the lens placed directly on the end of the endoscope), and that validity and reliability were assessed against lateral-view cineradiographic images, which do not reflect the three-dimensional nature of the system. Furthermore, Ibuki et al. (1983) admitted that their technique was too cumbersome to be used clinically.

Karnell, Ibuki, Morris, and Van Demark (1983) devised a rating system to standardize judgments of endoscopic images. The VP area was represented as a box, having a lower velar border, two lateral pharyngeal wall borders, and an upper posterior pharyngeal wall border. Movements of each wall were assigned a number based on the extent of movement relative to the total range of movement. The authors concluded that, with some restrictions, judgments of the VP mechanism made from endoscopy images are reliable and valid. Their restrictions included the necessity to obtain a view that encompasses all VP boundaries in a single view and the necessity for the examiner to have prior training in evaluating nasal endoscopy images. These reliability data must be interpreted in the same light as those of Ibuki et al. (1983), because the same side-viewing endoscope was used in both.

In 1990, an international working group was formed to attempt to standardize the reporting of nasal endoscopic examinations (Golding-Kushner et al., 1990). This group recommended that movement ratios as opposed to absolute values should be calculated. The group presented standardized qualitative and quantitative approaches to describing velar movement; lateral pharyngeal wall movement; posterior pharyngeal wall and Passavant's ridge; and the size, shape, and location of any velopharyngeal gap.

Endoscopy has grown to be a popular diagnostic tool since its first application to the study of the VP mechanism in the early 1970s. This growth is undoubtedly due, in part, to the fact that endoscopy offers the diagnostician a direct view of the VP mechanism in motion without the need for exposure to radiation. The main disadvantages of the technique rest in its invasiveness and the potential difficulties involved with completing the procedure on young children. The fact that interpretation of the data is subjective in nature and remains difficult to quantify must also be considered. However, D'Antonio, Marsh, Province, Muntz, and Phillips (1989) suggested that the judgments made from endoscopic images may be improved by using a panel of experienced clinicians, and Pigott and Makepeace (1982) suggested that endoscopy be used in conjunction with another diagnostic procedure. The latter authors argued that endoscopy and radiography complement each other because endoscopy provides a subjective view of "the real world," whereas radiography provides an objective view of "shadows." Pigott and Makepeace promoted simultaneous recording of nasal endoscopic and radiologic views to take advantage of the complementary information they provide. This view was reinforced by Albery, Bennett, Pigott, and Simmons (1982), who stated that simultaneous measurement will provide information on the size and shape of the orifice, and both the proportional and absolute movements of the soft palate and the lateral and posterior pharyngeal walls.

INDIRECT PRIMARY APPROACHES

Indirect primary approaches to studying the movement of the VP mechanism include phototransduction, electromyography, and movement transduction.

Phototransduction

The notion of using photoelectric technology in assessing VP function was first introduced by Ohala (1971), and expanded upon by Dalston (1982) and Moon and Lagu (1987). The technique is based on the principles of light transmission through a tube. A light source is placed on one side of the VP opening and a light sensor on the opposite side. The light sensor emits a voltage with magnitude dependent on the amount of light impinging on it. The distance between the light source and the detector is held constant (Figure 9.11).

The device described by Dalston (1982) employs two small (0.75-mm) fiberoptic fibers coupled to a light source and detector electronics, respectively. The fibers are inserted through the nasal cavity until the source fiber is positioned below the VP port and the detector fiber above. The fibers are small enough that they reportedly produce only slight dis-

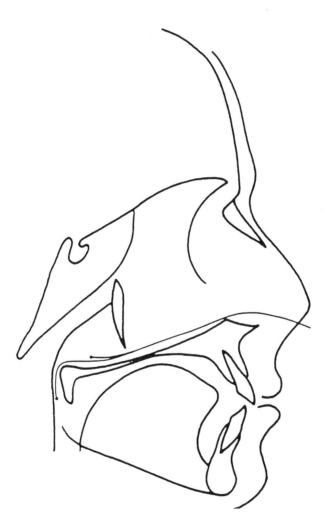

Figure 9.11   Placement of a phototransducer. (From "Photodetector Assessment of Velopharyngeal Activity" by R. Dalston, 1982, *Cleft Palate Journal, 19,* p. 4. Copyright 1982 by American Cleft Palate–Craniofacial Association. Reprinted with permission.)

comfort when passed through the inferior meatus of the nose. Topical anesthesia is not required in the majority of cases. The fibers weigh less than 1 g, and are not thought to interfere with VP function on that basis (Dalston, 1982). The fibers do have a rather large bending radius (i.e., stiffness). The effects of this property on function of the mechanism, however, have not been empirically tested. When the velum moves toward closure, the amount of light transmitted through the VP port is diminished, thus reducing the output of the detector. A typical trace is displayed in Figure 9.12.

Data collected using this device are relative; that is, one can interpret the opening size of the VP port in relation to maximal opening size, but not in terms of square millimeter area. Obviously, an important and desirable attribute of this type of device is linearity. Ohala (1971) stated emphatically that his original device is undoubtedly nonlinear. Dalston (1982) reported that the device output is related to VP opening size both directly and linearly. This statement is supported by the existence of a high correlation between detector output voltage and known simulated VP orifice areas (Jones & Moon, 1989).

The phototransducer is an interesting development in the battery of VP evaluation instruments. Although not a direct measure of VP movement, it is designed to provide quantifiable data regarding VP movement (e.g., Dalston & Seaver, 1990). It compares quite favorably with other instrumental measures of VP function. Dalston (1982) found

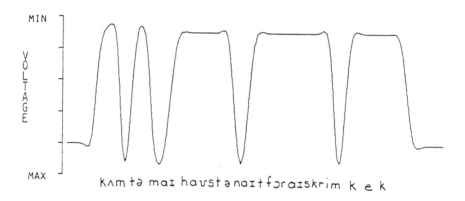

Figure 9.12 Sample phototransducer output obtained from a normal subject during production of the nonsense sentence, "Come to my house tonight from ice cream cake." Minimum and maximum voltage refer to closed and open position, respectively. (From "A Comparison of Photodetector and Endoscopic Evaluations of Velopharyngeal Functions" by M. Karnell, E. Seaver, and R. Dalston, 1988, *Journal of Speech and Hearing Research, 31,* p. 507. Copyright 1988 by American Speech–Language–Hearing Association. Reprinted with permission.)

a correlation of 0.907 between phototransducer output and orifice areas as determined using aerodynamic measures (to be discussed later). Zimmerman et al. (1987) evaluated the phototransducer against lateral-view cineradiography. They found that (a) the phototransducer output varied with opening and closing movements of the velum as seen on lateral-view cineradiography, (b) most phototransducer output changes occurred within 30 milliseconds of corresponding changes in velar position as seen using cineradiography, and (c) a highly positive relationship ($r > .80$) exists between magnitude of phototransducer output and extent of velar movement as measured from lateral cine traces. Although these results are promising, they are based on only two subjects. Finally, Karnell, Seaver, and Dalston (1988) developed a prototype system that may be used to collect endoscopy and phototransduction data simultaneously. The basic modification that permitted this development is substitution of the phototransducer light source by the endoscope light source. Their preliminary work revealed that the two techniques can be successfully coupled to provide both a direct view of the mechanism and objective data regarding its movement.

Electromyography

Electromyography (EMG) is used to study electrical activity associated with muscle contraction. Electrical activity within the muscle may be detected by inserting very fine wires into the muscle to pick up and conduct the electrical signals to signal conditioning and recording equipment outside the body. The wires, referred to as hooked-wire electrodes, are enclosed within a hypodermic needle. The needle is inserted into the muscle and, when removed, leaves the wires behind.

Although EMG has been used in the past in a research context to investigate VP muscle characteristics (Ashley, Brackett, & Lehr, 1985; Bell-Berti, 1976; Fritzell, 1979; Kuehn, Folkins, & Cutting, 1982), its use as a diagnostic tool has not materialized for a number of possible reasons. Although Fritzell (1979) suggested that needle electrode insertion is only minimally discomforting, others cite insertion discomfort as one reason why EMG remains a laboratory tool. A second major problem involves electrode placement: The combination of small size, relative inaccessibility, and possible malpositioning of muscles in speakers with cleft palates makes interpretation of EMG signals difficult. Finally, making inferences about movements of the velum based on observed EMG activity is tenuous. As stated by Kuehn et al. (1982), direction of muscle forces will undoubtedly change as velar position changes. Until a "quantitative model of velar biomechanics" is developed that takes into account interactions among all of the passive and active forces acting on the VP mechanism, moving from EMG activity to movement patterns of the normal and especially the disordered mechanism probably cannot be conducted with an appropriate degree of certainty (Kuehn et al., 1982).

Movement Transduction

A couple of attempts have been made to transduce VP movement using mechanical and electrical devices attached directly to VP structures. Moller, Martin, and Christiansen (1971) and Moller, Path, Werth, and Christiansen (1973) described a strain gauge transducer designed to track velar movement (Figure 9.13A). The device consists of an anchor to a maxillary second molar, and a bar/spring attachment placed into contact with the oral side of the velum in the midline. As the velum elevates, the spring sensor is moved. Velar movement is reflected in the electrical output of the strain gauge resistor. Adaptation to the device in the oral cavity was reportedly achieved readily, normal articulation was not interfered with, and physical discomfort was not a problem. When compared with radiographic measures of velar movement, a high level of agreement was achieved. The device was described as an "unobtrusive intraoral device to record velar movement continuously

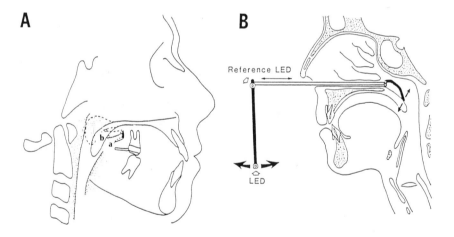

Figure 9.13 Approaches to the transduction of velar movement. (A) Schematic of strain gauge transduction system showing position at rest (a) and during production of /s/ (b). (From "A Technique for Recording Velar Movement" by K. Moller, R. Martin, and R. Christiansen, 1971, *Cleft Palate Journal, 8*, p. 266. Copyright 1971 by American Cleft Palate–Craniofacial Association. Reprinted with permission.) (B) Velotrace. (From "The Velotrace: A Device for Monitoring Velar Position" by S. Horiguchi and F. Bell-Berti, 1987, *Cleft Palate Journal, 24*, p. 105. Copyright 1987 by American Cleft Palate–Craniofacial Association. Reprinted with permission.)

during speech production" (Moller et al., 1971, p. 275). This displacement transducer system was used as a biofeedback device to increase velar elevation (Moller et al., 1973), but has not been used as an evaluation tool for assessing velar function.

A second mechanical–electrical device designed to collect data on velar position during speech is the velotrace (Bell-Berti & Krakow, 1991; Horiguchi & Bell-Berti, 1987). Whereas the Moller et al. (1971) device was placed intraorally, the velotrace (Figure 9.13B) is passed through the nose after application of topical anesthesia and decongestants. Movements of the velum are translated into linear movements of a push-rod, which, in turn, are translated into rotational movements of an externally positioned light-emitting diode (LED). A video camera is used to film the LED movements for later analysis. Horiguchi and Bell-Berti (1987) compared velotrace recordings with previously recorded endoscopic views, previously recorded velocity measures, and previously recorded measures of velar movement taken from lateral cineradiography. A different subject was employed for each measure, an approach that undoubtedly added some variability to the comparisons. Nonetheless, the authors concluded that the device accurately reflects velar movement during speech. Reported advantages of the system include no radiation and the ability to analyze movement on a frame-by-frame basis. Horiguchi and Bell-Berti also suggested that the device could be used with children; however, instrument and anatomical sizes obviously become a critical consideration.

A significant disadvantage of both the velotrace and the Moller et al. (1971) device is their ability to track velar movement only in the sagittal plane. Given the importance of analyzing the VP mechanism in all three of its dimensions, the diagnostic information obtained from these devices appears limited.

SECONDARY MEASURES

Using the categorization scheme of this chapter, secondary measures all fall under the category of indirect measures; that is, data collected using these techniques may be interpreted to make inferences regarding VP structure and function. They provide data about physiological events that are affected by VP movement. Secondary measures may involve either acoustic or aerodynamic phenomena. Acoustic measures include perceptual judgment, sound spectrography, sound pressure measurement, and accelerometry. Aerodynamic measures involve analysis of air pressure and airflow patterns in the nasal and oral cavities.

Acoustic Measures

Perceptual judgment. The ear was described earlier as the most basic and, in many respects, the most important diagnostic tool available to provide information about VP function. Although electronic devices have been and continue to be developed to transduce the physiological events associated with movement of the VP mechanism, most clinicians use the ear as the standard. Not surprisingly, more than 90% of the speech pathologists surveyed by Pannbacker et al. (1984) and Schneider and Shprintzen (1980) used listener judgments of nasality in assessing the status of the VP mechanism for speech.

A number of approaches ranging in complexity from screening tools to more elaborate multifactorial evaluations have been used in the perceptual analysis of VP incompetence (Kuehn, 1982; McWilliams et al., 1984). Historically, one of the more common screening approaches is to have the patient prolong the vowels /a/ and /i/ while the diagnostician occludes the nostrils (Moser, 1942). If the VP mechanism is competent, no change in nasality should be perceived compared with the unoccluded condition. In the case where VP valving is inadequate, addition of the nasal cavity to the vocal tract filter will produce a different resonance quality across the two conditions.

A second perceptual screening tool is based on articulatory performance. The *Iowa Pressure Articulation Test* (IPAT) (Morris, Spriestersbach, & Darley, 1961) was developed as a tool to discriminate between those with adequate and those with inadequate VP closure. The 43-item articulation test is loaded with fricatives, plosives, and affricates known to require impounding of oral air pressure for correct production. The selection of these items was based on an expectation that performance would reflect "differences in ability to impound such (air) pressure and, inferentially, ability to achieve VP closure" (p. 54). Although children with nasal air escape were likely to do poorly on the IPAT, so were those speakers with an adequate VP mechanism who misarticulate sounds for other reasons (e.g., lateral lisp). McWilliams et al. (1984) cautioned that observation of error type on this test is perhaps more important than the score itself. An additional aspect of this test that warrants comment is that, during test development, grouping of test subjects into adequate and inadequate was based on lateral still radiographs and wet spirometer ratios. Evidence now indicates that performance observed using these approaches may not accurately reflect actual performance during speech. No attempts have been made to reevaluate the IPAT against performance as observed using other instrumental approaches. The IPAT has been used recently to successfully differentiate between patients who required secondary management and those who did not (Karnell & Van Demark, 1986).

A more elaborate approach to evaluating VP function perceptually synthesizes speech performance on a number of parameters to derive a score that reflects the adequacy of the VP mechanism for speech (McWilliams et al., 1984; Philips, 1980). Nasal emission, facial grimace, nasal resonance, phonation, and articulation performance are assessed subjectively and scored on a standard form using weighted scores (Figure 9.14). A weighted score in excess of 7 is interpreted as indicative of VP incompetence.

Although subjective judgments comprise the basic diagnostic approach of many speech–language pathologists, their use has been criti-

	Value
Nasal Emission	
Inconsistent, Visible	_____1
Consistent, Visible	_____2
Audible	_____2
Nasal Turbulence	_____2
Facial Grimace	_____2
Nasal Resonance	
Mild Hypernasality	_____1
Moderate Hypernasality	_____2
Severe Hypernasality	_____3
Hypo-Hyper Nasality	_____2
Cul-de-Sac Resonance	_____2
Hyponasality	_____0
Phonation	
Mild Hoarseness	_____1
Moderate Hoarseness	_____2
Severe Hoarseness	_____3
Reduced Loudness	_____2
Strangled Voice	_____2
Articulation	
Omission of fricatives or plosives	_____1
Reduced intraoral pressure of fricatives	_____2
Lingual-Palatal sibilants	_____2
Omission of fricatives with hard glottal attack on vowels	_____3
Reduced intraoral pressure on plosives	_____3
Pharyngeal fricatives; snorts, inhalation or exhalation substitutions Glottal stops	_____3
Total	_____

Best estimate of efficiency of velopharyngeal valving mechanism using total (cumulative) score:

0	_____	Competent
1-2	_____	Competent to Borderline Competent
3-6	_____	Borderline to Borderline Incompetent
7+	_____	Incompetent

Figure 9.14 Global rating scale for perceptual assessment of velopharyngeal function. (From *Cleft Palate Speech* (p. 286) by B. McWilliams, H. Morris, and R. Shelton, 1984, Philadelphia: Decker. Copyright 1984 by B. C. Decker. Reprinted with permission.)

cized by numerous investigators. Judgments of nasality by individual listeners tend to be unreliable (Bradford, Brooks, & Shelton, 1964; Counihan & Cullinan, 1970). The sources of variability in listener judgments of VP function include lack of a preestablished standard (Counihan & Cullinan, 1970; Kuehn, 1982), articulation skills (Dalston & Warren, 1985; Spriestersbach, 1955), vocal pitch and intensity (Hess, 1959), and past experience of the listener (Dalston & Warren, 1985; Starr, Moller, Dawson, Graham, & Skaar, 1984). However, judgment reliability may be expected to improve with training (Bradford et al., 1964; Philips, 1980) and with the pooling of multiple-judge data (Counihan & Cullinan, 1970). Use of multiple judges may be especially useful when taking into account different listening conditions in which judgments must be made (Moller & Starr, 1984).

Clearly, listener judgments of speech proficiency must play a role in the assessment of VP function. However, a danger exists in using only a subjective evaluation based on what is heard. Those perceptions need to be supplemented with more standardized and objective views of the mechanism.

Spectrography.   Coupling the nasal cavity to the oral cavity may alter the resonance characteristics of the vocal tract and, hence, the output sound spectrum. A number of authors (Bloomer & Peterson, 1956; Curtis, 1969; Dickson, 1962; Hattori, Yamamoto, & Fujimura, 1958; Philips & Kent, 1984; Schwartz, 1971) have discussed the acoustic consequences of nasal–oral coupling.

Schwartz (1971) described four primary acoustic features associated with nasal–oral coupling during vowel production. The primary and most frequently observed feature is a reduction in intensity of the first formant. Other features, observed less consistently, include the presence of one or more antiresonances within the spectrum, the presence of extra resonances within the spectrum, and a shift in the center frequency of the formants. The traditional approach to studying these spectral changes involves the use of the sound spectrograph. Using a frequency filter system, the sound spectrograph produces a frequency × amplitude × time printout of the speech sample (Figure 9.15). Additionally, one can produce a frequency × amplitude display at a given instant in time (Figure 9.15). More recent approaches have been directed toward computer analyses of the spectral features of speakers with inappropriate nasal–oral coupling (Lindblom, Lubker, & Pauli, 1977).

Not surprisingly, few speech–language pathologists utilize spectrographic measures in the analysis of VP function. The difficulties involved with such an analysis are numerous. The correlates discussed above occur inconsistently. Spectrographic changes may not be readily dis-

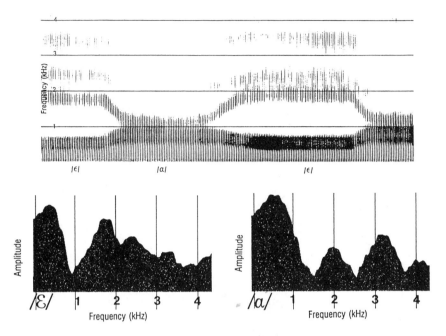

Figure 9.15 Output from sound spectrograph. Upper trace: broad band spectrogram of three vowels. Lower traces: amplitude × frequency spectra during two vowels. (From *Clinical Measurement of Speech and Voice* (p. 348) by R. Baken, 1987, Austin, TX: PRO-ED. Copyright 1987 by PRO-ED. Reprinted with permission.)

cernible unless the speaker has a highly significant level of VP incompetence (Bjork & Nylen, 1961). The techniques are time-consuming (Kuehn, 1982), measurements made are subject to error (Lindblom, 1962), and none of the traditional spectral measures can consistently differentiate between nasal and non-nasal speakers (Dickson, 1962).

Sound pressure measurement. A number of attempts have been made to measure nasal sound pressure level and relate it to oral sound pressure level (Shelton et al., 1969; Weiss, 1954). This approach is based on the premise that changes in the relative magnitudes of oral and nasal sound pressures will reflect the degree to which the oral and nasal tracts are coupled during speech production. Development work by Fletcher (1970, 1972) led to The Oral Nasal Acoustic Ratio (TONAR) and TONAR II instrumentation. The device is now commercially available as a computer-based system called the Nasometer™.

Simply described, the device consists of two microphones (nasal and oral), separated by a horizontal sound separator. Inputs from the nasal and oral microphones are individually conditioned (amplification, filtering, rectification) before the nasal signal is divided by the combined oral–nasal signal to derive a ratio. Thus, the absence of any nasal signal would result in a ratio of 0, whereas the absence of an oral signal would produce a ratio of 1. The output may be displayed in real time on a computer screen (Figure 9.16). A special feature built into this device is a filter system that limits the acoustic analysis to the speech frequency spectrum. Fletcher termed this nasal:oral–nasal ratio "nasalance."

Fletcher (1976) reported a high degree of agreement between nasalance values and group ratings of nasality ($r = 0.91$), and concluded that nasalance scores are a valid correlate of perceived nasality. Dalston and Warren (1986) also found a positive relationship ($r = .76$) between TONAR II scores and perceived nasality. Of 118 patients tested, only three had TONAR scores that indicated the need for prosthetic or surgical treatment when a speech assessment indicated only mild hypernasality. Three additional patients demonstrated nasalance scores not indicative of additional treatment when speech scores suggested that prosthetic or surgical treatment would be beneficial. However, Warren (1975) and McWilliams et al. (1984) cautioned against use of the device to provide objective data regarding VP function. Fletcher (1978) attempted to relate nasalance values with VP opening as assessed from lateral X-rays. He found a close correspondence between nasalance magnitude and VP closure in the range from touch closure to VP gap < 2 mm. Beyond this range (i.e., VP gap > 2 mm), "the relationship between the physiological and acoustical measurements became more tenuous" (p. 120).

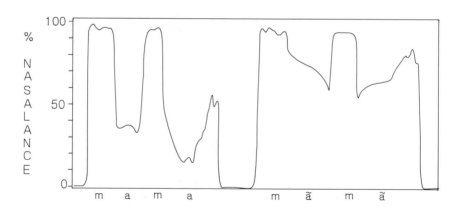

Figure 9.16 Sample output from nasometer during production of "mama" with normal resonance balance (left) and nasalization of vowels (right).

Dalston, Warren, and Dalston (1991) conducted an extensive (117 patients) comparison of acoustic (Nasometer), aerodynamic (orifice area calculation), and perceptual measures of velopharyngeal dysfunction. On the basis of their findings, Dalston et al. concluded that "the Nasometer can be used with considerable confidence in corroborating clinical impressions of hypernasality in the speech of patients seen for evaluation at craniofacial centers" (p. 187). They further suggested that the Nasometer may prove to be a useful tool for early identification of patients at risk for velopharyngeal problems as a consequence of continuing craniofacial growth.

With the possible exception of some patients with facial deformities that preclude proper fitting of the device, nasalance data can be collected easily and quickly. Although Schneider and Shprintzen (1980) reported utilization of TONAR by only 4% of their surveyed speech pathologists, its use will undoubtedly increase now that it is available commercially.

Accelerometry. As early as 1942, investigators were promoting the use of noninvasive instruments to detect head and neck tissue vibrations (Hultzen, 1942). The use of such instrumentation is based on the observation that acoustic energy present in the nasal cavity not only will be propagated outward into the air, but also will tend to vibrate the hard and soft tissues of the nose. Placement of a vibration-sensitive device such as a stethoscope (Moser, 1942) or an accelerometer (Stevens, Kalikow, & Willemain, 1975; Stevens, Nickerson, Boothroyd, & Rollins, 1976) over the nasal bone may be employed to "provide a measure of the degree of acoustic coupling through the VP opening" (Stevens et al., 1975, p. 594). Taken a step further, detection of nasal bone vibration in response to the presence of acoustic energy in the nasal cavity has been promoted as an objective correlate of nasality (Horii, 1980).

The accelerometric technique typically used today requires two accelerometers. One is placed on the nose (Figure 9.17). Because this accelerometer must transduce hard and soft tissue vibration, its positioning on the nose is important. Lippman (1981) compared accelerometer outputs from nine different placements. The position yielding the greatest accelerometer output was located on the upper side of the nose over the lateral nasal cartilage, just in front of the nasal bone. Attachment of the accelerometer to the nose is also important: The sensing surface of the device must remain flat against the nose, adequate (but not excessive) contact pressure must be maintained, and torque on the device must be kept to a minimum. Because the devices are typically quite light, careful use of double-sided tape between the accelerometer and the skin is usually sufficient. The second device is placed on the neck, overlying the thyroid lamina (Figure 9.17). In some cases, a standard microphone is used to obtain the oral signal (Edgerton et al., 1981).

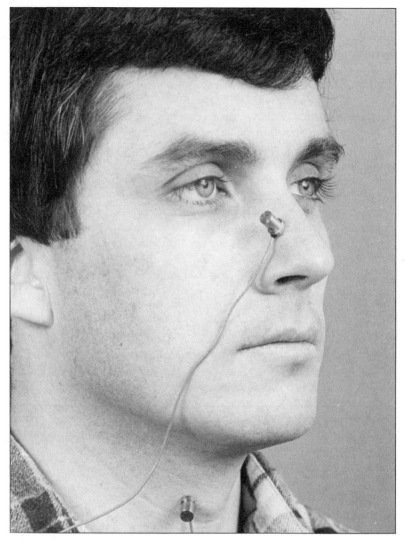

Figure 9.17 Placement of nasal and throat accelerometers for transduction of nasal bone vibration and derivation of nasal:throat accelerometer ratio.

The index of nasal coupling is taken as a ratio of nasal to oral or neck transducer output. The neck accelerometer is used as a reference to account for changes in vocal intensity that would elevate nasal accelerometer output without altering nasal coupling magnitude. Accelerometer output gains are adjusted so that, during a sustained production of /m/, a ratio of 1 is obtained—it is assumed that maximal transmission of acoustic energy into the nasal cavity takes place during that speech task. The ratio then may vary between 0 and 1. Various acronyms have been applied to this ratio, including HONC (Horii Oral Nasal Coupling; Horii, 1980), NAVI (Nasal Accelerometric Vibrational Index; Redenbaugh & Reich, 1985a), and NRI (Nasal Resonance Index; Edgerton et al., 1981).

During testing, the patient is asked to repeat words, sentences, and so forth. The nasal and oral signals are amplified, rectified, and smoothed before the nasal:oral ratio is calculated. The output of both channels and the resultant ratio (Figure 9.18) may be displayed in real time on an oscilloscope, computer screen, or other device, and recorded for further analysis if required. Because calculation of this nasality index requires the presence of an oral signal, the ratio will be calculated for vowels and voiced consonants, but not typically for unvoiced segments. However, one might see large ratio values if sufficient unvoiced energy occurs in the nasal tract. For example, a nasal snort might be expected to cause some vibration of the nasal soft tissues, but little change in oral cavity transducer output. Simultaneous audio recordings can prove to be useful in interpreting such signals.

Few comparative studies have been completed in attempts to relate accelerometer data to perceptual ratings of nasality, or to other instrumental measures of VP function. Using normal speakers who simulated hypernasal speech, Horii (1983) demonstrated an average correlation of 0.92 between mean nasal:oral ratios and perceived hypernasality scores. Redenbaugh and Reich (1985a, 1985b) utilized direct magnitude estimation and interval scaling estimates of perceived nasality to relate perceptual measures and accelerometer ratios. Although only 15 chil-

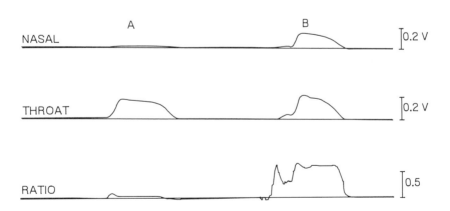

Figure 9.18 Nasal, throat, and nasal:throat accelerometer output recorded during production of /pa/. (A) Normal production. (B) Simulated hypernasality.

dren (12 with VP incompetence and 3 normal) were evaluated, moderate to high correlations were obtained. These authors concluded that nasal:oral accelerometer ratios "strongly reflect VP coupling behaviors and the resulting oral/nasal resonance balance" (Redenbaugh & Reich, 1985a, p. 280). They stated further that these data provide useful information regarding VP gestures. The small amount of data published to date would seem to indicate a significant relationship between accelerometer ratios and perceived nasality. The diagnostician should, however, be cautioned against interpreting this technique as an indicator of VP movement, as Redenbaugh and Reich (1985a, 1985b) suggest, for the same reasons discussed in the section on TONAR. An additional caution involves determination of nasal patency (Moon, 1990). The anatomic and physiological condition of the nasal passage appears to be an important variable in the detection of nasal tract acoustic energy using the accelerometric technique; that is, nasal:oral accelerometry ratios recorded from the more resistant side of the nose may be larger in magnitude than those recorded from the less resistant side of the nose.

Aerodynamic Measures

Because speech is an aerodynamic event, measurement of the airflows and air pressures associated with both normal and disordered speech production can be expected to provide useful diagnostic information. Measurement of vocal tract aerodynamics is not new. "Lo-tech" devices, such as a simple mirror that fogs when contacted with humidified air, have a long history in the analysis of speech production. However, technologic advances and refinements in electronic instrumentation have provided more precise and accurate devices that may be used to record airflow and air pressure signals during speech production.

Airflow detection. Perhaps the least sophisticated approach to studying the aerodynamics of VP function is, as stated above, the mirror test. The rationale for this test is that a lowering of the velum will allow passage of air into the nasal cavity that might serve as an indicator of nasalization (Baken, 1987). The presence of this humidified air stream will fog a mirror placed just under the nares. This crude approach is of questionable utility. Although it may differentiate gross VP incompetence from normal, the more important diagnostic determination of less obvious incompetence is beyond its capability.

An equally crude variation of the mirror test is a device called the "See-Scape." A flexible air tube positioned in the patient's naris is connected to a vertically oriented rigid tube housing a small piece of styrofoam. Air movement in the tube (i.e., nasal airflow) will displace the styrofoam float upward. Like the mirror test, this device is sensitive only to the presence or absence of nasal airflow. It provides no data regarding how much airflow is occurring (other than gross differences), where the air leak is occurring, or how large the air leak is (Glaser & Shprintzen, 1979). Quantitative measures of airflow rates associated with speech production require the use of more sophisticated equipment. Airflows are typically transduced by placing a known resistance in the airstream and measuring the pressure drop across the resistance. The pressure drop across the constant resistance will be linearly related to the flow through or around the resistance. The most common type of resistance employed is a fine wire mesh screen, although a honeycomb of narrow tubes has also been used. These resistances are incorporated into a pneumotachograph having an air inlet, air outlet, resistance component, and pressure-sensing ports (see Baken, 1987, for a more detailed explanation). The pneumotachograph may be coupled to the subject with some type of mask or with a length of tubing. A number of articles provide examples of different subject–instrument interfaces (e.g., Kastner, Putnam, & Shelton, 1985; Warren, 1984).

Laine, Warren, Dalston, and Morr (1988) demonstrated the use of airflow rate transduction using the pneumotachograph as a screening tool for VP incompetence. Based on data collected from 211 subjects, Laine et al. suggested that nasal airflow rates in excess of 125 cc/ second during production of /p/ in "hamper" are almost always associated with VP incompetence. Using this criterion, 15% of their diagnoses were considered misses, whereas only 4% were considered false positives. They did caution, not surprisingly, that this screening approach is not as sensitive with more subtle cases as it is with obvious instances of VP incompetence.

Air pressure detection. One of the simpler air pressure transduction tools is the oral manometer. Basically, the patient blows into (or sucks on) a tube connected to the manometer apparatus, which in turn displays the applied pressure on a gauge. This device is well known for its application in obtaining a nose-open:nose-closed pressure ratio (Morris, 1966). A ratio of 1 is thought to be indicative of VP adequacy; that is, no oral pressure is lost to the nasal cavity during the nose-open condition. In the presence of VP incompetence, oral pressure will be vented to the atmosphere via the nasal cavity during the nose-open condition, but not during the nose-closed condition, yielding a ratio less than 1. Morris (1966) suggested that these ratios may be interpreted as evidence of VP functional adequacy during a nonspeech task. As demonstrated by McWilliams and Bradley (1965), however, performance on this type of task may not accurately reflect a patient's performance during connected speech. Nonetheless, the oral manometer has traditionally been a popular diagnostic tool. According to Schneider

and Shprintzen (1980), it is employed by 47% of the speech pathologists surveyed.

Warren (1979) introduced a VP function screening device utilizing
air pressure signals that could be used during speech production. Named
the PERCI (Palatal Efficiency Rating Computed Instantaneously), this
device calculates the ratio between oral and nasal air pressures recorded
during the production of the consonant /p/. Air pressures are transduced
with an electronic pressure transducer. The transducer accepts a pressure signal, usually from a small tube placed somewhere in the vocal
tract or in close proximity to it, and produces a voltage signal with magnitude linearly related to the magnitude of input pressure (see Baken,
1987, for a more detailed explanation). Based on data collected from over
75 speakers, Warren concluded that oral:nasal pressure differentials in
excess of 3 cm H_2O were associated with adequate VP closure, whereas
a pressure difference of less than 1 cm H_2O indicated incomplete VP
closure. Differential pressure values between 1 and 3 cm H_2O are associated with borderline VP adequacy. In a follow-up study of 515 patients,
Morr, Warren, Dalston, and Smith (1989) demonstrated that pressures
greater than 3 cm H_2O were generally associated with adequate closure,
whereas pressures less than 3 cm H_2O were generally associated with
inadequacy. Like airflow screening, differential pressure screening may
be useful in differentiating normal from grossly abnormal, but is somewhat less sensitive in borderline or marginal cases, where accurate
diagnoses are most important and most difficult to achieve.

Orifice area estimation. The aerodynamic measurement techniques
presented thus far provide information only about the presence or
absence, and in some cases the magnitude, of airflow or air pressure
in the nasal and oral cavities. They do not, however, provide any information about the structure of the VP port itself. Warren and DuBois
(1964) first described a pressure–flow technique for estimating the cross-
sectional area of the VP orifice. Their technique is based upon a modification of the theoretical hydraulic principle and assumes that the area
of an orifice can be determined if the differential pressure across the
orifice is measured simultaneously with the rate of airflow through it.
Orifice area is calculated using the equation:

$$\text{Orifice area} = \frac{\text{rate of airflow through orifice}}{k\sqrt{2\left(\dfrac{\text{orifice differential pressure}}{\text{density of air}}\right)}}$$

Airflow rate is detected using a tube sealed into one naris and connected to a pneumotachograph–pressure transducer system (Figure 9.19). Orifice differential pressure is detected using two small tubes. The reference pressure tube is sealed into the other naris. The second pressure tube is held in the oral cavity. Both tubes are connected to a differential pressure transducer. By referencing oral pressure to pressure in the nasal cavity, the pressure drop across the VP orifice is measured. Patients are typically asked to repeat the CV syllable [pa] or the word "hamper." Airflow and pressure waveforms recorded during production of /pa/ with a normal and simulated incompetent VP mechanism are shown in Figure 9.20. Pressure and flow values are measured at the peak of nasal airflow during the bilabial plosive. These values may then be inserted into the equation to calculate cross-sectional area. Area values may also be obtained from a graph or chart as described by Moon and Weinberg (1985).

Based on orifice area data collected from a large number of patients, Warren (1976) grouped patients into categories of VP function. Patients

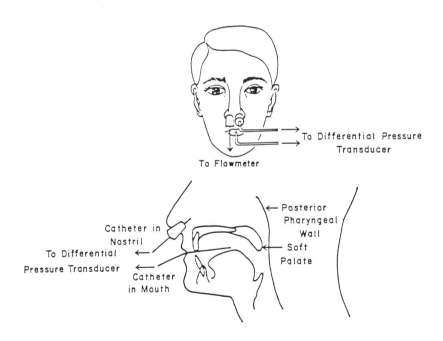

Figure 9.19 Orientation of airflow and air pressure sensing tubes for estimation of velopharyngeal orifice cross-sectional area. (From "Aerodynamics of Speech Production" by D. Warren, 1976, in N. Lass (Ed.), *Contemporary Issues in Experimental Phonetics* (p. 113). New York: Academic Press. Copyright 1976 by Academic Press. Reprinted with permission.)

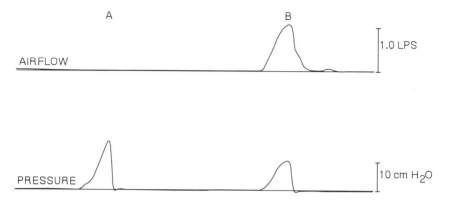

Figure 9.20   Nasal airflow and orifice differential pressure traces recorded during production of /pa/. (A) Normal production. (B) Simulated VP incompetence.

may be described as having adequate VP closure (areas less than 0.05 cm²), adequate/borderline closure (0.05 to 0.09 cm²), borderline/ inadequate closure (0.10 to 0.19 cm²), or inadequate closure (greater than 0.20 cm²). An explanation for these cutoff values was provided by Laine et al. (1988). The cutoff of 0.05 cm² was chosen for adequate closure because normal speakers without clefts do not demonstrate greater areas. The cutoff of 0.20 cm² was chosen for inadequacy because the orifice differential pressure is close to 0 above this value. The two categories lying between these extremes were assigned on an arbitrary basis, although Laine et al. assert that they are supported by both aerodynamic and perceptual data.

The pressure–flow technique is a potentially powerful tool in the evaluation of VP incompetence. It is relatively easy to apply, and provides quantitative data regarding the functional condition of the VP mechanism. The reliability of this technique as an estimator of VP orifice area has been studied in numerous investigations using a plastic vocal tract model (Lubker, 1969; Smith, Moon, & Weinberg, 1984; Smith & Weinberg, 1982). In general, the technique has been proven to provide accurate estimates of cross-sectional VP orifice area, at least in the model. A definitive evaluation of its reliability when applied to the human vocal tract has yet to be completed. Pressure–flow data have been shown to correlate reasonably well ($r = 0.80$) with listener judgments of nasality, and with nasalance scores ($r = 0.74$) (Dalston & Warren, 1986).

A somewhat less supportive view is held by others (McWilliams et al., 1981; Muller & Brown, 1980). Muller and Brown's apprehension is based, in part, on the fact that the technique was derived and tested on a model having a flat circular orifice when, in fact, the VP orifice is more three-dimensional. McWilliams et al. (1981) demonstrated an overall rate of agreement of only 23% between categorizations of VP incompetence based on pressure–flow data and those based on video-fluoroscopy.

A second VP orifice area estimation technique, described by Hixon, Bless, and Netsell (1976), takes a somewhat different approach. The technique is based on a simple airflow balancing procedure (Figure 9.21). Forced oscillatory airflow is supplied simultaneously to the patient's nasal cavity (via a nasal mask) and to a rigid walled model of the nasal and oral cavity having an adjustable orifice that mimics the VP port. The model's and patient's oral cavities are interfaced with separate pneumotachograph–pressure transducer systems. These outputs are relayed to a balance meter for comparison. As oscillatory airflow is supplied to both the patient and the model, and the model's VP orifice is manipulated until the balance meter reads zero, indicating that the model orifice cross-sectional area is equal to that of the patient.

This approach, although elegant in concept, suffers from some significant drawbacks. First, the VP mechanism must be held essentially motionless or static so that the model orifice can be adjusted. Second, patients must be selected who have low nasal airway resistance. Given that most patients present with elevated nasal resistance occurring as a result of septal deviation, vomerine spurs, and so forth, the technique appears to have limited utility. Hixon et al. (1976) addressed this drawback by pointing out that this approach will provide an estimate of the "effective" VP–nasal area; that is, the approach takes into account both nasal and VP resistance that contributes to aerodynamic events and their consequences during speech production.

Aerodynamic measures have proven appealing for the study of speech production. They are noninvasive, typically requiring only a small tube placed in the oral cavity and some type of mask covering the nose, mouth, or both. The systems are easy to calibrate with appropriate equipment and take little time to set up for data collection. They are, however, somewhat expensive. Furthermore, the equipment array may be intimidating to those less experienced in instrumentation. This expense may explain why pressure–flow approaches are used by relatively few speech pathologists (Pannbacker et al., 1984; Schneider & Shprintzen, 1980).

SUMMARY

It should be readily apparent from the information presented that VP function is a multifaceted and complex constellation of physiological

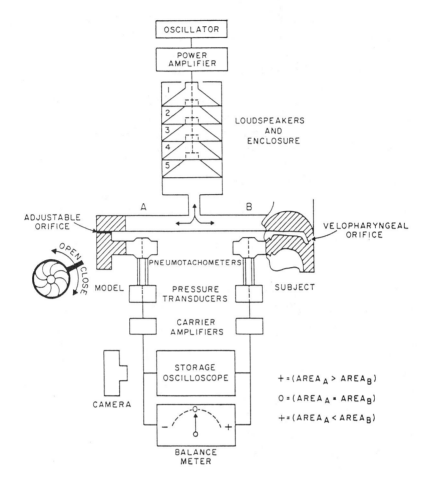

Figure 9.21 Airflow balancing procedure for measuring velopharyngeal cross-sectional area during vowel production. (From "A New Technique for Measuring Velopharyngeal Orifice Area During Sustained Vowel Production: An Application of Aerodynamic Forced Oscillation Principles" by T. Hixon, D. Bless, and R. Netsell, 1976, *Journal of Speech and Hearing Research, 19,* p. 602. Copyright 1976 by American Speech–Language–Hearing Association. Reprinted with permission.)

events. To date, no one tool is available that can evaluate all aspects of VP function. Instead, various devices have been designed to transduce the individual component events that take place during attempts at speech production. As stated at the outset, the bottom line is the perceptual judgment of the functional adequacy of the mechanism. Data collected using supplemental approaches and tools must ultimately be related to that perception and, of equal importance, to the underlying VP events that give rise to that perception.

Assuming for the moment that all of the tools discussed in this chapter are reasonably valid and reliable, one might ask which one is best. McWilliams et al. (1981) suggested that multiview videofluoroscopy is the method of choice. Although this technique might not appeal to everybody, many diagnosticians would probably agree that one of the direct primary approaches would be most useful because they allow visualization of the mechanism. Furthermore, they may be used by the clinician to form a bridge between perception and kinematics. Other tools provide objective data regarding perceptual phenomenon (e.g., accelerometry, TONAR), but cannot be used as easily to form the bridge referred to above. Still others provide objective data that have been used to infer structural characteristics of the VP mechanism (e.g., pressure–flow devices), but remain one step removed from observation of the mechanism itself. As discussed earlier, the techniques differ in other features as well: Some involve exposure to ionizing radiation. Some involve insertion of instruments into the oral and/or nasal cavity. Some are attached to an external body surface and are not invasive. Some are much more costly than others. Some are appropriate only in a medical clinic setting, whereas others might be used in school or other clinic settings.

However, which tool is best is not the important question to ask. The more critical question is "what combination of different measurements and assumptions will provide the most insight about any particular experimental or clinical question?" (Folkins & Moon, 1991). Stated differently,

> Treatment decisions should not be made on the basis of input from any single source of information concerning patient status. The greater the variety of valid information that can be obtained about patient performance, the more likely it is that an accurate assessment will be made. Of course, it is reasonable to suppose that there is a practical limit beyond which further assessment will provide little or no additional useful information. However, that limit has not yet been identified. (Dalston & Warren, 1986, p. 114)

REFERENCES

Albery, E., Bennett, J., Pigott, R., & Simmons, R. (1982). The results of 100 operations for velopharyngeal incompetence—Selected on the findings of endoscopic and radiologic examination. *British Journal of Plastic Surgery, 35,* 118–126.

Ashley, M., Brackett, I., & Lehr, R. (1985). A descriptive study of the relationship of intraoral air pressure to EMG activity of the levator palatini during CV syllables. *Folia Phoniatrica, 37,* 66–74.

Baer, T., Gore, J., Boyce, S., & Nye, P. (1987). Application of MRI to the analysis of speech production. *Magnetic Resonance Imaging, 5,* 1–7.

Baken, R. (1987). *Clinical measurement of speech and voice.* Austin, TX: PRO-ED.

Bell-Berti, F. (1976). An electromyographic study of velopharyngeal function in speech. *Journal of Speech and Hearing Research, 19,* 225–239.

Bell-Berti, F., & Krakow, R. (1991). Anticipatory velar lowering: A coproduction account. *Journal of the Acoustical Society of America, 90,* 112–123.

Bensen, J. (1977). A checklist for evaluating palatal closure. *Plastic and Reconstructive Surgery, 60,* 45–48.

Bjork, L., & Nylen, B. (1961). Cineradiography with synchronized sound spectrum analysis: A study of velopharyngeal function during connected speech in normals and cleft palate cases. *Plastic and Reconstructive Surgery, 27,* 397–412.

Bloomer, H., & Peterson, G. (1956). A spectrographic study of hypernasality. *Cleft Palate Bulletin, 6,* 10–12.

Bradford, L., Brooks, A., & Shelton, R. (1964). Clinical judgment of hypernasality in cleft palate children. *Cleft Palate Journal, 1,* 329–335.

Bzoch, K. (1968). Variations in velopharyngeal valving: The factor of vowel changes. *Cleft Palate Journal, 5,* 211–218.

Carrell, J. (1952). A cinefluorographic technique for the study of velopharyngeal closure. *Journal of Speech and Hearing Disorders, 17,* 224–228.

Cohn, E., Rood, S., McWilliams, B., Skolnick, M., & Abdelmalek, L. (1981). *Barium sulfate coating of the nasopharynx in lateral view videofluoroscopy.* Paper presented at the annual meeting of the American Speech–Language–Hearing Association, Los Angeles.

Counihan, D., & Cullinan, W. (1970). Reliability and dispersion of nasality ratings. *Cleft Palate Journal, 7,* 261–270.

Croft, C., Shprintzen, R., Daniller, A., & Lewin, M. (1978). The occult submucous cleft palate and the musculus uvulae. *Cleft Palate Journal, 15,* 150–154.

Croft, C., Shprintzen, R., & Rakoff, S. (1981). Patterns of velopharyngeal valving in normal and cleft palate subjects: A multi-view videofluoroscopic and nasendoscopic study. *Laryngoscope, 91,* 265–271.

Curtis, J. (1969). The acoustics of nasalized speech. *Cleft Palate Journal, 6,* 380–396.

Dalston, R. (1982). Photodetector assessment of velopharyngeal activity. *Cleft Palate Journal, 19,* 1–8.

Dalston, R., & Seaver, E. (1990). Nasometric and phototransductive measurements of reaction times among normal adult speakers. *Cleft Palate Journal, 27,* 61–67.

Dalston, R., & Warren, D. (1985). The diagnosis of velopharyngeal inadequacy. *Clinics in Plastic Surgery, 12,* 685–695.

Dalston, R., & Warren, D. (1986). Comparison of TONAR II, pressure flow, and listener judgments of hypernasality in the assessment of velopharyngeal function. *Cleft Palate Journal, 23,* 108–115.

Dalston, R., Warren, D., & Dalston, E. (1991). Use of nasometry as a diagnostic tool for identifying patients with velopharyngeal impairment. *Cleft Palate–Craniofacial Journal, 28,* 184–189.

Daniloff, R., Schuckers, G., & Feth, L. (1980). *The physiology of speech and hearing: An introduction.* Englewood Cliffs, NJ: Prentice-Hall.

D'Antonio, L., Marsh, J., Province, M., Muntz, H., & Phillips, C. (1989). Reliability of flexible fiberoptic nasopharyngoscopy for evaluation of velopharyngeal function in a clinical population. *Cleft Palate Journal, 26,* 217–225.

Dickson, D. (1962). An acoustic study of nasality. *Journal of Speech and Hearing Research, 5,* 103–111.

Dickson, D. (1975). Anatomy of the normal velopharyngeal mechanism. *Clinics in Plastic Surgery, 2,* 234.

Dunn, V., & Ehrhardt, J. (1984). Magnetic resonance imaging. *University of Iowa Communication, 1,* 1–5.

Edgerton, M., Sadove, M., Compton, M., Bull, G., Blomain, E., McDonald, W., & Bralley, R. (1981). Nasal vibration analysis: A noninvasive objective technique to evaluate the speech of patients with palatopharyngeal disorders. *Plastic and Reconstructive Surgery, 68,* 153–157.

Eisenbach, C., & Williams, W. (1984). Comparing the unaided visual exam to lateral cinefluorography in estimating several parameters of velopharyngeal function. *Journal of Speech and Hearing Disorders, 49,* 136–139.

Fletcher, S. (1970). Theory and instrumentation for quantitative measurement of nasality. *Cleft Palate Journal, 7,* 601–609.

Fletcher, S. (1972). Contingencies for bioelectric modification of nasality. *Journal of Speech and Hearing Disorders, 37,* 329–346.

Fletcher, S. (1976). Nasalence vs. listener judgments of nasality. *Cleft Palate Journal, 13,* 31–44.

Fletcher, S. (1978). *Diagnosing speech disorders from cleft palate.* New York: Grune & Stratton.

Folkins, J. (1988). Velopharyngeal nomenclature: Incompetence, inadequacy, insufficiency, and dysfunction. *Cleft Palate Journal, 25,* 413–416.

Folkins, J., & Moon, J. (1991). Approaches to the study of speech production. In J. Bardach & H. Morris (Eds.), *Multidisciplinary management of cleft lip and palate.* Philadelphia: Saunders.

Fritzell, B. (1979). Electromyography in the study of velopharyngeal function—A review. *Folia Phoniatrica, 31,* 93–102.

Gilbert, S., & Pigott, R. (1982). The feasibility of nasal pharyngoscopy using the 70 Storz–Hopkins nasopharyngoscope. *British Journal of Plastic Surgery, 35,* 14–18.

Glaser, E., & Shprintzen, R. (1979). See-Scape: Instrument and manual. *Cleft Palate Journal, 16,* 213–214.

Golding-Kushner, K. J., et al. (1990). Standardization for the reporting of nasopharyngoscopy and multiview videofluoroscopy: A report from an international working group. *Cleft Palate Journal, 27,* 337–348.

Harrington, J. (1970). A cinefluorographic study of the pharyngeal flap mechanism. *Cleft Palate Journal, 7,* 129–138.

Hattori, S., Yamamoto, K., & Fujimura, O. (1958). Nasalization of vowels in relation to nasals. *Journal of the Acoustical Society of America, 30,* 267–274.

Hawkins, C., & Swisher, W. (1978). Evaluation of a real-time ultrasound scanner in assessing lateral pharyngeal wall motion during speech. *Cleft Palate Journal, 15,* 161–166.

Hess, D. (1959). Pitch, intensity, and cleft palate voice quality. *Journal of Speech and Hearing Research, 2,* 113–125.

Hirschberg, J. (1986). Velopharyngeal insufficiency. *Folia Phoniatrica, 38,* 221–276.

Hixon, E. (1949). *An X-ray study comparing oral and pharyngeal structures of individuals with nasal voices and individuals with superior voices.* Unpublished masters thesis, University of Iowa, Iowa City.

Hixon, T., Bless, D., & Netsell, R. (1976). A new technique for measuring velopharyngeal orifice area during sustained vowel production: An application of aerodynamic forced oscillation principles. *Journal of Speech and Hearing Research, 19,* 601–607.

Honjo, I., Mitoma, T., Ushiro, K., & Kawano, M. (1984). Evaluation of velopharyngeal closure by CT scan and endoscopy. *Plastic and Reconstructive Surgery, 74,* 620–627.

Horiguchi, S., & Bell-Berti, F. (1987). The Velotrace: A device for monitoring velar position. *Cleft Palate Journal, 24,* 104–111.

Horii, Y. (1980). An accelerometric approach to nasality measurement: A preliminary report. *Cleft Palate Journal, 17,* 254–261.

Horii, Y. (1983). An accelerometric measure as a physical correlate of perceived hypernasality in speech. *Journal of Speech and Hearing Research, 26,* 476–480.

Hultzen, L. (1942). Apparatus for demonstrating nasality. *Journal of Speech and Hearing Disorders, 7,* 5–6.

Ibuki, K., Karnell, M., & Morris, H. (1983). Reliability of the nasopharyngeal fiberscope (NPF) for assessing velopharyngeal function. *Cleft Palate Journal, 20,* 97–104.

Iglesias, A., Kuehn, D., & Morris, H. (1980). Simultaneous assessment of pharyngeal wall and velar displacement for selected speech sounds. *Journal of Speech and Hearing Research, 23,* 429–446.

Jones, D., & Moon, J. (1989). *Response characteristics of the velopharyngeal photodetector to known orifice cross-sectional areas.* Paper presented at the annual meeting of the American Cleft Palate Association, San Francisco.

Karnell, M., Folkins, J., & Morris, H. (1985). Relationships between the perception of nasalization and speech movements in speakers with cleft palate. *Journal of Speech and Hearing Research, 28,* 63–72.

Karnell, M., Ibuki, K., Morris, H., & Van Demark, D. (1983). Reliability of the nasopharyngeal fiberscope (NPF) for assessing velopharyngeal function: Analysis by judgment. *Cleft Palate Journal, 20,* 199–208.

Karnell, M., & Morris, H. (1985). Multiview endoscopic evaluation of velopharyngeal physiology in 15 normal speakers. *Annals of Otology, Rhinology and Laryngology, 94,* 361–365.

Karnell, M., Seaver, E., & Dalston, R. (1988). A comparison of photodetector and endoscopic evaluations of velopharyngeal functions. *Journal of Speech and Hearing Research, 31,* 503–509.

Karnell, M., & Van Demark, D. (1986). Longitudinal speech performance in patients with cleft palate: Comparisons based on secondary management. *Cleft Palate Journal, 23,* 278–288.

Kastner, C., Putnam, A., & Shelton, R. (1985). Custom-fabricated masks for aero-mechanical measures. *Cleft Palate Journal, 22,* 197–204.

Kelsey, C., Minifie, F., & Hixon, T. (1969). Applications of ultrasound in speech research. *Journal of Speech and Hearing Research, 12,* 564–575.

Kuehn, D. (1979). Velopharyngeal anatomy and physiology. *Ear, Nose, Throat Journal, 58,* 59–66.

Kuehn, D. (1982). Assessment of resonance disorders. In N. Lass (Ed.), *Speech, language, and hearing* (Vol. 2). Philadelphia: Saunders.

Kuehn, D., & Dolan, K. (1975). A tomographic technique of assessing lateral pharyngeal wall displacement. *Cleft Palate Journal, 12,* 200–209.

Kuehn, D., Folkins, J., & Cutting, C. (1982). Relationships between muscle activity and velar position. *Cleft Palate Journal, 19,* 25–35.

Kuehn, D., & Moll, K. (1976). A cineradiographic study of VC and CV articulatory velocities. *Journal of Phonetics, 4,* 303–320.

Laine, T., Warren, D., Dalston, R., & Morr, K. (1988). Screening of velopharyngeal closure based on nasal airflow rate measurements. *Cleft Palate Journal, 25,* 220–225.

Lindblom, B. (1962). Accuracy and limitations of Sonagraph measurements. In *Proceedings of 4th International Congress of Phonetic Sciences,* pp. 188–202.

Lindblom, B., Lubker, J., & Pauli, S. (1977). An acoustic–perceptual method for quantitative evaluation of hypernasality. *Journal of Speech and Hearing Research, 20,* 485–496.

Lippman, R. (1981). Detecting nasalization using a low-cost miniature accelerometer. *Journal of Speech and Hearing Research, 24,* 314–317.

Loney, R., & Bloem, T. (1987). Velopharyngeal dysfunction: Recommendations for use of nomenclature. *Cleft Palate Journal, 24,* 334–335.

Lubker, J. (1968). An electromyographic–cinefluorographic investigation of velar function during normal speech production. *Cleft Palate Journal, 5,* 1–18.

Lubker, J. (1969). Velopharyngeal orifice area: A replication of analog experimentation. *Journal of Speech and Hearing Research, 12,* 218–222.

Lubker, J. (1975). Normal velopharyngeal function in speech. *Clinics in Plastic Surgery, 2,* 249–259.

Lubker, J., & Moll, K. (1965). Simultaneous oral–nasal air flow measurements and cinefluorographic observations during speech production. *Cleft Palate Journal, 2,* 257–272.

Lubker, J., & Morris, H. (1968). Predicting cinefluorographic measures of velopharyngeal opening from lateral still x-ray films. *Journal of Speech and Hearing Research, 11,* 747–753.

Mason, R., & Warren, D. (1980). Adenoid involution and developing hypernasality in cleft palate. *Journal of Speech and Hearing Disorders, 45,* 469–480.

McWilliams, B., & Bradley, D. (1965). Ratings of velopharyngeal closure during blowing and speech. *Cleft Palate Journal, 2,* 46–55.

McWilliams, B., & Girdany, B. (1964). The use of Televex in cleft palate research. *Cleft Palate Journal, 1,* 398.

McWilliams, B., Glaser, E., Philips, B., Lawrence, C., Lavorato, A., Beery, Q., & Skolnick, M. (1981). A comparative study of four methods of evaluating velopharyngeal adequacy. *Plastic and Reconstructive Surgery, 68,* 1–10.

McWilliams, B., Morris, H., & Shelton, R. (1984). *Cleft palate speech.* Philadelphia: Decker.

McWilliams-Neely, B., & Bradley, D. (1964). A rating scale for evaluation of videotape recorded x-ray studies. *Cleft Palate Journal, 1,* 88.

Moll, K. (1960). Cinefluorographic techniques in speech research. *Journal of Speech and Hearing Research, 3,* 227–241.

Moll, K. (1964). Objective measures of nasality. *Cleft Palate Journal, 1,* 371–374.

Moller, K., Martin, R., & Christiansen, R. (1971). A technique for recording velar movement. *Cleft Palate Journal, 8,* 263–276.

Moller, K., Path, M., Werth, L., & Christiansen, R. (1973). The modification of velar movement. *Journal of Speech and Hearing Disorders, 38,* 323–334.

Moller, K., & Starr, C. (1984). The effects of listening conditions on speech ratings obtained in a clinical setting. *Cleft Palate Journal, 21,* 65–69.

Moon, J. (1990). The influence of nasal patency on accelerometric transduction of nasal bone vibration. *Cleft Palate Journal, 27,* 266–270.

Moon, J., & Lagu, R. (1987). Development of a second-generation phototransducer for the assessment of velopharyngeal activity. *Cleft Palate Journal, 24,* 240–243.

Moon, J., & Smith, W. (1987). Application of cine CT technology to the assessment of velopharyngeal function. *Cleft Palate Journal, 24,* 226–232.

Moon, J., & Weinberg, B. (1985). Two simplified methods for estimating velopharyngeal orifice area. *Cleft Palate Journal, 22,* 1–10.

Morr, K., Warren, D., Dalston, R., & Smith, L. (1989). Screening of velopharyngeal inadequacy by differential pressure measurements. *Cleft Palate Journal, 26,* 42–45.

Morris, H. (1966). The oral manometer as a diagnostic tool in clinical speech pathology. *Journal of Speech and Hearing Disorders, 31,* 362–369.

Morris, H., Spriestersbach, D., & Darley, F. (1961). An articulation test for assessing competency of velopharyngeal closure. *Journal of Speech and Hearing Research, 4,* 48–55.

Moser, H. (1942). Diagnostic and clinical procedures in rhinolalia. *Journal of Speech Disorders, 7,* 1–4.

Mourino, A., & Weinberg, B. (1975). A cephalometric study of velar stretch in 8- and 10-year-old children. *Cleft Palate Journal, 12,* 417–435.

Muller, E., & Brown, W. (1980). Variations in the supraglottal air pressure waveform and their articulatory interpretation. *SMCL Preprints,* Spring–Summer. Madison, WI: Speech Motor Control Laboratory, University of Wisconsin.

Neiman, G., & Simpson, R. (1975). A roentgencephalometric investigation of the effect of adenoid removal upon selected measures of velopharyngeal function. *Cleft Palate Journal, 12,* 377–389.

Ohala, J. (1971). *Monitoring soft palate movements in speech.* Paper presented at the meeting of the Acoustical Society of America, Washington, DC.

Pannbacker, M., Lass, N., Middleton, G., Crutchfield, E., Trapp, D., & Scherbick, K. (1984). Current clinical practices in the assessment of velopharyngeal closure. *Cleft Palate Journal, 21,* 33–37.

Parush, A., & Ostry, D. (1986). Superior lateral pharyngeal wall movements in speech. *Journal of the Acoustical Society of America, 80,* 749–756.

Peterson, G., & Barney, H. (1952). Control methods used in the study of vowels. *Journal of the Acoustical Society of America, 24,* 175–184.

Philips, B. (1980). Perceptual evaluation of velopharyngeal competency. *Annals of Otology, Rhinology, and Laryngology,* Suppl. 69, 153–157.

Philips, B., & Kent, R. (1984). Acoustic–phonetic descriptions of speech production in speakers with cleft palate and other velopharyngeal disorders. In N. Lass (Ed.), *Speech and language: Advances in basic research and practice* (Vol. 11). New York: Academic Press.

Pigott, R. (1980). Assessment of velopharyngeal function. In M. Edwards & A. Watson (Eds.), *Advances in the management of cleft palate.* London: Churchill.

Pigott, R., & Makepeace, A. (1982). Some characteristics of endoscopic and radiological systems used in elaboration of the diagnosis of velopharyngeal incompetence. *British Journal of Plastic Surgery, 35,* 19–32.

Redenbaugh, M., & Reich, A. (1985a). Correspondence between an accelerometric nasal/voice amplitude ratio and listeners' direct magnitude estimations of hypernasality. *Journal of Speech and Hearing Research, 28,* 273–281.

Redenbaugh, M., & Reich, A. (1985b). *Perceptual validation of nasal/voice accelerometry using equal-appearing-interval scaling.* Paper presented at the annual meeting of the American Speech–Language–Hearing Association, Washington, DC.

Ryan, W., & Hawkins, C. (1976). Ultrasonic measurement of lateral pharyngeal wall movement of the velopharyngeal port. *Cleft Palate Journal, 13,* 156–164.

Schneider, E., & Shprintzen, R. (1980). A survey of speech pathologists: Current trends in the diagnosis and management of velopharyngeal insufficiency. *Cleft Palate Journal, 17,* 249–253.

Schwartz, M. (1971). Acoustic measures of nasalization and nasality. In W. Grabb, S. Rosenstein, & K. Bzoch (Eds.), *Cleft lip and palate: Surgical, dental, and speech aspects.* Boston: Little, Brown.

Schwartz, M. (1975). Developing a direct, objective measure of velopharyngeal inadequacy. *Clinics in Plastic Surgery, 2,* 305–308.

Seaver, E., & Kuehn, D. (1980). A cineradiographic and electromyographic investigation of velar positioning in non-nasal speech. *Cleft Palate Journal, 17,* 216–226.

Shaw, R., Folkins, J., & Kuehn, D. (1980). Comparison of methods for measuring velar position from lateral-view cineradiography. *Cleft Palate Journal, 17,* 326–329.

Shelton, R., Arndt, W., Knox, A., Elbert, M., Chisum, L., & Youngstrom, K. (1969). The relationship between nasal sound pressure level and palatopharyngeal closure. *Journal of Speech and Hearing Research, 12,* 193.

Shelton, R., Brooks, A., & Youngstrom, K. (1964). Articulation and patterns of palatopharyngeal closure. *Journal of Speech and Hearing Disorders, 29,* 390–408.

Shelton, R., Brooks, A., Youngstrom, K., Diedrich, W., & Brooks, R. (1963). Filming speed in cineradiographic speech study. *Journal of Speech and Hearing Disorders, 6,* 19–26.

Shelton, R., & Trier, W. (1976). Issues involved in the valuation of velopharyngeal closure. *Cleft Palate Journal, 13,* 127–137.

Shprintzen, R. (1983). An invited commentary on "Reliability of the nasopharyngeal fiberscope (NPF) for assessing velopharyngeal function." *Cleft Palate Journal, 20,* 105–107.

Simpson, R., & Chin, L. (1981). Velar stretch as a function of task. *Cleft Palate Journal, 18,* 1–9.

Simpson, R., & Colton, J. (1980). A cephalometric study of velar stretch in adolescent subjects. *Cleft Palate Journal, 17,* 40–47.

Skolnick, M. L. (1969). Video velopharyngography in patients with nasal speech, with emphasis on lateral pharyngeal wall motion in velopharyngeal closure. *Radiology, 93,* 747–755.

Skolnick, M. L. (1970). Videofluoroscopic examination of the velopharyngeal portal during phonation in lateral and base projections—A new technique for studying the mechanics of closure. *Cleft Palate Journal, 7,* 803.

Skolnick, M. L. (1975). Velopharyngeal function in cleft palate. *Clinics in Plastic Surgery, 2,* 285.

Skolnick, M. L., & McCall, G. (1972). Velopharyngeal competence and incompetence following pharyngeal flap surgery: Videofluoroscopic study in multiple projections. *Cleft Palate Journal, 9,* 1–12.

Skolnick, M., McCall, G., & Barnes, M. (1973). The sphincteric mechanism of velopharyngeal closure. *Cleft Palate Journal, 10,* 286–305.

Smith, B., Moon, J., & Weinberg, B. (1984). The effects of increased nasal airway resistance on modeled velopharyngeal orifice area estimation. *Cleft Palate Journal, 21,* 18–21.

Smith, B., & Weinberg, B. (1982). Prediction of modeled velopharyngeal orifice areas during steady flow conditions and during aerodynamic simulation of voiceless stop consonants. *Cleft Palate Journal, 19,* 172–180.

Spriestersbach, D. (1955). Assessing nasal quality in cleft palate speech of children. *Journal of Speech and Hearing Disorders, 20,* 266–270.

Starr, C., Moller, K., Dawson, W., Graham, J., & Skaar, S. (1984). Speech ratings by speech clinicians, parents, and children. *Cleft Palate Journal, 21,* 286–292.

Stathopoulos, E., & Weismer, G. (1985). Oral air flow and intraoral air pressure: A comparative study of children, youths, and adults. *Folia Phoniatrica, 37,* 152–159.

Stevens, K., Kalikow, D., & Willemain, T. (1975). A miniature accelerometer for detecting glottal waveforms and nasalization. *Journal of Speech and Hearing Research, 18,* 594–599.

Stevens, K., Nickerson, R., Boothroyd, A., & Rollins, A. (1976). Assessment of nasalization in the speech of deaf children. *Journal of Speech and Hearing Research, 19,* 393–415.

Stringer, D., & Witzel, M. (1989). Comparison of multi-view videofluoroscopy and nasopharyngoscopy in the assessment of velopharyngeal insufficiency. *Cleft Palate Journal, 26,* 88–91.

Subtelny, J. (1957). A cephalometric study of the growth of the soft palate. *Plastic and Reconstructive Surgery, 19,* 49–62.

Subtelny, J., & Koepp-Baker, H. (1956). The significance of adenoid tissue in velopharyngeal function. *Plastic and Reconstructive Surgery, 17,* 235–250.

Subtelny, J., McCormack, R., Subtelny, J., & Cichoke, A. (1960). Cineradiographic and pressure-flow analysis of speech before and after pharyngeal-flap surgery. *Plastic and Reconstructive Surgery, 44,* 336–344.

Taub, S. (1966). The Taub oral panendoscope: A new technique. *Cleft Palate Journal, 3,* 328–346.

Thompson, A., & Hixon, T. (1979). Nasal air flow during normal speech production. *Cleft Palate Journal, 16,* 412–420.

Trefler, M. (1985). Computed tomography. In T. Thompson (Ed.), *A practical approach to modern imaging equipment.* Boston: Little, Brown.

Van Demark, D., Kuehn, D., & Tharp, R. (1975). Prediction of velopharyngeal competency. *Cleft Palate Journal, 12,* 5–11.

Vannier, M. (1984). Nuclear magnetic resonance imaging. *Postgraduate Medicine, 76,* 159–170.

Wada, T., Yasumoto, M., Ikeoka, N., Fujika, Y., & Yoshinaga, R. (1970). An approach for the cinefluorographic study of articulatory movements. *Cleft Palate Journal, 7,* 506–522.

Warren, D. (1975). The determination of velopharyngeal incompetence by aerodynamic and acoustical techniques. *Clinics in Plastic Surgery, 2,* 299–304.

Warren, D. (1976). Aerodynamics of speech production. In N. Lass (Ed.), *Contemporary issues in experimental phonetics.* New York: Academic Press.

Warren, D. (1979). PERCI: A method for rating palatal efficiency. *Cleft Palate Journal, 16,* 279–285.

Warren, D. (1982). Aerodynamics of speech. In N. Lass, L. McReynolds, G. Northern, & D. Yoder (Eds.), *Speech language and hearing.* Philadelphia: Saunders.

Warren, D. (1984). A quantitative technique for assessing nasal airway impairment. *American Journal of Orthodontics, 86,* 306–314.

Warren, D., & DuBois, A. (1964). A pressure-flow technique for measuring velopharyngeal orifice area during continuous speech. *Cleft Palate Journal, 1,* 52–71.

Warren, D., & Hofmann, F. (1961). A cineradiographic study of velopharyngeal closure. *Plastic and Reconstructive Surgery, 28,* 656.

Webster's Seventh New Collegiate Dictionary. (1965). Springfield: G. C. Merriam.

Weiss, A. (1954). *Oral and nasal sound pressure levels as related to judged severity of nasality.* Unpublished doctoral dissertation, Purdue University, West Lafayette, IN.

Williams, W., & Eisenbach, C. (1981). Assessing velopharyngeal function: The lateral still technique versus cinefluorography. *Cleft Palate Journal, 18,* 45–50.

Willis, C., & Stutz, M. (1972). The clinical use of the Taub oral panendoscope in the observation of velopharyngeal function. *Journal of Speech and Hearing Disorders, 37,* 495–502.

Yules, R., & Chase, R. (1971). Secondary techniques for correction of palatopharyngeal incompetence. In W. Grabb, S. Rosenstein, & K. Bzoch (Eds.), *Cleft lip and palate: Surgical, dental, and speech aspects.* Boston: Little, Brown.

Zimmerman, G., Dalston, R., Brown, C., Folkins, J., Linville, R., & Seaver, E. (1987). Comparison of cineradiographic and phototransduction techniques for assessing velopharyngeal function during speech. *Journal of Speech and Hearing Research, 30,* 564–569.

Zwitman, D., Sonderman, J., & Ward, P. (1974). Variations in velopharyngeal closure assessed by endoscopy. *Journal of Speech and Hearing Disorders, 39,* 366.

CHAPTER 10

Articulation Assessment Procedures and Treatment Decisions

Judith E. Trost-Cardamone
and John E. Bernthal

Trost-Cardamone and Bernthal discuss the phonological problems of children with cleft palate speech in relation to phoneme acquisition and the occurrence of compensatory articulations. They advocate that speech treatment be based on careful assessment and note the importance of the degree of velopharyngeal adequacy in determining treatment strategies.

1. *Why do the authors consider the speech sound site deviations in persons with cleft palate to be phonological disorders?*
2. *What four speech characteristics cause cleft palate speech to be perceptually deviant and phonologically distinctive?*
3. *What are the main goals of a phonological evaluation?*
4. *Why should efforts to correct compensatory articulations include teaching children to make stops, fricatives, and affricates at contrasting places of articulation?*
5. *When a child has a repaired cleft palate that appears to accomplish velopharyngeal closure on an inconsistent basis, what speech treatment activities should be considered?*

Perhaps the most common speech disorder seen in persons with cleft palate is a disordered speech sound system, which frequently impairs speech intelligibility. Disorders that affect speech sound systems have traditionally been labeled in the speech–language pathology literature as *articulation disorders*. However, during the late 1970s and early 1980s, people began to use terms such as *phonological disorders* or *phonological disabilities* to describe these problems.

This change in terminology has become more common with the availability of linguistically based procedures for analyzing disordered speech sound systems. Locke (1983a) pointed out that, to some practitioners, this was merely a change in labeling the speech disorder. For others, the term *articulation* referred to only peripheral motor activity, whereas the term *phonologic* referred to the speaker's knowledge of the sound system and the rules that governed it. Stoel-Gammon and Dunn (1985) stated that phonology

> refers to the organization and classification of speech sounds that occur as contrastive units within a given language, and in another sense it is used as a general term referring to all aspects of the study of speech sounds, including speech perception and production, as well as cognitive and motor aspects of speech. (p. 3)

When clinicians now use the term articulation disorders for all children with disordered or delayed speech sound systems, we assume their usage of the term extends to all phonological disorders, and not only to peripheral production difficulties. It has long been recognized that articulation or phonological disorders can be caused by so-called higher level cognitive or linguistic impairments, as well as by motor control difficulties. An example of such a higher level disorder might be a child who collapses two phonemes into a single sound class because he or she does not make the distinctions needed to separate the phonemes into two sound classes.

Locke (1983b) and Shriberg and Kwiatkowski (1982) recommended that all disorders affecting the sound systems of language be termed phonological disorders. In defense of this position, Locke pointed out that distinguishing among the levels of phonology is difficult and that phonological disorders may frequently represent interactions among several phonological levels. Shriberg and Kwiatkowski (1982) recommended the term because it is more generic than articulation disorders.

At this point, the reader is probably asking, "What is the purpose of such an introduction when the phonological disorders seen in the individual with a cleft palate with or without cleft lip (CP ± CL) can, in most instances, be assumed to be directly related to structural problems associated with the cleft, and thus be viewed as articulation disorders?" We feel that such a position is too simple an explanation for a complex problem and might frequently be incorrect. We have chosen to label and approach the speech sound system disorders seen in individuals with cleft palate as phonological disorders for several reasons:

1. The term phonological disorders has been accepted as a holistic term that includes both phonetic (speech gesture) and phonemic (rule system) "levels" of impairment, and incorporates both segmental and linguistic or process-based diagnostic and treatment approaches.

2. The child with a cleft palate may have difficulties other than structural problems that may interact and account for the phonological delay or disorder. For example, what effect, if any, does an unoperated cleft have on the baby's early perceptual speech learning? Does the cleft alter motor speech development? Definitive data are not available on the effects of early chronic middle ear effusions on phonological perception or motor speech learning in children with phonologic systems that deviate from the norm. However, published data on the relationship between early otitis media with effusion (OME) and later speech adequacy implicates the auditory effects of OME as a primary source of both delayed and disordered phonological acquisition patterns for some children (Churchill, Hodson, Jones, & Novak, 1988; Paden, Novak, & Beiter, 1987; Shriberg & Smith, 1983). We suspect that several such factors interact to create the misarticulations observed in speakers with cleft palate.

3. Some children with CP ± CL may have developmental phonological disorders exclusively or in addition to specific speech patterns associated with structural deviations related to the cleft. Similarly, some children may have problems that are primarily linguistic in nature.

Before leaving this discussion, we wish to point out a couple of caveats. First, the analysis of a child's sound system in terms of phonological patterns or processes provides descriptions of the child's behavior, but does not provide explanations of why it occurs. The identification of phonological processes does not allow one to infer causality or to explain the disorder. When clinicians attempt to ascribe higher linguistic explanations to a child's use of phonological patterns or processes, they should do so with extreme caution.

On the other hand, certain patterns in the speech of individuals with phonological disorders can be attributed to phonetic factors and explanations. In the case of individuals with palatal clefts, there are frequently direct causal relationships between phonetic factors and the structural deviations associated with clefting. The observation of nasal emission consistently accompanying pressure consonants and of excessive and pervasive hypernasality in a child with a documented inadequate velopharyngeal valving mechanism is likely to indicate a phonetic problem with a structural explanation. In other instances, a clear causal relationship may be difficult or impossible to determine. The observation that a child with an oronasal fistula deletes stops and fricatives in postvocalic position while substituting glottal stops and pharyngeal fricatives in prevocalic position does not allow an easy phonetic explanation for the pattern of final consonant deletion. In summary, then, the application of a phonological pattern analysis should be viewed only as a descriptive device and will usually provide very little aid in the explanation of the error pattern.

SPEECH PRODUCTION PROBLEMS ASSOCIATED WITH CLEFT PALATE

Early Acquisition

Not all youngsters with cleft palates have phonological disorders. Normal, or near-normal, phonological acquisition in children with palatal clefts has become more likely in recent years, compared with even a decade ago. Although minimal data document why this has occurred, both speech–language pathologists and plastic surgeons have attributed these results to definitive closure of the cleft palate at earlier times (during the second 6 months of life) (Dorf & Curtin, 1982; Kuehn & Trost-Cardamone, 1988; O'Gara & Logemann, 1988). Such early surgery, when successful, allows for both a more normal oral structural environment and a competent velopharyngeal closure mechanism, and can be timed to accommodate a child's acquisition of speech sounds in first-word contexts.

In addition, recent reports have addressed the importance of surgical closure that is timed to maximize certain sensitive periods in the child's acquisition of the sound system (Kemp-Fincham, Kuehn, & Trost-Cardamone, in press; Trost-Cardamone, 1990a). Table 10.1, adapted from Oller (1980), outlines the several stages in the development of phonetic control during the first year of life. The late end of the expansion stage and the full reduplicated babbling stage are cited as sensitive periods during which the infant gains practice with speech motor controls and associated sensorimotor subroutines that underlie coordinated articulatory gestures. An open palate and absent velopharyngeal valving mechanism during these stages of development would likely alter the baby's perceptual and motor learning. The permanence of such early mislearning and its impact on later representational speech sound acquisition is not well understood. Based on normal acquisition patterns and schedules, compensatory articulation patterns are more likely to develop when palate repair is not accomplished successfully by the time a child engages in first-word productions. For some children, this may be before 12 months of age, and for others several months later. Based

TABLE 10.1

Stages of Normal Development of Phonetic Control

Normal Infant's Age	Characteristic of Vocalizations	Metaphonological Characteristic of Mature Languages
0–1 month—Phonation stage	Vocalizations with normal phonation but limited resonance produced with a closed or near-closed mouth	Introduction of normal phonation in nonreflexive vocalizations
2–3 months—Gooing stage	Velar consonant-like sounds; some "primitive" syllabification may be detected; sound similar to rounded back vowels [u]	Vocalizations with closure; alternation between opening and closure of the vocal tract
4–6 months—Expansion stage	Child gains increasing control of both laryngeal and oral articulatory gestures	
	• Fully resonant nuclei—adultlike vowels	Use of resonance capacity providing possibility for contrasts of resonance types
	• Raspberries; vocalization (bilabial trills)	Front as opposed to back; further manipulation of vocalizations during closure
	• Squealing and growling	Pitch contrasts introduced
	• Yelling	Amplitude contrasts
	• Ingressive-egressive sequences with vocalization	Further control of vocal breath stream
	• Marginal babbling—consonant-like and vowel-like features but lacking regular syllabic timing	Alternation of *full* opening and closure of the vocal tract

(Table continues)

TABLE 10.1 *Continued*

Normal Infant's Age	Characteristic of Vocalizations	Metaphonological Characteristic of Mature Languages
7–10 months— Canonical stage	Reduplicated babbling—true syllabic productions with a true consonant and vowel often chained in sequences [bababa]	Timing constraints on relationship of openings and closures (vocalic transitions)
11–12 months— Variegated babbling stage	Variegated babbling—continued use of adultlike syllables with increasing varied consonants [wətʌ]	Contrasts of consonantal and vocalic type

Note. Adapted from "The Emergence of the Sounds of Speech in Infancy" by D. K. Oller, 1980, in *Child Phonology: Vol. 1. Production* (p. 102) by G. Yeni-Komshian, J. Kavanagh, and C. A. Ferguson (Eds.), New York: Academic Press. Copyright 1980 by Academic Press. Adapted with permission.

solely on chronological age, palate repair that is delayed beyond 18 months would place most children at risk for developing compensatory strategies that become a part of the child's phonological rule system and may require long-term speech remediation.

Misarticulations Associated with Cleft Palate

Certain phonological patterns are commonly observed in individuals with palatal clefts. Four characteristics in particular cause cleft palate speech to be perceptually deviant and phonologically distinctive. These are (a) hypernasal resonance perceived during production of vowels, consonant glides, and liquids; (b) nasal air emission—the nasal airflow that distorts production of pressure consonants (i.e., stops, fricatives, and affricates); (c) weak pressure consonants associated with diminished intraoral air pressure; and (d) compensatory articulatory gestures observed to occur at several loci in the vocal tract. Trost-Cardamone (1990c) classified these attributes collectively as cleft palate misarticulations and noted that, whereas hypernasal resonance, nasal emission, and weak-pressure consonants cause *phonetic distortions,* compensatory gestures cause *phonetic substitutions.* Hypernasal resonance, nasal air emission, and weak-pressure consonants are frequently reduced or eliminated by surgical or prosthetic management. In contrast, presurgical compensatory articulations often persist postoperatively, even when adequate velopharyngeal valving can be achieved. Speech remediation for the speaker with cleft palate requires an appreciation of compensatory productions with respect to their phonetic parameters and error substitution patterns.

Although unanswered questions remain regarding the nature and origins of compensatory articulation gestures associated with cleft palate, a sizable body of clinical data is available. These data have revealed the following general characteristics:

1. *Phonetically,* compensatory articulations are (a) used as substitutions for pressure consonants and (b) predominately errors in *place* of articulation; the manner of production is usually preserved. The well-known substitutions of glottal stops for stop consonants and pharyngeal fricatives for sibilant fricatives are representative examples in which manner of production is maintained but place of production is changed.

2. Most compensatory articulations represent a pattern of (lingual) *articulatory backing* in which the place of articulation tends to be posterior in the oral cavity relative to that seen in standard English (Brooks, Shelton, & Youngstrom, 1965, 1966; Lawrence & Philips, 1975; McWilliams & Philips, 1979; Powers, 1962; Trost, 1981). The development and learning of backed articulations has several potential

explanations, including (a) pharyngeal and glottal valving of the articulators, where success is more likely because the point of articulation is below the level of the defect (Bzoch, 1971; Lawrence & Philips, 1975; Morris, 1979); (b) valving in the area of defect, so that the tongue is used to occlude the cleft or fistula, establishing a "place compromise" for anterior and posterior pressure consonants (Trost, 1981; Trost-Cardamone, 1987); (c) attempted use of the tongue as a "lingual assist" to occlude or valve the inadequate velopharyngeal port, causing obligatory backing for many speech sounds; and (d) the consequences of early chronic conductive hearing loss associated with OME (Hubbard, Paradise, McWilliams, Elster, & Taylor, 1985; Trost-Cardamone, 1990b).

Table 10.2 lists seven types of compensatory articulations, their general places of production, and corresponding phonetic symbols. Detailed descriptions of these productions in terms of perceptual speech characteristics, articulatory gestures, and radiographic documentation have been provided elsewhere (Trost, 1981; Trost-Cardamone, 1986, 1987). These error types are considered later in this chapter. As a group, compensatory articulations tend to occur either as sound replacements (substitutions) and/or as abnormal coarticulations. As used here, the term *coarticulation* denotes aberrant or maladaptive simultaneous articulatory maneuvers, as in [t̰], where there is one manner of production (stop), with simultaneous valving at two places of production (glottal and tip alveolar), and where the deviant place (glottal) is the effective one for manner (Trost, 1981; Trost-Cardamone, 1986, 1987). Trost (1984) reported on certain patterns in compensatory error substitutions and coarticulations observed in a group of speakers with repaired CP ± CL. Several trends were revealed from these data. Of six types of compensatory articulations studied, glottal stops were the most frequently produced and were used to replace all English pressure consonants. Whereas glottal stops, pharyngeal fricatives, and posterior nasal fricatives occurred as substitutions and coarticulations, as in /ʔ/ for /b/ and /b̰/, respectively, mid-dorsum palatal stops and pharyngeal stops were produced only as substitutions. It follows that compensatory articulations were produced more often as substitutions than as coarticulations. Pharyngeal fricatives either replaced or occurred as simultaneous articulations with the sibilant fricatives; some speakers produced pharyngeal affricates for the oral affricates as in /ʔʕ/ for /tʃ/. Pharyngeal stops replaced only /k/ and /g/, and mid-dorsum palatal stops replaced only /t/, /d/, /k/, and /g/. Based on these data, Trost concluded that the errors were mainly in-class in terms of manner of production, with the exception of glottal stops, which were used to replace stops, fricatives, and affricates. Interestingly, glottal stops have a frequent, but transient,

TABLE 10.2

Compensatory Articulations, Their Places of Production,
and Corresponding Phonetic Symbols

Compensatory Articulation	Place of Production	Phonetic Symbol	
		Unvoiced	Voiced
Glottal stop	Glottis, vocal fold valving		/ʔ/
Pharyngeal fricative	Lingual base approximates PPW	/ʕ̥/	/ʕ/
Pharyngeal affricate	Combines glottal stop + pharyngeal fricative gestures	/ʔʕ̥/	/ʔʕ/
Pharyngeal stop	Lingual base contacts PPW	/ʡ̥/	/ʡ/
Velar fricative	Posterior lingual dorsum contacts posterior palate	/χ/	/ɣ/
Mid-dorsum palatal	Lingual mid-dorsum contacts mid-palate	/ɛ/	/ɟ/
Posterior nasal fricative	Velum/uvula approximates PPW of nasopharynx; back tongue may elevate in attempt to assist in velopharyngeal closure	/△/	

Note. PPW = posterior pharyngeal wall.

presence in the normal child's phonetic inventory in the second 6 months of life (Locke, 1983b; Stoel-Gammon, 1988). Trost (1984) suggested that, in the context of clefting, these aberrant glottal productions could persist and become compensatory gestures because of constraints posed by the cleft.

Stopping is a phonological process that occurs in normal phonological acquisition. The presence of glottal stopping in the speech of youngsters with palatal clefts suggests that the young child with a cleft palate may indeed be following the norm, but that the abnormal oral and velopharyngeal structures prevent the phonemic representation(s) from being executed. Thus, the stopping pattern may persist because of the structural problem rather than dropping out as occurs in normal phonological acquisition. Glottal stops in the child with a cleft palate are typically compensatory and sometimes may reflect attempts to use normal phonological (stop) patterns. The data reported in Chapter 8 appear to support this hypothesis.

In addition to the seven compensatory articulations listed in Table 10.2, other atypical backed articulations have been observed in speakers with cleft palates. These articulations include back-velar substitutions for /l/, /r/, and /n/, resulting in [L], [Я], and [ŋ], respectively. Posterior shifts of the liquids /l/ and /r/ and the nasal /n/ in the child with a cleft may result from attempting to capture airflow or use the back of the tongue to help seal the velopharyngeal port. These productions, particularly [Я] and [L], also occur in the speech of children and adults without clefts. Their presence cannot always be assumed to represent compensatory behavior.

Some of the atypical productions classified as compensatory in speakers with cleft palates have been observed to occur in the disordered sound systems of youngsters without clefts. For example, the use of glottal stops to replace some or most consonants, and not merely the high-pressure consonants, is not uncommon in the phonetic repertoire of the phonologically deviant child. In fact, glottal replacement and stops substituted for glides have been suggested as idiosyncratic phonological processes in the speech of children with phonological disorders. Likewise, posterior nasal fricatives or "snorts" have been reported in the phonology of speakers without clefts (Edwards & Bernhardt, 1973; Hall & Tomblin, 1975; Trost-Cardamone, 1988). Trost (1981; Trost-Cardamone, 1988, 1990c) described a pattern of a phone-specific nasal emission in speakers without clefts, in which the nasal air escape distorts only certain consonants, especially sibilant fricatives and affricates, in the absence of hypernasality. Peterson (1975) reported similar characteristics in speakers with repaired palatal clefts. Even pharyngeal stops have been documented in the phonetic inventory of a phonologically impaired child without a cleft (Trost-Cardamone, 1985).

ASSESSMENT OF SOUND SYSTEMS IN INDIVIDUALS WITH CLEFT PALATES

The phonological assessment of a child with a cleft palate requires the speech–language pathologist to have knowledge of the structural deviations in the child's oral cavity that might contribute to deviant phonological patterns. This information includes the status and sphincteric pattern of velopharyngeal speech closure (Croft, Shprintzen, & Rakoff, 1981; Skolnick, McCall, & Barnes, 1973; Skolnick, Shprintzen, McCall, & Rakoff, 1975), the presence of any oronasal fistulae, and the dental and occlusal status. In addition, the palatine tonsils may sometimes cause velopharyngeal inadequacy. Using videonasendoscopy to examine the velopharyngeal sphincter, MacKenzle-Stepner, Witzel, Stringer, and Laskin (1987) and Shprintzen, Sher, and Croft (1987) showed that tonsillar tissue can proliferate up and behind the velum and thereby obstruct or impede velopharyngeal closure. Such tonsils, however, may not appear large on intraoral inspection (see Chapter 7). Speakers with consistent hypernasality and nasal air emission who show no obvious intraoral signs of palatal clefting are suspect for such an etiology. The sphincteric pattern of velopharyngeal closure can be determined only by superior or base views of the port, as obtained through nasendoscopy and videofluoroscopy. Discussion of the merits and importance of instrumental assessment is not within the purpose of this chapter, but is covered in Chapter 9.

The primary clinical task for the speech–language pathologist is to assess the child's phonological status and then infer the effects of structural deviations on the phonological behavior observed. The assessment of phonological behavior varies relative to the child's chronological age, and linguistic and cognitive functioning. Obviously, assessment procedures for a 14-month-old child who has acquired approximately 30 words differ from the procedures used with a 2-year-old who is using three- and four-word sentences, or from those used with a 6-year-old child who is using complete sentences.

A Protocol for Phonological Assessment

The material in this section offers guidelines for assessing the child's phonological status. Although the focus is on the preschool youngster, the suggestions are intended to be flexible and modifiable according to each patient's age and overall development. Such an assessment usually is done within the context of an overall communication evaluation that includes other aspects of speech and language behavior, such as syntax, pragmatics, semantics, voice, fluency, and the related procedures of hearing testing, oral cavity examination, and perceptual judgment. The primary purpose for assessing phonological behavior is to determine whether an individual needs intervention and, if so, the direction of such treatment.

To make these decisions, the clinician samples the client's speech through a variety of sampling procedures and then analyzes the data to determine the need and possible direction of intervention. Because of the importance that surgical timing may have on influencing the acquisition of speech sounds by a baby with a cleft palate, we recommend that the speech–language pathologist begin observation/intervention sessions with the child prior to initial palate repair and continue to follow the child until adequate velopharyngeal function and developmentally appropriate phonological behavior are achieved. The main goal in all evaluations is to distinguish speech errors that may be due to faulty velopharyngeal closure or other structural deviations from speech errors that are compensatory or developmental in nature.

Obtaining the Speech Sample

The type and size of the speech sample that serves as the data base for the analysis is important in a phonological assessment. Although a complete discussion of this topic is beyond the scope of the chapter, Edwards (1983) identified issues of potential importance concerning the size and type of the language sample used to determine phonological status. Specifically, she listed the importance of the following: (a) spontaneous production versus imitation; (b) isolated words versus phrases and continuous speech; (c) syntactic pragmatic and prosodic variables; (d) phonetic context, word length, complexity, and familiarity; (e) specific stimuli versus no set stimulus items; (f) number of attempts at each sound versus number of chances to apply each process; (g) word versus syllable positions; (h) one rendition of each lexical item versus multiple productions; (i) size of sample; and (j) type of transcription. This complex issue requires the clinician to make a series of compromises and judgments, especially during clinic visits, where time is often limited. Our general guidelines include taking several speech samples, as discussed in the following sections.

Connected speech.   A standard procedure in most assessments is an evaluation of productions during connected speech. A connected speech sample gives the examiner a notion of the speaker's overall intelligibility and the consistency of individual speech sound productions, as well as the effect of context and natural prosodic patterns. Some speech–language pathologists recommend a spontaneous speech sample as the exclusive data base (Shriberg & Kwiatkowski, 1980; Stoel-Gammon & Dunn, 1985). We suggest that a connected speech sample be a part of the test battery, but that other samples also be included. The preferred methodology for obtaining a connected speech sample is to engage the client in spontaneous conversation. If this cannot be accomplished, alternative procedures, such as response elicitation to picture stimuli, telling a story following the clinician's model, or having the child read a passage, can be used.

The clinician also needs to determine the size of the corpus. Obviously, the clinician needs a sample of sufficient size to obtain a representative sample of the child's phonology and to analyze other aspects of the child's language. We recommend a sample of approximately 100 words in which the child's intended words are known.

For the child with marginal velopharyngeal closure, a spontaneous speech sample may demonstrate a velopharyngeal valving problem that can be missed in single-word utterances, which make fewer timing demands on velopharyngeal function. For the unintelligible child, the exclusive use of spontaneous speech sampling may be difficult unless the intended lexical items can be determined. However, for the very young child (18 months or younger), a play situation in which spontaneous speech is sampled may be the only option other than some object naming or imitation following an adult model. In our experience, speech sampling with the very young child is best done monthly or bimonthly, and should involve the mother or other caregivers to obtain observations and document speech behaviors in more natural settings, outside of the clinic or office.

Sound inventories. A second useful format is a speech sound inventory in which the client names words in response to picture stimuli. These instruments typically sample consonants and consonant clusters in word-initial and word-final positions. The specific sounds included in such inventories vary, but usually include those sounds that have a high frequency of errors in children's speech. For a child with a cleft palate in whom velopharyngeal closure may be a concern, items should be selected to test the child's performance on pressure consonants (stops, fricatives, and affricates). One instrument that tests these consonants is the *Iowa Pressure Articulation Test,* a subtest of the *Templin–Darley Test of Articulation* (Templin & Darley, 1969). Another instrument that contains a high percentage of pressure consonants is the *Bzoch Error Patterns Diagnostic Articulation Tests* (Bzoch, 1979). In addition, Trost-Cardamone (1990c) recommended some specialized sampling contexts useful for documenting hypernasality and nasal air emission to determine patterns of phonetic distortion errors. These contexts include syllabic (CV) repetitions of all obstruent (pressure) consonants in the child's inventory and sustained phonations of high vowels /u/ and /i/, contrasting productions with the nares occluded and unoccluded. Such clinical tasks can often distinguish among the various sources of nasal air emission (e.g., velopharyngeal port, anterior or posterior fistulae), and phone-specific patterns. Repeated productions of a stop consonant + vowel pattern are particularly useful in hearing compensatory coarticulations. These patterns are discussed in more detail in our discussion of phonological analysis.

Stimulability. A third sample to be included in the test battery is stimulability testing. These samples are based on the child's imitation of an adult model, which may include both auditory and visual cues, and may consist of isolated sounds, syllables, words, or phrases that contain the adult form of the target speech sound. Imitation of words may suggest that the child has the necessary articulatory gesture to produce a sound that does not typically appear in his or her phonetic repertoire. Such testing may represent the child's maximum performance on such segments.

Transcription and scoring. Although clinicians continue to use the traditional method of scoring speech sound productions as substitutions, omissions, and distortions, we strongly recommend that such scoring not be used in assessing the speech of children with cleft palates. We recommend, instead, that the clinician use the International Phonetic Alphabet (IPA), including a set of diacritics (markers) that add detail to the broad phonetic symbols. Several close or narrow transcription notation systems can be used. The reader who desires notation information in addition to that provided in Table 10.2 is referred to Edwards (1986) and Shriberg and Kent (1982). The clinician should record as much phonetic detail as his or her transcription skills allow. Phonetic detail can assist the clinician in identifying phonological patterns and speech sound errors that are likely caused by velopharyngeal insufficiency or other structural factors.

Table 10.3 lists five possible error productions of the word "show." These different forms illustrate the importance of careful phonetic transcription. Error Production 1 in the table reflects an insufficient velopharyngeal mechanism (no fistula is present), and other pressure consonants are characterized by nasal emission. Error Production 4 depicts velopharyngeal insufficiency, as well as compensatory replacement of /s/ with a pharyngeal fricative.

We urge that the clinician record speech samples on audiotape using high-quality equipment so that he or she can play them back as often as is required to accurately transcribe the child's utterances. Included on the recording should be a "gloss" of what the clinician believes the child intended to say. An audio recording of the child will be of value not only in obtaining accurate transcriptions, but also as a baseline measure to assess change in the child's speech and language following intervention.

Finally, we recommend that the clinician establish a standard protocol for assessment. A standard protocol is a useful tool to establish a baseline for later assessment. A comparison of the child's speech production on the same stimuli pre- and postintervention is critical in assessing surgical intervention, as well as other interventions. This advice has merit with all types of disorders, but is most compelling with the population with cleft palates.

In summary, we recommend that the phonological test battery include a sample of approximately 75 to 100 words; a standard picture or word articulation test, including a subtest of pressure consonants; a syllable repetition task; and a test of stimulability. The transcription should be done live, whenever possible, and should include whole-word transcriptions with as much phonetic detail as the clinician can provide. All samples should be audiotaped for further transcription refinement and to assure a baseline record of the child's phonological status.

TABLE 10.3
Five Potential Errors in Saying "Show,"
with Corresponding Narrow Phonetic Transcription

Target Word	Error Production	Explanation
Show: /ʃoʊ/	1. [ʃ̃õʊ̃]	Nasal emission on /ʃ/; hypernasality on /oʊ/
	2. [ʢoʊ]	Pharyngeal fricative substitution for /ʃ/
	3. [ʢ͡ʃoʊ]	Pharyngeal fricative compensatory coarticulation with /ʃ/
	4. [ʢ̃õʊ̃]	Pharyngeal fricative substitution for /ʃ/; nasal emission on /ʢ̸/; hypernasality on /oʊ/
	5. [t̃õʊ̃]	Substitution of [t] for [ʃ] (phonologic process of stopping); nasal emission on /t/; hypernasality on /oʊ/

Note. Modified from "Effects of Velopharyngeal Incompetency on Speech" by J. E. Trost-Cardamone, 1986, *Journal of Childhood Communication Disorders, 10,* pp. 31–49.

Analyzing the Speech Sample

Following administration of the assessment protocol, the clinician analyzes the data to determine (a) the presence of cleft palate misarticulations and any noncleft (developmental or other) contributions to the disorder; (b) whether the child should be seen for treatment, and the direction it should take; (c) the need for instrumental assessment; and (d) whether (further) physical management is indicated.

Overall intelligibility. One of the clinician's first analysis procedures is to make a perceptual judgment of overall intelligibility. Speech intelligibility is a subjective judgment made by a listener and is the most frequent factor cited by listeners when rating speech. Speech intelligibility ratings are influenced by a variety of factors (e.g., hypernasal resonance and nasal air emission), but a major influence is the percentage of words in a speech sample understood by the listener. Speech intelligibility represents a continuum ranging from unintelligible (where the message is not understood) to totally intelligible (where all words in the message are understood). The intelligibility ratings of a child with a cleft palate are affected by a number of factors that do not typically affect the child with a normal vocal tract. For example, the child with velopharyngeal inadequacy is likely to have speech characterized by hypernasal resonance, compensatory articulatory gestures, nasal emission of air, and weak-pressure consonants. These factors tend to make the child's speech less intelligible. In fact, a low intelligibility rating may be less of a factor in determining whether this child should receive speech instruction than would such ratings in the case of a child with a normal oral mechanism. For example, the child who is scheduled for pharyngeal flap surgery in the future may not be a candidate for speech instruction until after the surgical procedure even though the child's speech intelligibility might be relatively low.

When compensatory articulations coexist with velopharyngeal inadequacy, however, caution is in order. Data suggest that, in some individuals, compensatory gestures may interfere with velopharyngeal closure. The videofluoroscopic data of Henningson and Isberg (1986) showed that the use of compensatory placements can alter otherwise adequate velopharyngeal speech closure. Similar data have come from clinical studies in which videonasedoscopy has been applied in biofeedback therapy (Hoch, Golding-Kushner, Siegel-Sadowitz, & Shprintzen, 1986; Witzel, Tobe, & Salyer, 1988). These data support the use of direct instrumental assessment prior to making decisions concerning secondary surgery.

Comparison of productions to developmental norms. A second factor that is frequently used to determine whether a child is a candidate for speech instruction is the appropriateness of the sound productions relative to the child's age. Traditionally, norms have been used to compare a child's speech sound productions with those of normally developing children to determine whether the speech sound productions are typical for the child's age. More recently, the presence of phonological patterns in a child's speech has been compared with the ages at which such patterns tend to no longer be used by a normal child during the phonological acquisition period. A comparison of performance against a normative standard is important for the child with a cleft palate, but the way in which such data are interpreted must be modified in many instances. For example, a child with a cleft may not produce bilabial stops (usually mastered early in the developmental sequence) because he or she is unable to build up the necessary intraoral air pressure because of an anterior palatal fistula. In this case, developmental data on bilabial stops would not be a significant factor in deciding whether to provide speech services to that child. The clinician should also keep in mind that in using the data from any large group study, individual subject data are obscured. Nevertheless, certain sound segments tend to be mastered earlier than others, and if segments normally acquired early are not present and their absence cannot be attributed to the structural deviation, developmental data will contribute to the treatment decisions.

Phonetic inventory. The clinician should identify all consonant single-tons and consonant clusters that the child produced correctly in the sample. All correct productions should be documented by position in words, the context in which such productions occurred, and the consistency with which such productions occurred. In the case of segments that were produced in manner or place that did not match the adult standard, the clinician should record the position and context in which they occurred, the consistency in which they occurred, and the exact phonetic description of the error.

Phonological pattern analysis. An important part of the analysis procedure is the organization of the speech sound errors into a meaningful picture. The clinician should review the test data and categorize errors according to commonalities or patterns. Frequently, these error patterns affect entire sound classes. For example, the child with an existing oronasal fistula may have an error pattern that distorts production of obstruents (pressure consonants). On the other hand, a pattern of gliding of liquids, as in /w/ for /r/, may not be related to structural problems associated with the cleft. These analysis procedures are important to understanding a child's phonological status.

A difficult issue for the clinician is to distinguish between those error patterns that are developmental in nature and those that may have a structural or physiological explanation as a result of the cleft. The clinician must be aware of common patterns that may have a physiological basis in children with cleft palate. The following articulatory patterns are sometimes seen in children with cleft palates and are not typically seen in children with structurally intact and functional oral and pharyngeal mechanisms:

1. *Consonant distortions associated with nasal emissions*—It is feasible to differentiate three error patterns associated with nasal emission, and different interventions may be in order for each.
   - *Nasal emission because of a persistence of velopharyngeal inadequacy.* When nasal emission is due to velopharyngeal inadequacy, the speaker exhibits nasal emission distortion during production of all pressure consonants and pervasive hypernasality accompanying production of vowels and of the vocalic consonants /l/, /r/, /j/, /w/.
   - *Nasal emission due to oronasal fistulae.* When nasal emission is the result of an oronasal fistula, there is a relationship between the location of the fistula and the consonants affected (Trost-Cardamone, 1986, 1990c). When the fistula is located posteriorly near the juncture between the hard and soft palate, /k/, and /g/ are likely to be distorted, and there may be little effect on the production of consonants produced at the anterior portion of the oral cavity. The more anterior pressure consonants, especially /t/, /d/,

/s/, /z/, /p/, and /b/, are likely to be distorted when a fistula is located in the anterior portion of the oral cavity, such as in the area of the incisive foramen.

- *Nasal emission that is phone specific.* This pattern may occur in the absence of clefting or other velopharyngeal impairment. This disorder typically does not affect an entire class of sounds and rarely has hypernasality associated with it. In these instances, the problem is likely the result of faulty learning and does not require surgical intervention, but can usually be treated with speech therapy (Trost-Cardamone, 1988). Unfortunately, this pattern is not always diagnosed appropriately and is often assumed to be due to a submucous cleft palate. Such youngsters may undergo unnecessary (and unsuccessful) surgery or prolonged and unprofitable speech instruction.

Because of the distinctly different treatments required in relation to these sources of nasal air escape, it is critical that the speech–language pathologist be able to identify and distinguish among language error patterns.

2. *Vowel distortions secondary to hypernasality*—These patterns warrant little discussion or explanation. It is important for the clinician to separate the hypernasal resonance deviations on vowels and vocalic consonants from the aerodynamic consequences of deficient velopharyngeal valving (i.e., nasal airflow and weak-pressure consonants).

3. *Compensatory articulations*—Several types of compensatory articulations are presented earlier in this chapter. With respect to treatment planning and in order to select appropriate intervention procedures, the clinician must be able to distinguish between productions that are used as substitutions and those that occur as coarticulations.

4. *Atypical backed articulations*—These patterns also have been addressed earlier in this chapter. The presence of such productions in the speaker's inventory, with or without coexisting compensatory articulations, should be analyzed to determine whether they are part of a phonological pattern of backing, or whether they represent selective articulatory substitutions.

Phonological analysis procedures have been published by several authors (Hodson, 1986; Ingram, 1981; Khan & Lewis, 1986; Shriberg & Kwiatkowski, 1980; Weiner, 1979). In these procedures, error patterns are described as phonological processes. Phonological patterns or processes are defined as systematic sound changes or simplifications that affect a class of sounds. The specific patterns or processes identified with these assessment procedures vary, and often process-based approaches yield little useful data on organic–structural or physiological disorders. For compensatory articulations in particular, and organic disorders in general, we recommend a place–manner–voicing analysis procedure similar to that described by Elbert and Gierut (1986).

Chapter 8 in this text and the report by Estrem and Broen (1989) provide data on phonological patterns observed in young children with cleft palate. In addition to material presented here, those data can be used by the clinician to help determine whether the phonological patterns identified in a particular child are characteristic of those seen in phonologically normally developing children, or in children with developmentally delayed phonology, or in children with cleft palate. Severe limitations are inherent in any attempt to describe the organization of the phonological system, even in structurally intact 11- to 15-month-old children who have relatively few words. Until a child has a working vocabulary of at least 50 words, the identification of the child's phonological patterns and phonetic inventory of English speech sounds is usually unreliable. Even normally developing children differ substantially in their phonetic preferences, word selection, and stability of word shapes (Vihman, 1988).

The assessment of toddlers may require several sessions and/or audiotapings of the parent–child interactions in the home. Phonological status often cannot be determined until the child has more connected speech. The stops are the earliest class of pressure consonants in the infant's inventory and are usually present in the speech of structurally intact children at 10 to 14 months of age. In contrast, the fricatives and affricates—speech sounds that constitute more than half of the consonants most likely to be replaced by compensatory productions by children with clefts—are mostly absent even in phonologically normal children at the beginning of the second year. However, none of the pressure consonants (obstruents) in English are normally produced in association with nasal air emission at any age. Therefore, even the baby who undergoes palatal repair at a young age, and whose consonant output consists primarily of stops, nasals, and glides and whose word shapes are predominantly open (CV) syllables ("car" → [kɑ]) and syllable reduplications ("water" → [wɑwɑ] or "cookie" → [kiki]), should not have nasal emission of air during pressure consonant production if there is structural and functional integration of the mechanism.

A judgment of the adequacy of velopharyngeal closure and reasonable judgments concerning the need for secondary surgery usually can be made even in toddlers if they produce oral stops and fricatives. Judgments of compensatory articulations and the permanence of the phonetic inventory are difficult to make and may not be reliable in the young child. For example, some youngsters may not yet be targeting sibilant fricatives and affricates, so the absence of pharyngeal fricatives or affricates is not informative. However, some youngsters may have a sizable pressure consonant inventory and appear to demonstrate velopharyngeal inadequacy. In such instances, the possible interaction between compensatory gestures and velopharyngeal closure needs to be carefully evaluated, usually with the aid of instrumental assessment.

In choosing phonological patterns and target segments for the initiation of treatment, the clinician should be aware of normal acquisition data because these data have application to children who have clefts (Grunewell, 1981; Hodson & Paden, 1981; Locke, 1983b; Prather, Hedrick, & Kern, 1975; Smit, 1986; Stoel-Gammon, 1987; Stoel-Gammon & Dunn, 1985). Unfortunately, there is a dearth of information concerning phonological acquisition in children with CP ± CL. In Chapter 8, Broen and Moller speak to these issues and report data on phonological patterns in children with clefts. They also make a plea for the collection of additional data on early phonological development in children with cleft palate. Several characteristics of normal phonological development appear to be established:

1. Open syllables (CV) and syllable reduplication are common phonological patterns that modify syllable structures used by children. Final consonant deletion and syllable reduplication are also common patterns in young children with cleft palates. These patterns are not usually seen in the phonologically normal child after about 30 months.
2. Singleton consonants are usually produced correctly by the child before consonant clusters. However, sometimes a specific cluster may facilitate production of a single consonant.
3. Most nasals, stops, and glides are usually acquired fairly early. Fricatives, affricates, and liquids are usually acquired later, and the time required for mastery is usually longer than for nasals, stops, and glides.
4. Generally, front placements precede back placements, labials precede alveolars, alveolars precede palatals, and velars are typically acquired last.
5. Stops are typically used in word-initial position before word-final or word-medial positions.
6. Many fricatives are produced correctly in word-final position prior to correct production in word-initial or word-medial positions.
7. Phonetic productions that are nonphonemic (for English) drop out of the child's consonant production repertoire toward the end of the first year.
8. Vowels are usually mastered by age 3, and by age 4, the normal child is producing most consonant sounds correctly.

9. Young children vary a great deal in their phonetic preferences, word selection, and stability of their word shapes. Children's patterns trend toward uniformity with age and increased knowledge of the language.

SPEECH TREATMENT DECISIONS

Establishing Diagnostic Baselines

Effective speech management depends upon comprehensive and reliable assessment. In the child with CP $\pm$ CL or related velopharyngeal inadequacy, assessment involves both clinical and instrumental procedures (see Chapter 9). It should provide data on the status and potential of the velopharyngeal closure mechanism, any oral structural deviations (including fistulae), hearing status, and a comprehensive speech–language assessment. Based upon these diagnostic baselines, appropriate speech treatment decisions can be made. Although malocclusion and specific dental deviations are secondary agents of impaired articulation in youngsters with CP $\pm$ CL, the resulting speech impairments usually are relatively minor (Trost-Cardamone, 1990a) and frequently are resolved through developmental (growth) changes in dentofacial relationships and direct orthodontic, prosthodontic, and/or orthognathic surgery interventions.

Our main focus in the remainder of this chapter is on treatment of compensatory articulations and the efficacy of various treatment alternatives for cleft palate misarticulations, since these are exceptional characteristics that distinguish the treatment of the misarticulating children with cleft palate from their phonologically impaired peers. The following discussion presumes that any nasal air emission caused by oronasal fistulae is either minimal or has been eliminated by surgery or prosthetic obturation and that otologic and hearing problems have been documented and are being appropriately managed.

Speech Errors: Deciding How to Treat Them

Velopharyngeal closure and phonological error patterns. In a child with repaired CP $\pm$ CL, the relationship between velopharyngeal closure and phonological error patterns can take several forms. Understanding this relationship is essential to appropriate choice of treatment. Table 10.4 presents hypothetical cases and outlines several of the more common speech pattern–velopharyngeal closure relationships seen in individuals with cleft palate, as well as recommended treatments. As shown in the table, postoperative velopharyngeal closure can be adequate, inadequate, inconsistently (questionably) adequate, or marginal.

TABLE 10.4

Treatment Decisions Based on Velopharyngeal Status and Phonological Error Patterns

Velopharyngeal Status	Phonologic Error Pattern(s)	Recommended Treatment(s)
Case 1. Repaired and adequate	Compensatory substitutions; no hyper-nasality or nasal emission	Articulation instruction to modify compensatory placements
Case 2. Repaired (or no cleft) and adequate	Phone-specific nasal air emission affecting /s, z, ʃ/ ± /tʃ, dʒ/	Behavioral (articulation) instruction to eliminate pattern
		Biofeedback therapy, using videonasendoscopy, if necessary (Witzel, Tobe, & Salyer, 1988)
Case 3. Repaired and inadequate	Pervasive and moderate to severe hyper-nasality and nasal emission across phonetic contexts; no compensatory articulations	Further physical repair, surgical or prosthetic
		Postoperative reassessment
Case 4. Repaired and inconsistently (questionably) adequate	Compensatory articulations accompanied by nasal emission; marginal or adequate closure on orally articulated pressure consonants	Articulation instruction to modify compensatory articulation placements; watch for changes in nasal emission with establishment of oral placements
		Pre- and posttreatment videonasopharyngoscopy
		Nasopharyngoscopy biofeedback instruction to modify pharyngeal and/or glottal compensatory articulations
		Speech training appliance to close velopharyngeal port and facilitate compensatory articulation modifications

(Table continues)

TABLE 10.4 *Continued*

Velopharyngeal Status	Phonologic Error Pattern(s)	Recommended Treatment(s)
Case 5. Repaired and marginally adequate	Mild nasal emission and hypernasality across phonetic contexts; no compensatory articulations	Videonasopharyngoscopy biofeedback instruction to modify sphincteric closure pattern (Siegel-Sadewitz & Shprintzen, 1982) Combined videonasopharyngoscopy and bulb reduction instruction to close velopharyngeal gap (McGrath, 1988)

Associated perceptual speech patterns vary from compensatory substitutions and no perceptible hypernasality or nasal emission, to pervasive nasal emission and hypernasality with no compensatory articulations, to velopharyngeal inadequacy specifically associated with compensatory postures and not observed on oral consonant productions, and so forth. This table is not meant to be used as a menu for a "cookbook approach" to treatment. Rather, it is offered as a guide for considering these important physiological relationships. In particular, the reader is urged to note how the different treatment alternatives vary in relation to the interaction between velopharyngeal closure status and articulatory error patterns.

An additional treatment variable is the presence or absence of compensatory articulations. Hoch et al. (1986) pointed out that the postoperative velopharyngeal insufficiency in patients who use pharyngeal and glottal compensatory articulations differs in pattern and consistency from that observed in speakers with clefts whose hypernasality and nasal emission exists in the context of oral pressure consonant productions. We concur with this position and advocate the use of speech instruction to modify some compensatory gestures prior to making decisions regarding secondary surgery. Depending upon its severity, submucous cleft palate (occult or classical) could present articulatory patterns similar to those presented for Cases 3, 4, or 5. Likewise, velopharyngeal insufficiency associated with tonsillar obstruction or postoperative adenoidectomy might show articulatory patterns similar to those described in Cases 3 and 5. Often, tonsillectomy or secondary surgery (pharyngeal flap, sphincter pharyngoplasty) is necessary in such cases where the problem exceeds marginal closure/mild speech severity levels.

Modifying compensatory articulations.   Although we do not know the extent to which early oral structural deviations associated with cleft palate interfere with acquisition of underlying phonological representations, the child with compensatory substitutions has problems with place features at the surface level. For this reason, the clinician should focus instruction on teaching place contrasts within the vocal tract, for the stops, fricatives, and affricates. Correction of compensatory articulations frequently involves shifting or expanding the child's places of articulation. Typically, this includes moving posterior and inferior placements forward and upward, as, for example, in modifying a pharyngeal fricative /ʕ/ for /s/ substitution. Because some children lack the articulatory gestures for correct productions, they may need to be taught how to make the target sound. Estrem and Broen (1989) suggested, on the basis of data from very young children, that some speakers with cleft palate prefer to articulate at the peripheral ends of the vocal tract, making little or no speech use of the middle and posterior palate. Thus, in remediation, auditory modeling usually does not provide sufficient cues to facilitate the desired placement modifications. Mirror work, tactile cues, and even schematic or diagrammatic representation of placement information are frequent treatment strategies, especially in the early stages of speech management. If compensatory coarticulations exist as when a child produces a glottal stop in conjunction with the lip movements for a /b/ (i.e., [ʔb] instead of producing a normal /b/, it is recommended that correct oral placement be established initially; then glottal (vocal fold) valving can be eliminated before adding voicing. Teaching voiceless homorganic oral fricatives first in establishing oral stops has been reported to be a useful technique for breaking up compensatory coarticulations (Trost, 1981).

Direct work on place of articulation or modification or articulatory gestures is obviously a phonetic activity. Once articulatory placements have been established in the child's production repertoire, then mastery of the phonemic pattern may be an appropriate goal. Treatment can be delivered through a number of approaches or combinations of approaches, including traditional segmentally based treatment. When multiple errors occur, treatment based on pattern analysis (Bernthal & Bankson, 1988; Elbert & Gierut, 1986; Hodson & Paden, 1981; Weiner, 1979) may be preferred. Irrespective of the type of compensatory substitution(s) or coarticulation(s) used by the child, the management goals and procedures are usually similar. The goals of placement work are threefold: (a) to teach the child (speaker) where to produce the correct target, (b) to establish internal mechanisms for correct target selection and perceptual–motor self-monitoring, and (c) to facilitate learning generalization and carryover.

Hoch et al. (1986, p. 317) described techniques for eliminating compensatory errors associated with velopharyngeal insufficiency. With respect to target phoneme selection, they recommended that training begin with phones that are stimulable, have an anterior place of production, are highly visible, and are developmentally appropriate. They also recommended that voiceless phones be established before voiced, particularly when error patterns involve glottal stop substitutions. They advocated the use of whispered speech to facilitate oral valving and reduce or eliminate glottal valving.

In addition to developmental considerations, the clinician should select target segments or focus on patterns that might contribute most to reduced intelligibility. For example, if a 5-year-old uses pharyngeal fricatives to replace /s/, and also produces glottal stops for /k/ and /g/ and substitutes /w/ for /l/ (gliding of liquids), /s/ might be an early focus because of its relatively high frequency of occurrence and important grammatical role in spoken English. Even if the child at first produces a (developmentally acceptable) /θ/ and /ð/ or frontal lisp pattern on /s/ and /z/, such oral fricatives are more intelligible than the compensatory pharyngeal or glottal replacements, and usually can be modified to /s/ and /z/ productions.

Compensatory substitution patterns tend to be fairly consistent across phonetic contexts, with minimal variability across word contexts. This is in marked contrast to the normally developing speech of 2- and 3-year-olds and to the impaired speech of the structurally intact, but phonologically delayed, child. These children frequently show a wide range of phonetic ability to produce targets, but their phonemic behavior typically displays variability across contexts.

SUMMARY

The treatment of children with CP ± CL involves special considerations when compared with phonologically delayed children who have structurally intact oral mechanisms. A major consideration for the child with a cleft is the interaction of velopharyngeal closure and the phonological patterns observed. This relationship frequently influences the nature of phonological management. For example, when velopharyngeal closure is inadequate and nasal emission and hypernasality are present, additional physical management, surgical or prosthetic, may be the most appropriate treatment decision, with speech instruction delayed until physical management is completed. In contrast, for the youngster who has a repaired cleft with adequate velopharyngeal closure, but still has nasal emission of air on selected phones (a phone-specific pattern), treatment utilizing a traditional phonetic approach to instruction that focuses on phonetic placement and/or biofeedback using videonasendoscopy may be the treatment of choice. A second area for treatment that is a frequent target for children with clefts is the modification of compensatory articulations, which usually requires moving the place of articulation forward and upward. Once oral articulatory placements have been established, then the focus of instruction usually is on pattern analysis, and the approaches used are similar to those used with the phonologically delayed child who has a structurally intact oral mechanism. For some youngsters with both velopharyngeal inadequacy and compensatory articulations, speech instruction with or without the use of velopharyngeal biofeedback techniques may eliminate the use of compensatory articulations and satisfactorily modify velopharyngeal closure. For others, both speech treatment and physical management may be required.

REFERENCES

Bernthal, J. E., & Bankson, N. W. (Eds.). (1988). *Articulation and phonological disorders* (2nd ed.). Englewood Cliffs, NJ: Prentice-Hall.

Brooks, A. R., Shelton, R. L., & Youngstrom, K. A. (1965). Compensatory tongue–palate–posterior pharyngeal wall relationships in cleft palate. *Journal of Speech and Hearing Disorders, 30,* 166–173.

Brooks, A. R., Shelton, R. L., & Youngstrom, K. A. (1966). Tongue palate contacts in persons with palatal defects. *Journal of Speech and Hearing Disorders, 31,* 14–25.

Bzoch, K. R. (1971). Categorical aspects of cleft palate speech. In W. C. Grabb, S. W. Rosenstein, & K. R. Bzoch (Eds.), *Cleft lip and palate: Surgical, dental and speech aspects.* Boston: Little, Brown.

Bzoch, K. R. (1979). Measurement and assessment of categorical aspects of cleft palate speech. In K. R. Bzoch (Ed.), *Communicative disorders related to cleft lip and palate* (2nd ed.). Boston: Little, Brown.

Churchill, J. D., Hodson, B. W., Jones, B. W., & Novak, R. E. (1988). Phonological systems of speech disordered clients with positive/negative histories of otitis media. *Language, Speech and Hearing Services in Schools, 19,* 100–107.

Croft, C. B., Shprintzen, R. J., & Rakoff, S. J. (1981). Patterns of velopharyngeal valving in normal and cleft palate subjects: A multi-view videofluoroscopic and nasendoscopic study. *Laryngoscope, 91,* 265–271.

Dorf, D. S., & Curtin, J. (1982). Early cleft repair and speech outcome. *Plastic and Reconstructive Surgery, 70,* 74–79.

Edwards, M. L. (1983). Issues in phonological assessment. In J. Locke (Ed.), Assessing and treating phonological disorders: Current approaches. *Seminars in Speech and Language, 4.* New York: Thieme-Stratton.

Edwards, M. L. (1986). *Introduction to applied phonetics: Laboratory workbook.* Austin, TX: PRO-ED.

Edwards, M. L., & Bernhardt, B. (1973). *Phonological analyses in the speech of four children with language disorders.* Unpublished manuscript, Stanford University.

Elbert, M., & Gierut, J. (1986). *Handbook of clinical phonology: Approaches to assessment and treatment.* Austin, TX: PRO-ED.

Estrem, T., & Broen, P. A. (1989). Early speech productions of children with cleft palate. *Journal of Speech and Hearing Research, 32,* 12–23.

Grunewell, P. (1981). The development of phonology: A descriptive profile. *First Language, 3,* 161–191.

Hall, P., & Tomblin, J. (1975). Case study: Therapy procedures for remediation of a nasal lisp. *Language, Speech and Hearing Services in Schools, 6,* 29–32.

Henningson, G. E., & Isberg, A. M. (1986). Velopharyngeal movement patterns in patients alternating between oral and glottal articulation: A clinical and cine radiographical study. *Cleft Palate Journal, 23,* 1–9.

Hoch, L., Golding-Kushner, M., Siegel-Sadowitz, V. L., & Shprintzen, R. J. (1986). Speech therapy. In B. J. Williams (Ed.) Current methods of assessing and treating children with cleft palates. *Seminars in Speech and Language, 7,* 313–325.

Hodson, B. W. (1986). *The assessment of phonological processes–Revised.* Austin, TX: PRO-ED.

Hodson, B. W., & Paden, E. P. (1981). Phonological processes which characterize unintelligible and intelligible speech in early childhood. *Journal of Speech and Hearing Disorders, 46,* 369–373.

Hubbard, T., Paradise, J., McWilliams, B. J., Elster, B., & Taylor, F. (1985). Consequences of unremitting middle ear disease in early life: Otologic, audiologic and developmental findings in children with cleft palate. *The New England Journal of Medicine, 312,* 1529–1534.

Ingram, D. (1981). *Procedures for the phonological analysis of children's language.* Baltimore: University Park Press.

Kemp-Fincham, S. I., Kuehn, D. P., & Trost-Cardamone, J. E. (1990). Speech development and the timing of primary palatoplasty. In J. Bardach & H. L. Morris (Ed.), *Management of cleft lip and palate* (pp. 736–745). New York: Grune and Stratton.

Khan, L. M., & Lewis, N. P. (1986). *Khan–Lewis phonological analyses.* Circle Pines, MN: American Guidance Service.

Kuehn, D. P., & Trost-Cardamone, J. E. (1988). *Speech development and the timing of primary palatoplasty.* Paper presented at the annual meeting of the American Cleft Palate Association, Williamsburg, VA.

Lawrence, C., & Philips, B. J. (1975). A telefluoroscopic study of lingual contacts made by persons with palatal defects. *Cleft Palate Journal, 12,* 85–94.

Locke, J. L. (1983a). Clinical phonology: The explanation and treatment of speech sound disorders. *Journal of Speech and Hearing Disorders, 48,* 339–341.

Locke, J. L. (1983b). *Phonological acquisition and change.* New York: Academic Press.

MacKenzie-Stepner, K., Witzel, M. A., Stringer, D., & Laskin, R. (1987). Velopharyngeal insufficiency due to hypertrophic tonsils. *International Journal of Pediatric Otolaryngology, 14,* 57–63.

McGrath, C. O. (1988). *Prosthetic management strategies for velopharyngeal dysfunction.* Study session given at the annual meeting of the American Cleft Palate Association, Williamsburg, VA.

McWilliams, B. J., & Philips, B. J. (1979). Velopharyngeal incompetence. In *Audioseminars in Speech Pathology.* Philadelphia: Saunders.

Morris, H. L. (1979). Abnormal articulation patterns. In K. R. Bzoch (Ed.) *Communicative disorders related to cleft palate* (2nd ed.). Boston: Little, Brown.

O'Gara, M. M., & Logemann, J. L. (1988). Phonetic analyses of the speech development of babies with cleft palate. *Cleft Palate Journal, 25,* 122–134.

Oller, D. K. (1980). The emergence of the sounds of speech in infancy. In G. H. Yeni-Komshian, J. F. Kavanagh, & C. H. Ferguson (Eds.), *Child phonology: Volume 1. Production.* New York: Academic Press.

Paden, E. P., Novak, M. A., & Beiter, A. L. (1987). Predictors of phonological inadequacy in young children prone to otitis media. *Journal of Speech and Hearing Disorders, 52,* 232–242.

Peterson, S. J. (1975). Nasal emission as a component of the misarticulation on sibilants and affricates. *Journal of Speech and Hearing Disorders, 40,* 106–114.

Powers, G. (1962). Cinefluorographic investigation of articulatory movements of selected individuals with cleft palate. *Journal of Speech and Hearing Research, 5,* 59–69.

Prather, E. M., Hedrick, D. L. & Kern, C. A. (1975). Articulation development in children aged two to four years. *Journal of Speech and Hearing Disorders, 40,* 179–191.

Shprintzen, R. J., Sher, A., & Croft, C. B. (1987). Hypernasal speech caused by tonsillar hypertrophy. *International Journal of Pediatric Otolaryngology, 14,* 45–56.

Shriberg, L. D., & Kent, R. D. (1982). *Clinical phonetics.* New York: Macmillan.

Shriberg, L. D., & Kwiatkowski, J. (1982). Phonological disorders: I. A diagnostic classification system. *Journal of Speech and Hearing Disorders, 47,* 226–241.

Shriberg, L. D., & Smith, A. J. (1983). Phonological correlates of middle ear involvement in speech-delayed children: A methodological note. *Journal of Speech and Hearing Research, 26,* 293–297.

Shriberg, L. D., & Kwiatkowski, J. (1980). *Natural process analysis.* New York: Wiley.

Siegel-Sadewitz, V. L., & Shprintzen, R. J. (1982). Nasopharyngoscopy of the normal velopharyngeal sphincter: An experiment of biofeedback. *Cleft Palate Journal, 19,* 194–200.

Skolnick, M. L., McCall, G. N., & Barnes, M. (1973). The sphincteric mechanism of velopharyngeal closure. *Cleft Palate Journal, 10,* 286–305.

Skolnick, M. L., Shprintzen, R. J., McCall, G. N., & Rakoff, S. J. (1975). Patterns of velopharyngeal closure in subjects with repaired cleft palate and normal speech: A multiview videofluoroscopic analysis. *Cleft Palate Journal, 12,* 369–376.

Smit, A. B. (1986). Ages of speech sound acquisition: Comparisons and critiques of several normative studies. *Language, Speech and Hearing Services in Schools, 17,* 175–186.

Stoel-Gammon, C. (1987). Phonological skills of 2-year-olds. *Language, Speech and Hearing Services in Schools, 18,* 323–329.

Stoel-Gammon, C. (1988). Prelinguistic vocalizations of hearing impaired and normal hearing subjects: A comparison of consonantal inventories. *Journal of Speech and Hearing Disorders, 53,* 302–315.

Stoel-Gammon, C., & Dunn, C. (1985). *Normal and disordered phonology in children.* Austin, TX: PRO-ED.

Templin, M. C., & Darley, F. L. (1969). *The Templin–Darley tests of articulation* (2nd ed.). Iowa City: Bureau of Educational Research and Service, University of Iowa.

Trost, J. E. (1981). Articulatory additions to the classical description of the speech of persons with cleft palate. *Cleft Palate Journal, 18,* 193–203.

Trost, J. E. (1984). *Compensatory articulations: Error types, patterns, and treatment approaches.* Paper presented at the annual meeting of the American Cleft Palate Association, Seattle.

Trost-Cardamone, J. E. (1985). *Phonological process analysis: Its role in the diagnosis of the child with cleft palate.* Paper presented at the annual meeting of the American Speech–Language–Hearing Association, Washington, DC.

Trost-Cardamone, J. E. (1986). Effects of velopharyngeal incompetency on speech. *Journal of Childhood Communication Disorders, 10,* 31–49.

Trost-Cardamone, J. E. (1987). *Cleft palate misarticulations: A teaching tape.* Videotape produced by the Instructional Media Center, California State University, Northridge.

Trost-Cardamone, J. E. (1988). *Phone-specific nasal emission: A cleft palate sound-alike.* Paper presented at the annual meeting of the American Cleft Palate Association, Williamsburg, VA.

Trost-Cardamone, J. E. (1990a). Speech: Anatomy, physiology and pathology. In D. A. Kernahan & S. W. Rosenstein (Eds.), *Cleft lip and palate: A system of management.* Baltimore: Williams & Wilkins.

Trost-Cardamone, J. E. (1990b). Speech in the first year of life: A perspective on early acquisition. In D. A. Kernahan & S. W. Rosenstein (Eds.), *Cleft lip and palate: A system of management.* Baltimore: Williams & Wilkins.

Trost-Cardamone, J. E. (1990c). The development of speech: Assessing cleft palate misarticulations. In D. A. Kernahan & S. W. Rosenstein (Eds.), *Cleft lip and palate: A system of management.* Baltimore: Williams & Wilkins.

Vihman, M. M. (1988). Early phonological development. In J. E. Bernthal & N. W. Bankson (Eds.), *Articulation and phonological disorders.* Englewood Cliffs, NJ: Prentice-Hall.

Weiner, F. F. (1979). *Phonological process analysis.* Austin, TX: PRO-ED.

Witzel, M. A., Tobe, J., & Salyer, K. (1988). The use of nasopharyngoscopy biofeedback therapy in the correction of velopharyngeal closure. *International Journal of Pediatric Otolaryngology, 75,* 137–142.

CHAPTER 11

Behavioral Approaches to Treating Velopharyngeal Closure and Nasality

Clark D. Starr

Starr discusses research findings relating to the use of behavioral therapy techniques to modify velopharyngeal muscles, control of velopharyngeal muscles, and aspects of speech that affect listeners' perceptions of nasality. He concludes that research evidence supporting behavioral approaches is limited and conjectures about the characteristics of patients who might profit from behavioral therapy and the approaches that might be effective.

1. *Why does Starr believe that efforts to modify velopharyngeal muscles through exercise programs have been ineffective?*

2. *What types of feedback have been used in efforts to improve patients' control over their velopharyngeal closure mechanisms?*

3. *Is there evidence that patients can increase control of their velopharyngeal mechanisms under some conditions?*

4. *According to Starr, what are the characteristics of patients who are most likely to benefit from behavioral therapy?*

5. *What changes in speech have been shown to modify listeners' perceptions of the presence of nasality?*

In this chapter, behavioral approaches are defined and used in a broad sense. They include those in which patients attempt to develop control over velopharyngeal closure and nasality by making use of the structures and functions available to them. They involve diverse therapy activities, such as ear training, muscle exercises, and the use of acoustic and visual feedback systems. They do not include approaches that make use of surgery or speech prostheses that are permanently placed and designed to improve velopharyngeal closure and nasality.

The use of behavioral therapy in the management of nasality has been discussed previously by a number of authors (Cole, 1979; McWilliams, Morris, & Shelton, 1990; Ruscello, 1982), who have expressed concern with the extent to which speech clinicians employ these approaches, in the light of the limited support for their use in existing literature. I concur with these concerns. Behavioral approaches are probably inappropriate for the majority of hypernasal patients who have structural or functional deficits. However, I believe that some patients may be helped by these approaches and that clinicians should understand them to determine who will most likely benefit from their use and how they should be used.

When behavioral approaches are being considered, clinicians must deal with at least three issues:

1. *Muscle change.* Can these approaches bring about changes in velopharyngeal closure muscles? Can the potential of these muscles be changed by increasing their mass, strength, contractibility, or endurance?
2. *Muscle control change.* Can these approaches change patients' abilities to control their closure muscles? Will they improve coordination, rate, or consistency with which the muscles function for closure?
3. *Listener perceptual change.* Can these approaches be used to develop speech patterns that modify listeners' perceptions of nasality? Will changes in articulation, phonation, or resonance affect listeners' judgments of the presence of nasality in speech?

In the following sections, I discuss these issues, draw some conclusions, and speculate on the future of behavioral therapy in the treatment of nasality.

MUSCLE CHANGE

The occurrence of a cleft palate and subsequent surgical repair may result in a velopharyngeal mechanism that is fully capable of producing closure for speech. Similar circumstances may produce a mechanism in which the palate is too short or the muscles that elevate it are inappropriately positioned or too weak to accomplish closure. Patients in the latter situation will need to undergo further surgery or to be fitted with a speech prosthesis to produce the closure they need for speech. Unfortunately, all patients do not fit easily into one of these categories. Some appear to have palates that are almost normal in length or muscles that are almost normal in function. They may accomplish velopharyngeal closure during swallowing, blowing, or other nonspeech activities and come close to accomplishing it for speech. Some may even accomplish closure inconsistently for speech or accomplish it only on specific speech activities. Clinicians have speculated that these patients might be able to accomplish closure for speech consistently, if the strength, mass, contractibility, and/or endurance of their closure muscles could be increased. Based on these speculations, patients have been subjected to a wide range of muscle exercise programs in the hope of bringing about needed changes.

Effortful blowing and sucking have been suggested as ways to exercise closure muscles. Voluntary gagging and interrupted swallowing have been tried for the same purposes. Palates have been massaged in efforts to enhance muscle functions. Various devices have been used in attempts to improve the effectiveness of exercises (Lubit, 1969).

Formal studies of the effects of these approaches are limited. One study (Massengill, Quinn, Pickerell, & Levinson, 1968) attempted to evaluate the effects of blowing, sucking, and swallowing exercises on velopharyngeal closure of patients with surgically repaired cleft palate. Twice a day for 27 days, five patients did swallowing exercises, four did blowing exercises, and four did sucking exercises. Motion radiographic films, obtained pre- and posttherapy, were used to measure changes in velopharyngeal gap (the shortest distance between the palate and the posterior pharyngeal wall) during production of a sustained vowel. Significant gap changes were found for the swallowing exercise group and for some patients in the other groups. Measurement procedures did not allow the authors to determine specific muscle changes, and no attempt was made to see if the changes that occurred had a significant effect on speech.

In a similar study, Powers and Starr (1974) studied four patients with surgically repaired clefts and clinically significant degrees of hypernasality to investigate the effects of a combination of blowing, swallowing, and gagging exercises on velopharyngeal gap and nasality. The patients exercised three times a day for a 6-week period and were systematically rewarded for increases in effort. Lateral still radiographs of sustained vowels were made pre- and posttherapy and used to evaluate velopharyngeal gap. Speech recordings were made pre- and posttherapy and used to evaluate nasality. The authors found no evidence of changes in gap or nasality over the period of exercise. The method used to measure changes in velopharyngeal function in this study was limited. However, if muscle potential did change as a result of treatment, either the changes were insufficient to alter speech or the patients did not use them in ways that would improve speech.

Yules and Chase (1969) reported observable change in muscle mass during therapy. In this study, electrical stimulation was used to activate pharyngeal muscle function, presumably in an effort to help patients learn to control these muscles. According to the investigators, 2 of the 20 patients being treated developed hypertrophic pharyngeal muscles, and their hypernasality subsequently disappeared.

The results of these studies indicate that the value of muscle exercises has not been established sufficiently to warrant their use in therapy programs designed to modify hypernasality. If they have a role in therapy, three things must occur before their value can be established. First, procedures must be devised that will allow measurement of the adequacy of specific muscle function (i.e., mass, strength, contractibility, endurance). These measures are needed to determine which muscles are deficient and the nature of the deficiency. Second, exercise programs must be developed to treat the specific muscle deficiencies that are identified. Third, researchers must determine how to train patients to use new muscle competencies, if they are created. It appears improbable that continued efforts to use general exercise activities, without knowledge of their effects on specific muscles, will increase understanding or help patients. Furthermore, it seems unlikely that spontaneous changes in speech will occur if muscles are modified. Patients will have to learn how to use these new potentials. As noted in Chapter 6, speech appliance reduction programs appear to create significant changes in the function of velopharyngeal mechanisms, for some patients. However, it remains unclear whether the changes occur in the muscles themselves, or in the patients' control of them.

MUSCLE CONTROL CHANGE

As previously noted, speech clinicians are often confronted with patients who show evidence of an ability to obtain velopharyngeal closure in one set of circumstances and not in another. Some close for blowing and swallowing and almost close for speech. Some may even close for speech, but not consistently. These circumstances have led some clinicians to conclude that these patients may have the potential for closure during speech, but that they need to improve their control over closure muscles if they are to accomplish this task and sustain it. The validity of this conclusion has been questioned. Peterson (1973) suggested that differences exist in the neuromuscular patterns used to accomplish closure for speech and nonspeech activities and that nonspeech patterns may not be suitable for speech. Kuehn and Dalston (1988) suggested that the inconsistency of closure for speech may occur because closure muscles are operating at the limits of their potentials and that inconsistency is characteristic of muscles functioning under these conditions.

Muscle Control Therapy

Various techniques have been used in efforts to help patients learn to control their closure mechanisms. Some have focused on enhancing speakers' perceptions of the occurrence of their nasality. Some have provided direct or indirect visual feedback on muscle activity or airflow during closure. Others have used tactile stimulation to enhance sensory awareness of muscle function.

Perceptual and acoustic feedback therapy. Ear training is perhaps the oldest and most widely used approach to modifying nasality. Its use appears to be based on the assumption that patients must be able to perceive the occurrence of nasality before they can learn to control it. Ear training is usually accomplished by creating tasks in which patients learn to differentiate nasal from non-nasal speech segments and to identify the occurrence of nasal segments in their own speech. It often makes use of the variations in nasality that occur on specific phonemes, at different speaking rates, at different pitch and loudness levels, or on an unexplained basis. If variations include circumstances under which there is no nasality or a low level of nasality, patients are taught to identify these variations when they occur and to use them as goals or indicators of the level of control they should try to attain.

Simple devices are often used to enhance ear training:

- A plastic tube with one end placed under the nostril and the other by the patient's ear allows sound emitted from the nose to be directed to the ear. Presumably, this helps the patient isolate the occurrences of nasality in the complex speech signal.
- A small microphone, attached to an amplifier with an intensity meter, can be placed under the nares and used to amplify nasally emitted sound and provide visual evidence that nasality is present. This also may help the patient focus on nasality.
- An accelerometer may be attached to the surface of the nose and used in ways similar to the microphone. It picks up nasal tissue vibrations that occur in conjunction with nasally emitted sound. It has the advantage of not responding to other noise in the environment.

These devices may prove of aid in therapy, but they are limited in the extent to which they can be used to quantify the levels of nasality because they are affected by the speaker's overall loudness level. However, some of these devices have been incorporated into more complex instruments that attempt to quantify levels of nasality, control for speakers' loudness levels, and provide opportunities to record and analyze speakers' performances during and after therapy sessions.

One of these instruments is a Nasometer™ (Kay Elemetrics Corporation). It consists of a sound baffle (i.e., a plastic shelf) with microphones mounted on the upper and lower surfaces. A head gear holds the baffle against the upper lip so that one microphone is near the nostrils and the other is near the mouth. The outputs of the microphones are processed, filtered, and combined to provide a ratio of nasally emitted acoustic energy to orally emitted energy. A visual trace of the ratio can be presented on a monitor screen as the patient speaks and recorded for future analysis (for more information, see Chapter 9). The ratio has been referred to as nasalance by Fletcher (1970), who developed the Nasometer. Data on relationships between listener perceptions of nasality and nasalance, as measured by this instrument, are limited. However, data were obtained with an earlier version of the Nasometer, called TONAR II, which is no longer available. Fletcher (1976) reported data showing a correlation of .91 between TONAR II measures of nasalance and listener judgments of nasality. Dalston and Warren (1986) found a correlation of .76 between TONAR II measures and listener judgments of nasality. Both studies included patients with wide ranges of nasality, but neither looked at relationships of nasalance to different levels of nasality in individual patients.

Fletcher also reported on the use of TONAR II in several therapy studies. In his first report (Fletcher, 1972), he used TONAR II with two patients. One, a 23-year-old female, developed hypernasality following a tonsillectomy and adenoidectomy. After seven therapy sessions in which TONAR II was used to provide her with visible evidence of changes in her nasalance, she reduced her nasalance from 70% to below 15% and maintained this level at a 3-month follow-up. Fletcher noted that her habitual pitch level dropped 20 Hz during treatment. The second patient was a 23-year-old female who had a surgically repaired cleft palate and wore a speech bulb. According to Fletcher, she reduced her nasalance from 85% to 5% with TONAR-based therapy. He provided no information on the extent to which the gain was generalized or maintained.

In the same report, Fletcher indicated that he had used TONAR II in treatment programs for seven children between the ages of 5 and 15 years. He did not report on the effects of treatment on nasalance scores, but noted that four of the five did not demonstrate a potential for normal speech through TONAR-based therapy.

In a later study, Fletcher (1978) reported on the results of TONAR-based therapy with a group of 19 children between the ages of 5 and

15 years. They all had surgically repaired cleft palate and nasalance levels of 20% or higher. These patients were subjected to a 1-week intensive therapy program designed to determine the modifiability of their nasalance. Therapy focused on patients' performance on lists of sentences, and patients were systematically rewarded for producing the lists at lower nasalance levels. According to Fletcher, the group reduced their mean nasalance level from 40% to 31%. Eight of the patients reached the normal level of nasalance (i.e., 15%) on two sentence groups and were able to maintain this level. Five reached the normal level but were unable to maintain it, another five reduced their nasalance but did not reach the normal level, and one failed to produce any significant changes.

Fletcher's work is of interest because it represents the only reported systematic study of attempts to modify nasality through behavioral therapy. His findings are encouraging, but offer only limited evidence that the gains made by patients were clinically significant and lasting.

In a study similar to Fletcher's, Burrell (1989) used the Nasometer to determine the effects of behavioral therapy on two patients with mild inconsistent hypernasality, judged to be clinically significant. One patient, an 11-year-old male without a cleft, had a long history of clinically significant, but inconsistent hypernasality. He was treated 1 hour a day for 8 days, using three lists of sentences without nasal phonemes. Pretherapy, his mean nasalance levels on the three lists were 48%, 43%, and 40%. When the first list was treated, the nasalance level decreased to below 15% in 3 days. When the second list was treated, the nasalance level fell to below 20% in 3 days. Nasalance levels for the third list fell to below 20% with 2 days of treatment, but the decrease was not stable. Judgments obtained from a listener group indicated that nasality decreased significantly from the patient's high to low nasalance levels. Lateral videofluoroscopic evaluation indicated no palatal pharyngeal wall contact on eight of nine test sentences pretherapy and contact on all sentences posttherapy. The habitual pitch level of this patient dropped 20 Hz during therapy.

Burrell's second patient was an 18-year-old female with a surgically repaired cleft palate and a history of mild inconsistent hypernasality. Her pretherapy nasalance levels on the three sentence lists were 31%, 30%, and 26%. When the first sentence list was treated, it fell below 15% on the second day. The second list also fell below 15% on the second day, although it had not been treated. The third list, treated on the third day, fell below 15% during the first treatment session. Listener groups also judged this patient's nasality to have significantly decreased from her high to low nasalance performances, but neither frontal nor lateral videofluoroscopic films revealed observable changes in velopharyngeal function.

Burrell's study supports some of the findings reported by Fletcher, but it also falls short of demonstrating the long-term effects of changes observed during therapy. It does provide evidence of patients' ability to generalize nasality control learned with one set of sentences to other sets, and it provides some evidence that changes in velopharyngeal function occur in conjunction with decreases in nasality associated with behavioral therapy.

With the availability of the Nasometer in many clinics, it seems likely that more studies like those of Fletcher and Burrell will be carried out and reported. However, until more evidence is available, treatment programs of this type must be considered experimental.

Horii (1980) devised an instrument, similar to the Nasometer, that uses accelerometers to measure nasality. The accelerometers are placed on the external nasal surface and on the neck, where they respond to tissue vibrations that occur during speech. Their outputs are processed and combined to produce a nasal/oral index called HONC (Horii Oral Nasal Coupling). Horii and Lang (1981) reported finding a correlation of .81 between listener judgments of nasality and the HONC index, across normal speakers' simulations of different levels of nasality. Reich and Redenbaugh (1985) modified Horii's procedures and produced a ratio they call NAVI (Nasal Accelerometric Vibrational Index). They reported correlations of .90 and .91 between NAVI and listener judgments of nasality, for patients with varying degrees of hypernasality. Studies using HONC and NAVI as indices of nasality have not been reported at this time, although the instrumentation needed to carry out such studies is available and appears well suited for use in therapy.

Visual feedback therapy.   Some clinicians have speculated that patients might obtain better control over their velopharyngeal closure mechanisms if they could see them function. The simplest way to provide such a view is to place a mirror in front of the mouth and phonate. Unfortunately, this limits observations to views of the lower portion of the pharyngeal walls and the undersurface of the palate during sustained production of a few low back vowels. This view has been enhanced somewhat by the use of a rigid endoscope. This instrument consists of a tube with built-in light source and lens. When attached to a video camera and a monitor, it provides a view of the pharynx and undersurface of the palate, which can be seen easily by the patient and recorded for future analysis.

A significant improvement on these approaches is obtained through the use of a flexible fiber endoscope. This instrument is similar to the rigid endoscope, except that the tube is replaced by a long bundle of flexible fiber optic strands. The diameter of these bundles is small enough to allow them to be inserted through the nose. This provides a view of the upper pharynx and the upper surface of the palate. More importantly, the view is available during the production of all speech sounds.

At this time, techniques for making objective measurements from views obtained with endoscopes have not been developed to the point that they are usable in clinical activities. This means that patients and clinicians must make perceptual judgments of structures and functions viewed and any changes that take place. Although video recordings of endoscopic views allow evaluation of the reliability of observer judgments, their validity is difficult to establish.

The extent to which the elevation of the soft palate and contraction of the pharyngeal walls can be controlled with visual feedback has been evaluated in several studies of subjects with normal velopharyngeal mechanisms. Shelton, Harris, Sholes, and Dooley (1970) attempted to train four children and five adults to voluntarily elevate and lower their palates without producing audible speech. A mirror was used to provide visual feedback during practice sessions, and children were tested without feedback. Under test conditions, both groups were asked to elevate or lower their palates. The children responded correctly to approximately 85% of these requests, and the adults responded correctly to approximately 96%. In a subsequent study, Shelton, Paesani, McClelland, and Gradfield (1975) used an oral panendoscope (a type of rigid endoscope) to train three adults with normal mechanisms to elevate their palates on nonspeech tasks. In this study, subjects were able to elevate their palates and to imitate reflexive movements elicited from touch pressure cues provided by the investigators. Siegel-Sadewitz and Shprintzen (1982) carried out a study on an adult with a normal velopharyngeal mechanism. They provided her with visual feedback from a flexible fiber endoscope inserted through the nose. Her task was to learn to produce velopharyngeal closure with increased use of the pharyngeal walls. According to the authors, she practiced the task with visual feedback for six sessions. At that time, she was able to repeat short samples of connected speech with this new pattern or with her old pattern, without the aid of visual feedback.

These studies are of interest in that they support the notion that speakers can learn to exert some voluntary control over their velopharyngeal closure muscles with visual feedback, and that they may have some ability to modify their closure patterns. However, the limits of available voluntary control have not been defined.

Visual feedback techniques have been tried in studies of persons with velopharyngeal closure problems. Shelton, Beaumont, Trier, and Furr (1978) reported on the use of a rigid endoscope, attached to a video camera, in the treatment of two patients with velopharyngeal problems. The patients were provided an oral view of their pharynx and palate on a monitor, while they attempted to improve their velopharyngeal closure on speech and nonspeech tasks. According to the authors, both patients improved closure as therapy progressed, but the improvements did not become automatic. Analysis of pre- and posttherapy video recordings indicated that both patients had learned to modify closure in some, but not all, tasks.

Several studies using visual feedback have been carried out in Japan. Miyazaki, Matsuya, Yamaoka, and Nishio (1974) used nasally placed flexible fiber endoscopes in the treatment of 37 patients with velopharyngeal problems. Apparently, other forms of therapy were conducted in conjunction with the visual feedback treatment. Pretherapy, all patients' closure was evaluated on swallowing, blowing, and some speech tasks. According to the authors, after 6 months of therapy, 16 of the patients had developed closure that was judged to be the best or most adequate for them. The authors suggested that those who accomplished pretherapy closure for blowing were most likely to profit from therapy.

Yamaoka, Matsuya, Miyazaki, Nishio, and Ibuki (1983) carried out an extensive study in which fiber optic endoscopes were used to provide visual feedback. In this study, 59 patients with repaired clefts, persistent hypernasality, and long histories of speech therapy were treated during a 1-year program that involved visual feedback training, articulation therapy, and speech stimulation activities carried out in the patients' homes. Pre- and posttherapy video recordings and articulation tests were used to evaluate patients' progress. According to the authors, all 23 patients who demonstrated complete closure on swallowing, blowing, and some speech tasks prior to therapy, significantly improved their closure for speech with therapy. Only 7 of the 36 patients who did not show closure on blowing or speech tasks prior to therapy, made significant speech improvement during therapy.

Witzel, Tobe, and Salyer (1989) described the use of nasally placed fiber optic endoscopes in the treatment of three adult patients with cleft palates and persistent hypernasality following pharyngeal flap surgery. Therapy involved having patients view their closure mechanisms and experiment with nonspeech and speech activities in which closure or near closure was obtained. They were urged to be aware of the sensations accompanying these closure efforts. When they had gained some control over closure activity, therapy focused on attaining closure on single phonemes, syllables, and word productions. According to the authors, two patients progressed to the point where their nasality was normal during connected speech. A 1-year follow-up on one of these patients indicated that the gains made in therapy were still present. The third subject gained control over her closure mechanism by her fifth therapy session, but chose not to continue in therapy.

Although these studies present some evidence that patients increase control of their closure mechanisms in conjunction with visual feedback training, their findings are complicated by the fact that most patients who received visual feedback training were receiving other types of therapy simultaneously. It is of interest to note that pretherapy most of the patients who appeared to benefit from treatment had produced closure on some tasks and that blowing and speech appeared to be the best predictors of success. An increase in the availability of fiber optic endoscopes may lead to an increase in their use as feedback procedures for therapy. However, they are somewhat invasive and their use may be limited to older patients seen in medical settings.

In a single-subject study, Moller, Path, Werth, and Christiansen (1973) provided a somewhat different mode of visual feedback. They used an orally placed appliance, with an attached strain gauge transducer, to provide feedback on palatal elevation in the form of a tracing on a graphic level recorder. The tracing could be viewed by a patient during efforts to accomplish closure. A 12-year-old with velopharyngeal inadequacy was provided with this type of feedback for 15 therapy sessions. In each session, the clinicians set criterion levels for the visual trainings and rewarded the patient for attaining them. According to the authors, this subject learned to control his palatal movement with visual feedback. Pre- and posttherapy lateral still X-rays of a sustained /u/ showed that the subject had learned to increase palatal elevation, but that his velopharyngeal gap did not decrease. Based on X-ray evidence, the authors suggested that adenoid atrophy was occurring during the therapy period and that this may have accounted for the subject's failure to demonstrate a reduced velopharyngeal gap.

Airflow and air pressure feedback therapy.   Nasal air loss during speech has been shown to be related to hypernasality and inadequate velopharyngeal closure (Warren, 1979). Efforts have been made to devise instruments and procedures that measure this loss and can be used for diagnostic and treatment purposes. The instruments range from simple to complex. One simple device, the air paddle (Bzoch, 1979), consists of a thin plastic strip that can be held under the nostrils while patients produce non-nasal phonemes. Air escaping through the nose causes the paddle to move and tells the patient and the clinician that velopharyngeal closure is not complete. Another instrument is the Scape-scope (Shprintzen, McCall, & Skolnick, 1975). This device consists of a plastic tube that runs from a nasally placed plug, with a hole in it, to a clear plastic cylinder that contains a piston. Air escaping from the nose causes the piston to rise in the cylinder. This provides the patient and clinician with visible evidence of velopharyngeal inadequacy. These devices can be used to determine when nasal air loss occurs, but they provide only crude indications of the amount or the timing of the loss.

Shprintzen et al. (1975) used a Scape-scope (see Chapter 9) in a study to determine whether patients who had velopharyngeal closure during whistling and blowing could learn to achieve closure during speech. They used four patients who had failed to attain closure for speech through traditional therapy techniques, but who demonstrated closure on blowing and whistling tasks. Treatment procedures included having patients view the Scape-scope to observe their ability to attain closure for blowing and whistling. Next, they attempted to blow and whistle while simultaneously phonating. Again, they used the Scape-scope to identify nasal air loss. When patients could do these tasks, attempts were made to fade out the blowing and whistling during phonation. After patients had demonstrated they could maintain closure on vowels, they worked on consonant–vowel combinations. Finally, the use of the Scape-scope was faded out, and patients were urged to rely on their perceptions of nasality to control closure. The therapy program made use of reinforcements administered by the clinician.

According to the investigators, one adult patient with a repaired cleft palate, a pharyngeal flap, and severe hypernasality achieved normal resonance after 36 therapy sessions and had maintained gains at a 4-month follow-up. A 4-year-old with a cleft palate, slight hypernasality, and infrequent nasal air emission achieved normal resonance after 26 sessions. A 6-year-old with a cleft palate, a pharyngeal flap, and severe hypernasality also learned to control resonance in conversational speech. A 10-year-old patient without a cleft, but with severe hearing loss and hypernasality that had developed after an adenoidectomy, gained some control over nasality after 24 sessions, but did not learn to control it consistently during connected speech. Pre- and posttherapy videofluoroscopic evaluations indicated that an increase in palatal elevation and pharyngeal wall movement had occurred for all patients during speech.

The results reported in this study are impressive, in view of the observation that two of the patients had severe hypernasality pretherapy. The results support findings by Miyazaki et al. (1974) and Yamaoka et al. (1983), which suggest that closure in blowing may be predictive of success in therapy, and they add whistling as a predictive variable. Shprintzen (1989) reviewed this study and suggested that subsequent clinical experiences have indicated that patients who attain velopharyngeal closure on blowing and whistling are likely to attain closure on sustained /s/ or /f/ productions. He commented that velopharyngeal closure for patients in his previously reported study may not have been adequately determined, because their performance on sustained /s/ and /f/ was not evaluated. He further suggested that an appropriate therapy strategy for patients who attain closure on these sounds should include efforts to extend closure efforts to other voiceless pressure consonants.

Electrical stimulation therapy. A strategy tried by several investigators involves the use of electrical stimulation of muscles to help patients learn to control their velopharyngeal mechanisms. Presumably, the stimulation causes closure muscles to contract, and the patient is able to sense these movements and learn to control them voluntarily. As previously noted, this strategy may also serve to exercise muscles. The first study employing this strategy was carried out by Yules and Chase (1969), who treated 30 patients with velopharyngeal closure problems associated with surgically repaired cleft palate and other conditions. Patients were treated from 2 to 6 weeks in a program that involved placing electrodes on their posterior pillars and stimulating muscle function while they voluntarily attempted a series of speech and speechlike tasks. When the patients were able to successfully carry out the tasks on a voluntary basis, the electrical stimulation was withdrawn. Subsequently, acoustic feedback devices were used to help the patients sustain their newfound voluntary control over nasality. During the time they were undergoing electrical stimulation therapy, the patients were also involved in a home training program that included tactual stimulation and visual feedback as aids to sustaining their control over closure. Pre- and posttherapy cinefluorographic evaluations and airflow measures were used to assess patients' closure on selected tasks. Based on these measures, the authors concluded that 24 of the 30 patients learned to control velopharyngeal closure on speech tasks. These 24 were provided with additional speech therapy and, according to the authors, 14 attained normal nasality, 7 showed some improvement, and 3 did not progress.

Weber, Jobe, and Chase (1970) replicated this study using the same therapy approach and pre- and posttreatment measures. They began their study with 34 patients, but 18 withdrew because of failure to progress, and 9 of the remaining 16 did not return for posttreatment evaluations. According to the authors, 7 of the remaining patients learned to produce closure voluntarily, but had difficulty maintaining it in connected speech, and only 1 had a significant decrease in nasality.

In a related study, Peterson (1974) investigated responses to electrical and tactile stimulation in nine normal subjects, five patients with palatal pathology and adequate velopharyngeal closure, and five with palatal pathology and inadequate closure for speech. Peterson stimulated the palate at three locations and at varying voltages and tactile force levels. She used cinefluorography to evaluate the effects of electrical stimulation on soft palate function. She found that 11 of her subjects responded only sporadically to tactile or electrical stimulation. Five of the remaining subjects responded systematically to electrical stimulation, but only one of these was in the velopharyngeal incompetency group. Based on these findings, Peterson concluded that this approach has limited clinical value until procedures for its application have received further laboratory study.

Although the results of Yules and Chase's (1969) study are impressive, failures to replicate it and the difficulties encountered in applying electrical stimulation suggest that a great deal of additional work must be done before this approach can be justified.

LISTENER PERCEPTUAL CHANGE

Over many years, speech clinicians have been concerned with the variability of the hypernasality that exists in persons with clefts and the conditions under which it occurs. Because nasality has been measured by listener judgments of speech, it is difficult to determine whether these variations reflect changes in the acoustic energy that is being emitted nasally, or if they reflect changes in other aspects of speech which, in turn, make the presence of this acoustic energy that we perceive as nasality more or less acceptable to the listener. If the latter is true and existing nasality can be made more acceptable, this would seem to be a reasonable treatment goal for some patients.

In several early studies, close relationships were found between listener judgments of nasality and the severity of patients' articulation problems (McWilliams, 1954; Spriestersbach, 1955; Van Hattum, 1958). However, when listeners rated nasality of patients' speech and then rated the speech samples played backward on a tape recorder, the relationships diminished (Spriestersbach, 1955); that is, when the tapes were played backward so listeners could not hear the articulation errors, the severity of the patients' nasality was not found to be as closely related to the severity of their articulation problems. Based on these findings, it appears that listeners may be prone to perceive nasality as being less severe when speakers have good articulation skills. This conclusion has led speech clinicians to consider articulation therapy as a possible way of making existing nasality more acceptable. Systematic studies of the effects of articulation therapy on listener judgments of nasality for individual patients have not been carried out. However, it should be noted that in one study (Shelton, Chisum, Youngstrom, Arndt, & Elbert, 1969) lateral cinefluorography did not show that the gap between the soft palate and the posterior pharyngeal wall or the anterior movement of the posterior wall were affected by improvement in articulation that occurred in conjunction with therapy.

Other parameters of speech have been viewed in a similar manner. Investigators have examined the effects of pitch on speakers' perceptions of nasality. In a frequently quoted study, Hess (1959) found that when patients spoke at their normal pitch levels and at levels 1.4 times higher, listeners perceived the higher pitch levels as being less nasal. However, the extent to which the degree of decrease might be of clinical significance was not evaluated.

Spriestersbach (1955) studied relationships between the use of "effectiveness of pitch usage" and listener judgments of nasality in 50 patients with varying degrees of nasality. Effectiveness was determined by three experienced clinicians, and nasality was rated by 40 speech pathology students. Spriestersbach found a low negative relationship between the two variables when listener judgments were based on speech recordings played forward and no relationship when they were based on recordings played backward. His findings can be interpreted as suggesting that effective use of pitch does change listeners' perceptions of nasality to some extent, but that it does not change the amount of acoustic nasal energy in the patients' speech.

The effects of changes in intensity on listeners' nasality judgments also have been studied. Hess (1959) looked at the effects of intensity on nasality ratings for the same patients he used to study pitch change. He found that listeners judged that vowels produced at 75 dB were more nasal than those produced at 85 dB. Counihan and Cullinan (1972) looked at relationships between vocal intensity and vowel productions of 10 male and 10 female cleft palate speakers with oral manometer ratios (see Chapter 9) of .75 or less. Their speakers recorded four vowels at four intensity levels. When the recordings were rated by experienced listeners, only two vowels were found to be affected by the intensity changes. Females' productions of /u/ and males' productions of /a/ increased in nasality as intensity increased. Subsequently, the vowels were dubbed on a tape so they all appeared at the same intensity level. Listeners' ratings of the vowels under this condition indicated that nasality varied with intensity for only one vowel: The males' productions of /i/ became more nasal as intensity increased.

Moore (1976) carried out a similar study in which 26 speakers with cleft palates recorded a reading passage in a quiet background and with 85 dB of speech noise fed into their ears through earphones. Three stimulus tapes were constructed using 20-second samples from each reading. Tape 1 contained samples read at the original intensity levels. In Tape 2, the intensity of samples read in the noisy background was reduced to the level of the quiet samples. In Tape 3, the quiet sample was dubbed at its original intensity level and at the intensity level of the noisy sample. Listener ratings of Tapes 1 and 2 revealed no evidence that nasality varied with speech produced in different background noise levels. However, differences were found in Tape 3. When intensity levels in the quiet condition were amplified, listeners judged the speech to be more nasal.

Based on the findings of these studies, speakers' intensity levels appear to have minimal and probably varied effects on listeners' perceptions of the amount of nasality present. Efforts to determine whether the effects found are related solely to intensity or to other changes in speech that occur in conjunction with changes in intensity are not conclusive. All things considered, it does not appear wise to assume that intensity and nasality are related for most speakers with cleft palates or that, when a relationship is found, its nature will be predictable.

Another approach to modifying perceived nasality involves efforts to alter the oral resonance cavity. Although these alterations may not affect nasal resonance, it is presumed that they will affect oral resonance and lead to a balance between oral and nasal resonance that is more acceptable to listeners. It has been suggested that this can be accomplished by either lowering the posterior position of the tongue during speech or increasing the size of the mouth opening. Without specifying oral cavity changes, some clinicians have suggested that improvement in nasality can be accomplished by instructing patients to focus their voices in the facial mask or encouraging them to use a relaxed form of voice production. At the present time, no formal reports have been published of the effects of any of these procedures.

Finally, it should be noted that some speakers try to diminish their hypernasality by speaking with a soft, breathy, or somewhat harsh vocal quality. Again, the value of this approach has not been investigated. However, clinicians should be aware that this type of voice may be a consequence of laryngeal problems that develop in response to patients' efforts to control articulation or resonance in the presence of an inadequate velopharyngeal mechanism, and may complicate, rather than diminish, the problem. In general, it would not seem wise to modify vocal quality in an effort to control nasality.

CONCLUSIONS AND RECOMMENDATIONS

Most researchers question the use of behavioral treatment for hypernasality related to clefting, but most clinicians report that they use these approaches with some patients. The limited number of formal studies dealing with the effectiveness of this form of treatment does not provide clear evidence to support either group. However, existing studies do offer some evidence that some patients can modify hypernasality, to some extent, in response to some forms of behavioral treatment. Unfortunately, they do not provide convincing evidence that the modifications attained can be generalized to all speaking circumstances or that they are lasting. This leaves clinicians with the difficult task of deciding if, or when, they should use these approaches.

Based on the evidence available and personal experiences, I believe that in some circumstances behavioral treatment will benefit patients and that clinicians should consider it as an option. I also believe that the clinician and the patient must be aware that, when they engage in behavioral treatment for nasality, they are engaging in experimental therapy and that the benefits of the approach cannot be guaranteed. When clinicians choose to try behavioral treatment, they should take advantage of information obtained in past studies, along with the knowledge gained in other treatment areas, to design programs that can be monitored and evaluated.

Past studies offer some suggestions as to which patients are likely to respond to behavioral treatment and which strategies are likely to be effective. For example, studies and clinical reports suggest that behavioral treatment is most likely to be of help for patients who demonstrate some ability to accomplish velopharyngeal closure prior to the onset of treatment. Patients with mild to moderate degrees of nasality and those who can control nasality in some speech activities appear to be the best candidates. Evidence of an ability to accomplish closure in nonspeech activities, such as whistling and blowing, may also be a positive indicator. However, the ability to attain closure during swallowing is probably of limited value as an indicator of success in therapy.

The frequency and consistency with which positive indicators occur may be of importance, although this has not been thoroughly investigated. Other patient characteristics, such as maturity, intellect, desire to change, and the presence of other physical deficits, are likely to be of equal importance to those previously mentioned. At this time, it does not appear that the type of surgical procedure patients have undergone is of predictive value for behavioral treatment.

The relative value of different behavioral treatment options is difficult to evaluate, because only a few have been subjected to systematic study. Nevertheless, the results of studies that have been carried out provide some insights that may aid clinicians. For example, results suggest that treatment procedures designed to modify muscle status are not well understood and are difficult to evaluate. Treatment procedures designed to enhance motor control are somewhat easier to understand and more often appear to have met with some degree of success. Motor control studies seem to suggest that approaches that make use of visual or auditory feedback may enhance treatment, at least in the clinical setting. Treatment that relies on electrical or tactual stimulation appears difficult to implement and is probably impractical in most clinical settings. Treatments that attempt to modify speech in ways that alter listeners' perceptions of nasality are appealing, although their effectiveness has not been demonstrated. The improvement of articulation skills appears to be the most promising approach in this group. Efforts to modify pitch, intensity, and vocal quality should be undertaken with great care because they may serve to complicate rather than simplify patients' problems.

Although any of these approaches may involve the use of simple devices or clinicians' judgments to indicate changes in resonance or velopharyngeal closure, instrumentation that provides visual or acoustic feedback is likely to enhance the chances of success. This equipment is available for use in clinics and some school settings and is generally user friendly.

Finally, it seems clear that behavioral management of hypernasality and velopharyngeal problems is inappropriate for most patients with velopharyngeal problems and that more information is needed before clinicians can easily identify patients for whom it might be appropriate and decide on the methods they should use to implement it. This information is unlikely to come from large laboratory studies, but rather from documented reports of clinicians operating in a wide variety of settings. The skills they have developed for teaching other speech skills will serve them well in helping patients learn to control nasality. Very likely, the reports they generate will be in the form of single-subject research models and will incorporate some of the instrumentation referred to in this chapter.

ADDENDUM

This chapter has focused on the use of behavioral therapy in the management of hypernasality; however, persons with cleft palates may also have problems with hyponasality. Traditionally, hyponasality has been defined as a loss of nasal resonance on normally nasalized sounds (i.e., /n/, /m/, /ŋ/). This is generally considered to occur as a result of structural deviations in the nasal or pharyngeal cavities that occlude or partially occlude openings between the nasal and oral cavities. Deviations in the septum or turbinates, the presence of large adenoids, the swelling of nasal tissue, or the accumulation of large amounts of thick mucus may be responsible for the occurrence of hyponasality. Persons with clefts often demonstrate hyponasality after undergoing surgical procedures that involve the construction of pharyngeal flaps (see Chapter 3). Hyponasality may occur in patients who have no structural defects, but who do not exert appropriate control over their velopharyngeal mechanism. These patients often have severe hearing losses or neurological deficits.

The use of behavioral therapy to manage hyponasality has received very little attention in clinical and research literature. Most clinicians apparently do not believe that such therapy is an effective way to treat problems due to structural limitations. Its use appears to be more appropriate for patients with severe hearing losses or neurological deficits.

REFERENCES

Burrell, K. (1989). *The modification of nasality using Nasometer feedback.* Unpublished master's thesis, University of Minnesota, Minneapolis.

Bzoch, K. (1979). Measurement and assessment of categorical aspects of cleft palate speech. In K. Bzoch (Ed.), *Communicative disorders related to cleft lip and palate* (2nd ed.). Boston: Little, Brown.

Cole, R. (1979). Direct muscle training for the improvement of velopharyngeal closure. In K. Bzoch (Ed.), *Communicative disorders related to cleft lip and palate* (2nd ed.). Boston: Little, Brown.

Counihan, D., & Cullinan, W. (1972). Some relationships between vocal intensity and rated nasality. *Cleft Palate Journal, 9,* 101–108.

Dalston, R., & Warren, D. (1986). Comparison of Tonar II, pressure flow, and listener judgements of hypernasality in the assessment of velopharyngeal function. *Cleft Palate Journal, 23,* 108–115.

Fletcher, S. (1970). Theory and instrumentation for quantitative measurement of nasality. *Cleft Palate Journal, 7,* 601–609.

Fletcher, S. (1972). Contingencies for bioelectric modification of nasality. *Journal of Speech and Hearing Disorders, 37,* 329–346.

Fletcher, S. (1976). Nasalance vs listener judgments of nasality. *Cleft Palate Journal, 13,* 31–44.

Fletcher, S. (1978). Diagnosing speech disorders from cleft palate. New York: Grune & Stratton.

Hess, D. (1959). Pitch, intensity and cleft palate voice quality. *Journal of Speech and Hearing Research, 2,* 113–125.

Horii, Y. (1980). An accelerometeric approach to nasality measurement: A preliminary report. *Cleft Palate Journal, 17,* 254–261.

Horii, Y., & Lang, J. (1981). Distributional analyses of an index of nasal coupling (HONC) in simulated hypernasal speech. *Cleft Palate Journal, 18,* 279–285.

Kuehn, D., & Dalston, R. (1988). Cleft palate and studies related to velopharyngeal function. In H. Winitz (Ed.), *Human communication and its disorders— A review.* Norwood, NJ: Ablex.

Lubit, E. (1969). The Lubit palatal exerciser: A preliminary report. *Cleft Palate Journal, 6,* 120–133.

Massengill, R., Jr., Quinn, G., Pickerell, K., & Levinson, C. (1968). Therapeutic exercise and velopharyngeal gap. *Cleft Palate Journal, 5,* 44–47.

McWilliams, B. (1954). Some factors in the intelligibility of cleft palate speech. *Journal of Speech and Hearing Disorders, 19,* 524–527.

McWilliams, B., Morris, H., & Shelton, R. (1990). *Cleft palate speech* (2nd ed.). Philadelphia: Decker.

Miyazaki, T., Matsuya, T., Yamaoka, M., & Nishio, J. (1974). *A nasopharyngeal fiberscope.* Film presented at meeting of the American Cleft Palate Association, Boston.

Moller, K., Path, M., Werth, L., & Christiansen, R. (1973). The modification of velar movement. *Journal of Speech and Hearing Disorders, 38,* 323–334.

Moore, J. (1976). *The effects of noise and rate on the perception of nasality in cleft palate speech.* Unpublished master's thesis, University of Minnesota, Minneapolis.

Peterson, S. (1973). Velopharyngeal function: Some important differences. *Journal of Speech and Hearing Disorders, 38,* 89–97.

Peterson, S. (1974). Electrical stimulation of the soft palate. *Cleft Palate Journal, 11,* 72–86.

Powers, G., & Starr, C. (1974). The effects of muscle exercises on velopharyngeal gap and nasality. *Cleft Palate Journal, 11,* 28–35.

Reich, A., & Redenbaugh, M. (1985). Relation between nasal/voice accelerometric values and interval estimates of hypernasality. *Cleft Palate Journal, 22,* 237–245.

Ruscello, D. (1982). A selected review of palatal training procedures. *Cleft Palate Journal, 19,* 181–193.

Shelton, R., Beaumont, K., Trier, W., & Furr, M. (1978). Videoendoscopic feedback in training velopharyngeal closure. *Cleft Palate Journal, 15,* 6–12.

Shelton, R., Chisum, L., Youngstrom, K., Arndt, W., & Elbert, M. (1969). Effect of articulation therapy on palatopharyngeal wall and tongue posture. *Cleft Palate Journal, 6,* 440–448.

Shelton, R., Harris, K., Sholes, G., & Dooley, P. (1970). A study of nonspeech voluntary palate movements by scaling and electromyographic techniques. In J. Bosma (Ed.), *Second symposium on oral sensation and perception.* Springfield, IL: Thomas.

Shelton, R., Paesani, A., McClelland, K., & Gradfield, S. (1975). Panendoscopic feedback in the study of voluntary velopharyngeal movements. *Journal of Speech and Hearing Disorders, 10,* 232–244.

Shprintzen, R. (1989). Research revisited. *Cleft Palate Journal, 26,* 148–149.

Shprintzen, R., McCall, G., & Skolnick, L. (1975). A new therapeutic technique for the treatment of velopharyngeal incompetence. *Journal of Speech and Hearing Disorders, 40,* 69–83.

Siegel-Sadewitz, V., & Shprintzen, R. (1982). Nasopharyngoscopy of the normal velopharyngeal sphincter: An experiment of biofeedback. *Cleft Palate Journal, 19,* 194–200.

Spriestersbach, D. (1955). Assessing nasal quality in cleft palate speech of children. *Journal of Speech and Hearing Disorders, 20,* 266–270.

Van Hattum, R. (1958). Articulation and nasality in cleft palate speakers. *Journal of Speech and Hearing Research, 1,* 383–387.

Warren, D. (1979). PERCI: A method for rating palatal efficiency. *Cleft Palate Journal, 16,* 279–285.

Weber, J., Jobe, R., & Chase, R. (1970). Evaluation of muscle stimulation in the rehabilitation of patients with hypernasal speech. *Plastic and Reconstructive Surgery, 46,* 173–176.

Witzel, M., Tobe, J., & Salyer, K. (1989). The use of videonasopharyngoscopy for biofeedback therapy in adults after pharyngeal flap surgery. *Cleft Palate Journal, 26,* 29–34.

Yamaoka, M., Matsuya, T., Miyazaki, T., Nishio, J., & Ibuki, K. (1983). Visual training for velopharyngeal closure in cleft palate patients: A fiberscopic procedure (preliminary report). *Journal of Maxillofacial Surgery, 11,* 191–193.

Yules, R., & Chase, R. (1969). A training method for reduction of hypernasality in speech. *Plastic and Reconstructive Surgery, 43,* 180–185.

CHAPTER 12

Psychological Characteristics Associated with Cleft Palate

Lynn C. Richman and Michele J. Eliason

> *Richman and Eliason discuss the role of the psychologist in treating persons with clefts. They review literature related to parents' reactions to the birth of children with clefts; problems faced by children with facial disfigurements; the development of intellect, academic skills, and personalities in those with clefts; and their status as adults.*

> 1. *How might the distortion of facial appearance affect a patient's ability to communicate?*
> 2. *What are the four most common concerns of parents who have children with clefts? According to Richman and Eliason, how should they be dealt with?*
> 3. *In what ways do teachers' and parents' perceptions of the behavior of children with clefts appear to differ?*
> 4. *How do children with and without clefts appear to differ on IQ and reading test scores?*
> 5. *According to the authors, what two types of language learning disabilities appear to be present in children with clefts?*
> 6. *Is there a high incidence of psychopathology in persons with clefts? Do they have unique personalities?*
> 7. *Based on studies reviewed by the authors, how do persons with clefts differ from their peers in relation to marriage, education, and vocational attainment?*

The identification of a psychologist to serve on a cleft palate or craniofacial team requires some preliminary comments regarding the profession of psychology in general. Psychologists are trained in many different specialty areas, such as experimental, physiological, social development, educational, and clinical psychology. Because a psychologist involved with a cleft palate or craniofacial team needs to serve the developmental, emotional, and educational concerns relevant to craniofacial anomalies, individuals trained in clinical or applied educational psychology are likely to be considered. Psychological aspects of the condition include, for example, early parent concerns regarding guilt and acceptance, early childhood development (especially related to speech, language, and intellectual development), and emotional responses of the patient, family, and peers to possible facial disfigurement. Furthermore, problems related to speech and/or language impairment, as well as inhibition regarding class discussions or volunteering in class, frequently present significant educational problems.

A relatively new specialty is health psychology, frequently identified as pediatric psychology in child health settings. This specialty provides training in clinical, educational, and developmental psychology, as well as supervised experience within a health care setting. A health psychologist is especially appropriate to serve on a cleft palate or craniofacial team because the individual will have prior training and experience evaluating and treating children with medical and developmental problems. The psychologist should be trained in evaluating infants and toddlers because parents of children with craniofacial anomalies often have concerns regarding developmental and intellectual status. The psychologist should also have expertise in evaluation techniques used to assess children with speech, language, and hearing problems. Use of traditional tests of cognitive ability, which are usually verbal, may result in an underestimate of intellectual ability. Furthermore, evaluation of emotional responses to an observable disability requires training and experience in behavioral and personality assessment.

The American Psychological Association, the primary national organization of psychologists, is divided into over 40 specialty divisions. Divisional membership usually identifies special areas of interest and professional expertise. Pertinent divisions for individuals participating on a craniofacial team might include, but are not restricted to, the following: clinical (with subgroups of child clinical and pediatric), children and youth, educational, school, developmental, and health psychology. The clinical practice of psychology is governed in most states by formal licensure and usually requires a doctoral degree, as well as supervised clinical training at the postdoctoral level. Although credentials provide a general index for evaluating a qualified psychologist for a craniofacial team, experience and training in the assessment and treatment considerations previously mentioned are equally important. Psychologists with doctoral training have experience in research methodology and statistics because these are an integral component in the measurement of human behavior, intelligence, learning, and emotions.

The role of the psychologist on the cleft palate or craniofacial team will depend partially on the team's makeup. However, typical roles might include the following:

1. Consultation with parents who have an adverse emotional reaction to the birth of a child with a deformity
2. Developmental assessment during preschool years, especially when a delay in development may be related to speech deviation, hearing loss, or emotional withdrawal
3. Educational assessment during early elementary and adolescent years
4. Evaluation of behavior when children respond negatively to teasing or lack of acceptance by others
5. Personality evaluation, especially during adolescence or early adulthood when indications of withdrawal or acting out may be a response to the disability

In addition, the psychologist's input is frequently important in management decisions. For example, the timing of surgical intervention might be clarified by the psychologist's evaluation of emotional response to appearance. The psychologist may be asked to assist in the differential diagnosis of mental retardation, language disability, and severe emotional withdrawal when verbal skills are delayed. Another patient management decision that may involve the psychologist's input is parental or patient refusal of recommended treatment. The psychologist also provides objective assessment of development, behavior, intelligence, and personality to assure that management decisions are based on reliable measurement of the child's functioning, rather than on assumptions of parents, teachers, or others.

OVERVIEW OF PSYCHOLOGICAL ASPECTS OF CLEFT LIP AND/OR PALATE

Children with both cleft lip and palate are at risk for the development of psychological problems because of several factors. They frequently have a highly visible cosmetic deformity that may elicit negative reactions from parents, siblings, peers, teachers, and others. The face is a significant source of communication that provides the initial stimulus for the expression of the speaker's emotions, character, and personality

(Cohen, 1982). Atypical facial appearance may impair the ability of others to accurately interpret facial expression as a source of nonverbal communication. Cleft lip and palate represents a unique defect that can be "seen, felt, and heard" (Lis, Pruzansky, Koepp-Baker, & Kobes, 1956). Other risk factors for psychosocial concerns include a high incidence of early middle ear infections, with resulting fluctuating hearing loss; frequent hospitalizations and separation from family and friends; and speech deviations. These factors may be related to secondary psychological factors, including behavioral inhibition, lower school achievement, and self-consciousness regarding the perceptions of others. Psychosocial problems secondary to the disability may adversely influence the final habilitative process even more than the primary disability does (Lencione, 1980). There is a need for awareness of these psychological factors because an individual's behavior may be influenced more by self-perception of facial appearance and speech than by the "objective" assessment of these by professionals. These psychological influences may create life-long learning, emotional, and social effects (Richman & Eliason, 1986a, 1986b).

The discussion of psychosocial aspects is divided in this chapter into the following areas: (a) early parental reactions and developmental concerns, (b) parent–child interactions, (c) physical attractiveness variables, (d) intellectual ability and school achievement, (e) behavior and personality, and (f) psychological adjustment of adults with cleft lips and/or palates.

EARLY PARENTAL REACTIONS AND DEVELOPMENTAL CONCERNS

Giving birth to a child with a physical defect can be a traumatic, guilt-laden event. A wide variety of negative emotions have been described in parents' responses to infants with defects. They include grief, anxiety, confusion, depression, shock, anger, disbelief, inadequacy, resentment, withdrawal, and frustration (Clifford, 1973). Cohen (1982) categorized five stages of parental reaction, beginning with shock or disbelief, followed by sadness, denial, equilibrium, and finally reorganization. It has been suggested that the stress of the birth of a child with defects may lead to family disintegration in some cases, but in others may actually strengthen family bonds (Clifford & Crocker, 1971). Although the duration of the initial crisis period has been reported to vary from family to family, most studies, usually based on retrospective interviews, have found that rapid dissipation of the negative feelings occurs within a short period (Clifford, 1968; Slutsky, 1969).

The resolution of early negative reactions can be facilitated by professional intervention. Clifford (1968) reported that 75% of mothers of children with clefts involving the lip only or the lip and palate discovered the defect at birth, and an additional 20% were told the following day. In contrast, only 8% of the mothers of infants with cleft palates only were told of the defect at birth, and 14% were informed 1 day postpartum. Clifford and Crocker (1971) found a positive correlation between the time that elapsed before a professional discussed the cleft with the parents and the adjustment period for parental acceptance of the child's condition. They hypothesized that the parents of a child with such conditions may not fulfill the usual social rituals associated with a new baby, such as encouraging family and friends to visit the infant.

Based on interview data, Weachter (1959) identified 10 areas of parental concern expressed shortly after the birth of a child with a cleft. These are listed in order of frequency of occurrence:

1. The child's appearance
2. Desirability of immediate surgery
3. Speech development
4. Feeding
5. Reaction of the spouse
6. Reaction of siblings
7. Reaction of friends and family
8. Intellectual development
9. Financial problems
10. Recurrence of the defect in yet unborn children

Appearance variables are frequently the major concern of parents and are discussed in a later section. The desire for immediate surgery and concern over reactions of others are likely related to the child's appearance. Although speech development is a legitimate concern for parents, some parents with no prior knowledge of the cleft condition have expressed the belief that the child would not learn to speak or would be unintelligible. It is important to assess the parents' knowledge concerning cleft lip and palate shortly after birth and provide them with realistic expectations. Continued effort should be made to monitor parents' expectations and knowledge of various treatment considerations throughout the habilitation years.

Feeding problems may present psychological concerns because feeding a baby is usually a time of closeness and attachment for mother and infant. The nontraditional feeding methods required for some children with clefts may initially produce anxiety for mothers; however, in most cases, feeding is rarely a long-term problem. For extremely difficult to feed infants, it may be important to supplement the mother's and child's bonding experience independent of the feeding time when physical closeness can be a more pleasant interaction.

Another problem not frequently encountered in parents' reports, but likely to be a source of some concern, is the high incidence of middle ear infections. The additional stress on parents frequently awakened by an infant with ear pain may exacerbate other sources of stress in managing a child with a chronic medical condition. In addition, the child needs close monitoring of hearing status and perhaps repeated placement of ventilating tubes, adding to the frequency of hospital visits. The time off needed from work and the expense of this management may create further parental difficulties.

A frequently felt, but often unexpressed, parental concern is who might be responsible for the defect. A parent may think of other, perhaps quite distant, family members with the disorder and worry about whether the spouse will blame him or her. Less frequent, but quite dramatic when it occurs, is the mother's concern that she may have done something during pregnancy to create the condition. Although genetic counseling and information regarding reproduction and fetal development are beneficial, it is also important to assesss the parents' emotional response to this information. Many examples of parents' thoughts and feelings are provided by intensive interviews reported by Spriestersbach (1973). Based on these reports, it is apparent that positive, yet direct, questioning is needed to elicit these underlying thoughts.

Some parents are concerned that the child may be brain damaged or mentally retarded. This may be based on misconceptions related to perceptions of older acquaintances with unrepaired cleft or the physical proximity of the defect to the brain. Providing assurance regarding the incidence of mental retardation in the cleft population may not be reassuring if the parent has psychological fears related to many of society's superstitions. Introducing parents to other families who have children with clefts and normal intelligence and development may be more reassuring than professional counseling.

Because parents experience a variety of emotional reactions to the child with a cleft and have continued developmental concerns, it is important for the psychologist to determine which of these are realistic and typical. Parental concerns regarding appearance, surgical interventions, speech, and feeding are so common that counseling regarding these areas should occur with every parent of a child with a cleft lip and palate. Even though a parent may not verbalize a concern, underlying feelings can affect treatment. The professional should provide a direct, but supportive, interview regarding sensitive parental feelings that may have the potential to create long-term emotional problems, including possible negative reaction of a spouse, anxiety related to the nature of intercourse, and guilt regarding maternal care during fetal development. These are the least likely feelings to be expressed due to the sensitivity of the subject. However, if such feelings exist and remain unresolved, the effects may be disastrous to the family. The professional must also be alert to the possibility of denial of parental negative feelings toward the child; this may lead to projection of blame onto the child, a subtle form of rejection. Fortunately, the literature indicates that most parents of children with clefts or other craniofacial anomalies adjust to the management problems and are realistic in their concerns for the children. This process of adaptation can be facilitated by initial proactive counseling and information sharing by knowledgeable professionals, rather than waiting until parents express problems.

PARENT–CHILD INTERACTIONS

Attachment is defined as a unique relationship between two people that is specific and enduring. A mother must first accept her baby before an attachment or bond can occur. Brazelton (1963) suggested that an intrauterine mother–infant attachment is formed during pregnancy, whereby the mother fantasizes about her "perfect" child. Robson and Moss (1970) found that many mothers experience impersonal feelings toward their infants for the first few weeks, but during the second month when the baby exhibits visual fixation and smiling, maternal attachments are formed. If the baby has a facial characteristic or appearance similar to a family member, this aids the attachment process. Eye contact, touching, and holding of the child are important factors in forming the mother–infant bond, as are the compatibility of the mother's and child's temperaments. Although the fear of having a defective baby is experienced by many pregnant women, few are prepared for the emotional shock involved with the reality of an infant with a physical defect.

Slutsky (1969) interviewed 66 mothers of children with cleft lips and palates and found that 80% initially reacted with strong feelings of shock, hurt, disappointment, resentment, and even hysteria in a few cases. Emotional reactions to a facial defect are generally greater than to anomalies of other body parts, and the first sight of a cleft lip can be quite distressing for a new parent. Mothers of infants with clefts may be inhibited from touching or close physical contact with their babies (Rubin, 1963). Furthermore, facial deformity may be accentuated by increased attention to the face due to concerns about feeding, speech, and eruption of teeth.

In spite of many early concerns, parents of children with clefts generally demonstrate satisfactory adjustment and form positive parent–child attachments. Perhaps the improvement due to early medical–surgical interventions, increased emphasis on public awareness of the condition, and parental knowledge of other families with a similarly affected child, aid in the process of adjustment. MacDonald (1979) suggested that parental needs and stresses are variable during different periods in the child's development. Stressful periods include the birth experience and initial hospitalization, the beginning of expressive language, entry into school, and adolescent years. In most cases, periods of relative calm are reported, followed by traumatic events. It is interesting to note, however, that the life events reported by MacDonald produce mild stress for parents of any child, although the intensity of stress may be exacerbated for parents of a child with a facial deformity.

Richman and Harper (1978a) compared parental child-rearing practices as reported by children with clefts versus a group of control children without clefts. The children reported their perceptions of the parenting techniques used by their parents. The study examined reports of 68 children with clefts ranging in age from 9 to 18, and 68 matched controls. Findings revealed no significant differences between children with clefts and controls on parental acceptance/rejection or firm control/lax control measures. However, males with clefts perceived their mothers as exerting greater psychological control or intrusiveness than did male controls, suggesting some degree of overprotectiveness of mothers of males with clefts.

In summary, though many factors could interfere with healthy parent–child interactions, such as the stress of dealing with an "imperfect" baby, frequent hospitalizations, and visible deformity, the majority of families appear to experience healthy interactions. Many parent–child interactions that become impaired may be due to factors other than the cleft lip and/or palate and may merely be exacerbated by this condition. Objective information regarding parent–child interactions is sparse. Most reports are based on parental interview or, in some cases, interview of the child. The most comprehensive data are based on reports of both parent and child (Spriestersbach, 1973). The findings reveal many areas of concern that warrent further investigation. These include examination of family dynamics by comparing the behavior of the parents toward the child with a cleft with their behavior toward their children without a cleft. Further research is also needed to determine how concerns expressed by parents affect their behavior toward a child with a cleft compared with behavior of parents of a child without a cleft. An important question is whether the parents' expressed concerns affect parent–child interaction. If so, are these exaggerated effects of normal parental concerns regarding birth, appearance, development, and so on, or are they unique to the parent–child interactions of the family with a child with a cleft? A review of this topic can be found in Clifford's (1987) book.

PHYSICAL ATTRACTIVENESS VARIABLES

"Normal" Subjects

Physical appearance variables seem to convey as much information about an individual as actual behavior and personality traits. Research in social psychology in the past decade has revealed the strength of physical attractiveness in forming opinions about others (Berscheid & Walster, 1974). Nondisabled children of lesser attractiveness were rated by teachers as having lower achievement, less chance at higher education, and poor peer relationships than attractive peers (Clifford & Walster, 1973). Female college students rated an unattractive child who had committed a serious transgression more harshly than an attractive child who had committed the same act (Dion, 1972). Children rate unattractive peers as less friendly, not as smart, and as less desirable playmates (Dion, 1973; Langlois & Stephan, 1977). Rist (1970) found that less attractive children were more likely to be placed in low ability groups during the early elementary school years, but there were confounding factors in addition to attractiveness. Barocas and Black (1974) found that attractive children in third-grade classrooms were more often referred by their teachers for psychological and educational services. The referrals of attractive children tended to be of a "helpful" nature, whereas referrals of unattractive children were more often of a disciplinary nature. The authors interpreted these findings to suggest that more positive attention is paid to the more attractive students; thus their need for help is more likely to be noticed and to receive a positive response.

Observations of unattractive children in play suggest that they behave according to others' expectations (Snyder, Tanke, & Berscheid, 1977) or play with others of the same attractiveness level (Langlois & Downs, 1979). The latter study also found unattractive preschoolers to be more aggressive and active than attractive children. Dion and Berscheid (1974) reported that, compared with attractive peers, unattractive male preschoolers were considered more aggressive and unattractive female preschoolers more fearful. Most researchers have found no significant relationship between school achievement and attractiveness, with the exception of Lerner and Lerner (1977) who found a low, but significantly positive correlation between attractiveness and grade point average. However, a stronger relationship may exist between achievement and attractiveness for individuals with observable physical handicaps. If attractiveness variables influence interactions of nonhandicapped individuals, a facial deformity may create even greater difficulty in social interactions.

Attitudes Toward Children with Physical Disabilities

Livneh (1982) discussed the origins of negative attitudes toward people with disabilities and listed several possible factors in the development and maintenance of these negative reactions. These factors include

1. Sociocultural conditioning, with society's emphasis on beauty, youth, athletic prowess, productivity, and achievement.
2. Childhood influences, which involve parental beliefs, both verbal and behavioral, and child rearing practices that emphasize health and normalcy.
3. Psychodynamic explanations of negative attitudes, including the requirement of mourning, whereby people with disabilities should grieve the lost part or function and are expected to suffer. Some people associate disability with punishment for sin, or they fear social ostracism from being seen in the company of the disabled and guilt of being able-bodied.
4. Disability-related factors, including whether the disorder is functional or organic, level of severity, degree of visibility of the handicap, degree of cosmetic involvement, contagiousness, affected body part, and degree of curability.
5. Other miscellaneous factors, including aesthetic aversion, threat to body image, attitudes toward minority groups in general, and demographic and personality variables.

Richardson (1970, 1971a, 1971b) reported a series of investigations of children with and without handicaps at a summer camp. Children ranked drawings of children based on preference for friendship in the following order: (1) no handicap, (2) crutches and brace on one leg, (3) wheelchair bound, (4) hand missing, (5) facial disfigurement, and (6) obesity. These rankings are relatively consistent over the respondents' age, sex, and socioeconomic status. Females tend to rate facial disfigurement more negatively, whereas males rate functional disability more negatively (Richardson, 1970, 1971a). Unfortunately, Richardson (1971b) found that, even after peers had interacted with handicapped children during the summer camp experience, the rankings did not change.

Individuals with Cleft Lip and/or Palate

Podol and Salvia (1976) examined stereotypes associated with a cleft. Sixty speech pathology students, all of whom read the same case study of a 9-year-old female with a repaired cleft (type unspecified) viewed one of two pictures, one showing a cleft lip scar and one retouched to remove the scar. Those who saw the picture with a lip scar while listening to speech judged the speech as more nasal and were more likely to recommend speech therapy than those who listened to the same speech while observing the picture with the lip scar removed.

As mentioned earlier (Weachter, 1959), the child's appearance was often the parents' major concern soon after birth. Tisza and Gumpertz (1962) reported that parents were more upset by the appearance of a child with a cleft lip and palate than of a child with a cleft palate only. Slutsky (1969) also found more concern in parents of a child with a cleft lip and palate in the first year of life than in parents of a child with cleft palate only; however, in the second year, parents of a child with cleft palate only became more concerned because, as speech developed, their child's disability became more obvious to others.

Teachers' judgments of children's abilities are also affected by the severity of facial disfigurement. Richman (1978a) divided children with both cleft lips and palates into two groups: those with relatively normal facial appearance and those with moderate to severe disfigurement. The groups were formed on the basis of independent ratings by five professionals prior to the study. All children had also received individual intelligence tests prior to the study, and the teachers did not know the results. Teachers underestimated the ability of bright children with significant disfigurement and overestimated the ability of slower children with significant disfigurement. Children with relatively normal facial appearance received quite accurate estimates of intellectual ability by their teachers. It is not clear what effect unrealistic teacher expectations may have on actual child behavior, although some studies have suggested that less attractive individuals receive more punishment, have lower achievement, and are less friendly (Berscheid & Walster, 1974; Clifford & Walster, 1973; Dion, 1972, 1973).

Richman, Holmes, and Eliason (1985) compared two groups of adolescents with both cleft lip and palate who were divided by parent ratings on a behavior checklist into a well-adjusted group ($n = 18$) and a poorly adjusted group ($n = 18$). In addition to parents' ratings of behavior, the adolescents' teachers were asked to rate their facial appearance. The adolescents also completed self-ratings of behavior and appearance. It was found that well-adjusted adolescents' ratings of appearance and behavior were similar to those of teachers and parents, suggesting a realistic perception. The poorly adjusted group rated themselves as more attractive than did teachers and rated their behavior as more "normal" than did their parents. The authors suggested that poorly adjusted adolescents were not realistic in their perceptions, perhaps due to denial of facial disfigurement and resultant social withdrawal.

Summary

Although little research is available on peers', teachers', and others' preceptions of the child with a cleft lip and palate, research with other populations with physical stigmata suggests that a subtle negative reaction may impair the judgment of others in estimating a child's ability and behavior. The research available for children with cleft lip and palate indicates that teachers rate the children's behavior as more inhibited than parents do (Richman, 1978b), and teachers underestimate the intellectual ability of bright children with cleft lip and palate who have significant facial disfigurements (Richman, 1978a). Futhermore, the research suggests that school-age children are less likely to choose a child with a cleft lip and palate as a friend than to choose children with most other handicapping conditions. The relationships cited above do not provide enough evidence to determine specific effects of facial disfigurement on the judgment of others.

Isolating the possible negative effects of facial disfigurement on others is extremely difficult because judgments of others are based on many complex aspects of appearance and behavior. Many of the research paradigms used in nonhandicapped populations appear to be appropriate, such as examining judgments of the same individual under different facial appearance conditions while holding all other conditions constant. This, of course, is an extremely difficult task to design and must be done with picture alteration.

INTELLECTUAL ABILITY AND SCHOOL ACHIEVEMENT

Several previous studies have found slightly lower mean intelligence quotients (IQs) in groups of children with cleft lip and/or palate than in the general population, although the IQs of the groups with clefts fell within the average range (Billig, 1951; Estes & Morris, 1970; Lewis, 1961; Means & Irwin, 1954; Munson & May 1955). Goodstein (1961) and Ruess (1965) found that this lowered general intelligence could be attributed to deficits only on verbal skills, whereas nonverbal skills approximated the population mean. Estes and Morris (1970) suggested that a lack of early language stimulation in the home may account for this verbal deficit. Other factors that may influence verbal ability include history of fluctuating hearing loss related to middle ear infections, speech deficit, and behavioral inhibition (Richman & Eliason, 1986b).

The relationship between intelligence and type of cleft has also been investigated. Goodstein (1961) reported lower mean IQ in a group of children with cleft palate (CP) only than in groups with cleft lip and palate (CLP) or cleft lip only. Others attributed a similar finding of lower IQ in children with CP only to the higher frequency of other congenital anomalies in children with CP only, which might suggest a general defect in development (Lewis, 1961; McWilliams & Matthews, 1979). Lamb, Wilson, and Leeper (1973) reported results suggesting a sex × cleft type interaction and IQ. Those children in the lowest frequency by occurrence groups (female with CLP and males with CP only) were more likely to be "language deficient." It has also been proposed that younger children with clefts have impaired language skills that improve with age (Musgrave, McWilliams, & Matthews, 1975). This interpretation is based on data showing lower verbal ability for younger children with CLP and higher verbal ability for older children. However, this explanation does not account for the cleft type × sex differences in verbal ability. There has also been a report indicating that language skills of children with clefts decline with age (Kommers & Sullivan, 1979); however, this study was based on measures of written language and, therefore, cannot be compared with the other studies that used measures of spoken language.

Some studies have attempted to isolate specific cognitive disabilities in children with CLP. Brantley and Clifford (1979) compared a group of adolescents with cleft palate, a group with obesity, and a control group of adolescents on several cognitive measures of language, memory, and visual perception, and found no significant differences. However, there is some question whether all these tasks were actually intellectual or cognitive style measures, and the effects of IQ were not controlled. Brennan and Cullinan (1974) and Smith and McWilliams (1968) suggested that visual–perceptual–motor deficits are common among children with CLP, whereas Lamb, Wilson, and Leeper (1972) found no such deficits. Specific language deficits may account for some findings of poor visual–perceptual skills because some picture tasks require naming skill and some strategies used to solve visual–perceptual tasks rely on verbal mediation.

Several studies by Richman have suggested at least two types of language learning disability in children with CLP who demonstrate verbal deficits. Richman (1980) examined 57 children with clefts who had Verbal IQs less than Performance IQs on the *Wechsler Intelligence Scale for Children* (WISC). This study included examination of results from the *Hiskey–Nebraska Test of Learning Aptitude,* a test originally developed for deaf children which requires no spoken language on the part of the examiner or the child. However, it does test nonverbal language mediation skills and short-term memory. One group of children with clefts displayed below average performance on the Hiskey, indicating a specific verbal expressive deficit. The other group, however, demonstrated poor associative reasoning (verbal mediation) on the Hiskey, reflecting a general language disability. This group included a high number of males with CP only who also displayed a significant degree of academic underachievement.

A later study compared 24 children with CP only and 24 children with CLP (ages 8 to 12 years) who were matched for age, sex, and Verbal, Performance, and Full Scale IQs on the WISC (Richman & Eliason,

1984). The sample consisted of 14 males and 10 females in each group. The researchers administered the Hiskey and cognitive measures of associative reasoning, memory, visual–perceptual skills, and reading achievement. Results supported the finding that children with CP only are more likely to have pervasive language disability, whereas children with CLP have a milder verbal expressive deficit and higher reading achievement. The type of reading errors also differed between groups. The CP only group tended to make more whole-word, gestalt-type errors, and demonstrated poorer performance on guessing a word based on its initial letter. Children with CLP were more likely to make phonetic errors, reflecting peripheral speech problems interfering with phonics performance. Despite the lack of any finding of neuropsychological deficits, children with CLP had lower reading achievement than expected.

In a survey of the incidence of reading disability in a large sample of children with clefts (Richman & Eliason, 1985), the overall incidence of reading disability in the sample was 36%, compared with estimated figures of 10% to 20% in the general population. Children with CP only had an incidence of 48% compared with about 30% in children with CLP. This finding of more significant language and reading problems for children with CP only than for those with CLP has received further support (Richman, Michele, & Lindgren, 1988). In this latter study of 172 children, children with CP only had a high rate of reading disability at all ages, whereas the children with CLP had decreasing rates of reading disability from ages 6 to 13.

In summary, although early studies suggested that children with clefts have lower IQs than the general population, in most cases this can be attributed to only a verbal deficit. No other specific cognitive deficits have been consistently identified. The verbal deficit is identified in two subtypes of language disabled children with clefts. One form involves only a mild verbal expressive deficit with some effect on reading and school achievement. This problem may be developmental in nature. The other subtype involves a more pervasive language disorder with more profound effects on school achievement.

School achievement deficits have consistently been identified in children with cleft lip and/or palate (Kommers & Sullivan, 1979; Richman, 1976, 1980; Richman & Harper, 1978b) and remedial intervention is required for these children. More children (especially males) with CP only demonstrate a pervasive language disorder that warrants more extensive language evaluation and therapy. Futher research in language and other neuropsychological functions of children with clefts is warranted to determine whether there are indications of neurological impairment, especially in certain cleft type × sex subgroups.

BEHAVIOR AND PERSONALITY

Studies in several areas of disability have attempted to identify specific personality patterns related to specific types of disability; however, these have not been successful (Shontz, 1975). No significant psychopathology has been reported in the area of cleft palate. Although some studies have noted subtle variations of normal behavior, there are some inconsistencies in the findings. Elementary-age children with clefts have been found to have lower self-concept than controls (Kapp, 1979), but adolescents with clefts were found to have higher self-concept than controls in another study (Brantley & Clifford, 1979). However, the two different age groups and different self-esteem measures make comparisons between these studies difficult.

A study of *Minnesota Multiphasic Personality Inventory* (MMPI) findings of 52 adolescents with clefts (Harper & Richman, 1978) found no significant psychopathology. This study did note that the adolescents with clefts displayed excessive inhibition of impulse, increased self-concern, and ruminative self-doubts over interpersonal relationships. Females with clefts expressed more dissatisfaction with their life situations than did males. Richman (1983) also examined 30 adolescents with clefts and 30 controls (ages 15 to 18) regarding their self-perceived adjustment and concerns related to speech, social, and appearance factors. The MMPI and a structured interview were administered. No significant difference existed between control and the entire cleft sample on perceived educational satisfaction or social satisfaction. MMPI results showed that 16 of the profiles of adolescents with clefts were normal and 14 were abnormal. The adolescents with abnormal profiles expressed more concern over school, social, and appearance variables. Even well-adjusted adolescents expressed some concern over facial appearance, suggesting that facial concerns were related to normal adolescent concerns about appearance and body image. Results indicated that younger adolescents may be more concerned with speech, whereas older adolescents may worry more about appearance. Beder and Weinstein (1980) found that adolescents with orofacial anomalies scored higher than the norms on the inadequacy, anger, and sensitivity scales of the *Cornell Medical Index*. A study of children with clefts who were in elementary school also showed excessive inhibition of impulse (Richman & Harper, 1979).

Spriestersbach (1973), using structured parent interviews, found that parents perceived their children with clefts as less independent, less aggressive, and less confident than control children. Richman (1976, 1978b) and Richman and Harper (1978b), using behavior checklists, and Richman and Harper (1979), using self-rated personality measures, supported those findings. These studies indicated that children with clefts tend to score higher than normal children on internalizing factors (withdrawal, inhibition of impulse).

Richman (1978b) found a difference in teacher and parent ratings of children with CLP. Teachers viewed both male and female children with clefts as more inhibited in the classroom than other children, whereas parents rated their children's behavior as comparable to that of other children. This finding could be related to different behaviors in the different settings, or it could indicate that parents do not perceive inhibited behavior as a problem.

There appears to be some relationship between cleft severity and certain measures of personality. Children with milder degrees of facial deformity showed greater inhibition of impulse than children with more severe disfigurements (Harper, Richman, & Snider, 1980). This finding is contrary to the common assumption that more severe deformity leads to more withdrawal and passivity. It may be that the less severe disability creates more behavioral withdrawal to avoid calling attention to oneself, whereas the more severe disfigurement is more noticeable and unlikely to be overlooked.

Eliason and Richman (1987), in a study of children with CLP who ranged in age from 4 to 16, found behavioral differences related to age, sex, and cleft type. Female subjects with CP only showed higher conduct (acting-out) and personality (anxiety) scores than females with CLP. On the other hand, male subjects with CP only showed lower conduct scores, but equal personality scores to those with CLP. When age is considered, both males and females showed increases on both behavioral dimensions over time, in spite of a decrease in speech deviation. The reasons for age, sex, and cleft-type variations in behavior remain unclear, and further examination of these relationships is warranted.

Few studies have examined interventions to improve social skills and decrease the inhibition of children with clefts. However, one study indicates that interventions may be effective (Lochman, Haynes, & Dobson, 1981). During a summer camp experience, children with clefts became more socially responsive to peers and less passive regarding interpersonal interactions.

In summary, although the cleft palate population exhibits no increased incidence of psychopathology, several studies do indicate excessive inhibition. This pattern may be even more pronounced in mildly affected individuals than in those with more severe deformities. Furthermore, behavioral manifestations may be related to age, sex, and cleft type, without clear support for consistent generalizations. Children and adolescents with clefts appear to experience normal developmental stresses, which may be exacerbated by physical disfigurement, speech problems, and social responses of others.

PSYCHOLOGICAL ADJUSTMENT OF ADULTS WITH CLEFT LIP AND/OR PALATE

The same factors that contribute to maladjustment of children or adolescents with clefts—parental reactions, physical appearance variables, lowered academic expectations and school achievement, and behavioral inhibition—may also affect adjustment of adults with clefts. Clifford, Crocker, and Pope (1972) evaluated 98 adults who had undergone surgery by the same surgeon 22 or 27 years prior to the interview. Their satisfaction with employment, marriage, and accomplishments was high, although they had some continued concerns about appearance and speech. In general, however, this group perceived their clefts as having little influence on their lives.

In a comprehensive adult study, Peter and associates presented a four-part discussion of adult functioning in 196 individuals (ages 24 to 54) with cleft lip and/or palate, 190 of their siblings, and 209 random controls. Questionnaire data were gathered in four major areas: marriage, education, vocational and economic aspects, and social integration. Peter and Chinsky (1974a) reported that adults with clefts marry at a significantly lower rate than siblings or controls; 26.5% of the cleft group, 8.9% of the siblings, and 8.6% of the controls had never married. There was also a difference in age at first marriage; adults with clefts marry later (age 24.2) than siblings (21.7) or controls (21.2). Individuals with CLP marry later than individuals with CP only, perhaps reflecting the effects of cosmetic appearance. Although the divorce rate was highest for controls (who also married earliest), the divorce rate for individuals with clefts was higher than for their siblings. They also had significantly fewer children per marriage and were more likely to remain childless than siblings or controls.

Peter and Chinsky (1974b) reported that general educational attainment and school dropout rates did not differ between cleft and noncleft groups, although other studies have suggested a higher dropout rate for individuals with clefts (McWilliams & Paradise, 1973). Of the 196 persons with clefts, 26% had attended one or more years of college, compared with 29% of the siblings and 34% of the controls. This was not a statistically significant difference. Individuals with CLP were more likely to complete college than persons with CP only. Questionnaire responses comparing educational aspirations versus actual educational attainment indicated that a significantly greater number of persons with clefts had aspired to higher education than they actually obtained. Of those aspiring to higher education, individuals with CLP had lower aspirations than controls, whereas those with CP only did not differ from controls. Additionally, the rate of college attendance was slightly lower for individuals with clefts than for siblings or controls, but the college completion rate was comparable. However, persons with CLP were more likely to complete college than were those with CP only.

Peter, Chinsky, and Fisher (1975a) examined vocational and economic conditions of individuals with cleft lip and palate. In this phase of the study, the socioeconomic status (SES) scales of the U.S. Census Bureau were used to judge economic status of the groups. No differences were found in mean SES levels or occupational and educational status; however, income status did differ. Individuals with clefts earned less than siblings, although they did not differ from controls. Persons with clefts also earned less gross family income than either siblings or controls. Employment stability (continuous employment in one job) did not differ by overall groups; however, periods of unemployment were more frequent and of greater duration for persons with clefts than for either siblings or controls. Although controls felt more suited to their jobs, the groups did not differ in job satisfaction. Individuals with clefts tended to have higher aspirations for getting a better job than did controls. These results suggest that adults with clefts may experience less job satisfaction and income than others, even when they have similar educational levels. It is unclear whether this difference is related to objective work productivity differences or possible prejudices of employers.

Peter, Chinsky, and Fisher (1975b) evaluated the family and social integration of adults with clefts. Family interdependence measures showed that persons with clefts, regardless of marital status, were more likely to live with relatives and, of those who lived away from home, to visit relatives more often than siblings or controls. They were also more likely to settle in the same geographic area as their parents. When home activities were categorized as active or passive, individuals with clefts were more likely to engage in passive activities and reported more difficulty in meeting new people, reported fewer close friendships, and belonged to fewer community organizations than siblings or controls.

Peter and associates warned against literal interpretation of their results for several reasons. Self-report questionnaires of this type may by misleading due to a possible discrepancy between self-perceptions of behavior and actual behavior or to a social desirability effect, whereby individuals provide favorable interpretations of their situations. However, even with limitations of the method, it seems that, like children with cleft lip and/or palate, adults with clefts differ from controls in subtle ways. Although these adults report more social isolation, they express no significant signs of emotional maladjustment. Nevertheless, subtle expectation effects of employers or teachers cannot be disregarded. Richman and Harper (1980) found that young adults with clefts (mean age 18.5) experience less self-doubt and concern over social interactions than do adolescents with clefts (Harper & Richman, 1978). However, these young adults had received ongoing team care since infancy, which may have assisted them in developing maximum physical and psychological adjustment.

SUMMARY AND CONCLUSIONS

In this chapter, we discussed the major areas of psychological concern for individuals with clefts. Early concerns are largely parent based and include problems related to coping with the birth of a defective child and learning to adjust to a child's long-term disability. Parents are concerned about the infant's appearance and how others will react. They are concerned about feeding, speech, and intellectual development. They worry about how they will cope financially with the numerous surgeries and extensive orthodontic treatments, and they fear that the defect will occur in subsequent children. Many of these concerns can be dealt with effectively by the cleft palate or craniofacial team. Most parents quickly adjust to different feeding methods and can be reassured regarding the child's speech and mental development. Financial concerns are often overcome by insurance or state support. Genetic counseling provides the parents with empirical information about the nature of clefting and the risk figures for having another child with a cleft.

The issue of physical appearance is frequently not dealt with satisfactorily. All team members need to be sensitive to the variations of physical appearance that may remain for many patients, even after extensive treatment. Professionals should discuss realistic management goals with parents and children regarding appearance and speech performance. As many studies have shown, even minor deviations from normal appearance or speech may influence other people's perceptions of the child. These perceptions can result in the child's having more difficulty with social interactions and in lessened expectations by others (teachers, parents, employers). Use of pictures or real-life models after treatment may help persons with clefts and their families establish realistic goals. Professionals should also be aware that objective measures of appearance and speech may be less influential on the child's adjustment than self-perception of these variables. Hypersensitivity to minor deviations or denial of disfigurement need to be identified and dealt with.

Another issue that needs to be addressed by cleft palate management teams is the problem of underachievement and learning disability in children with clefts. Parent should be alerted to watch for signs of learning problems (especially in reading), and teachers should be informed of the child's abilities to avoid possible deterimental expectations related to the physical attractiveness stereotype. Because teachers may underestimate the abilities of children with facial disfigurements, they may attribute lower achievement to perceived lower ability level and, therefore, may not seek further diagnosis or treatment. Routine screening of a child's reading ability is a cost-effective means of identifying reading problems early and instituting remediation before the problem becomes more severe.

Behavioral symptoms of inhibition of impulse, which are frequent characteristics of children with clefts, may contribute to lower school achievement and less satisfactory social relations. Helping the child to cope with an altered facial appearance at an early age may aid later social adjustment. Cleft type, age, and sex seem to influence behavior, although these relationships need further study. In general, children with clefts show relatively good adjustment to their disability, with only minor variations of normal behavior. Adults with clefts appear to be similar to controls in social relationships, college completion rates, and levels of employment. Further studies are needed to examine those individuals with clefts who demonstrate adjustment problems, to determine more specific factors related to these problems.

In conclusion, the psychologist may serve a vital function on a cleft palate or craniofacial team in the areas of developmental, intellectual, and personality assessment; parent and/or child counseling; liaison work with schools; monitoring of possible psychological consequences of disability; and fostering of an atmosphere sensitive to normal child behavior. Although children's feelings, self-concepts, and school achievement difficulties may not be obvious in the clinic setting, these may be major factors in the habilitation process. For optimal results from treatment, the total child must be considered.

REFERENCES

Barocas, R., & Black, H. (1974). Referral rates and physical attractiveness in third grade children. *Perceptual and Motor Skills, 39,* 731–734.

Beder, O., & Weinstein, P. (1980). Explorations of the coping of adolescents with orofacial anomalies using the Cornell Medical Index. *Journal of Prosthetic Dentistry, 43,* 565–567.

Berscheid, E., & Walster, E. (1974). Physical attractiveness. In L. Gerkowitz (Ed.), *Advances in experimental social psychology* (Vol. 7). New York: Academic Press.

Billig, A. (1951). A psychological appraisal of cleft palate patients. *Proceedings of the Pennsylvania Academy of Science, 25,* 31.

Brantley, H., & Clifford, E. (1979). Cognitive, self-concept, and body-image measures of normal, cleft, and obese adolescents. *Cleft Palate Journal, 16,* 177–182.

Brazelton, T. (1963). The early mother–infant adjustment. *Pediatrics, 32,* 931–937.

Brennan, D., & Cullinan, W. (1974). Object identification and naming in cleft palate children. *Cleft Palate Journal, 11,* 188–195.

Clifford, E. (1968). *Effects of giving birth to a cleft lip–palate baby.* Paper presented at the Plastic Surgery Research Council, Durham, NC.

Clifford, E. (1973). Psychological aspects of orofacial anomalies: Speculations in search of data. *ASHA Reports, 8.*

Clifford, E. (1987). *The cleft palate experience: New perspectives on management.* Springfield, IL: Thomas.

Clifford, E., & Crocker, E. (1971). Maternal responses: The birth of a normal child as compared to the birth of a child with a cleft. *Cleft Palate Journal, 8,* 298–306.

Clifford, E., Crocker, E., & Pope, B. (1972). Psychological findings in the adulthood of 98 cleft palate children. *Journal of Plastic and Reconstructive Surgery, 50,* 234–237.

Clifford, M., & Walster, E. (1973). The effect of physical attractiveness on teacher expectations. *Sociology of Education, 46,* 248–258.

Cohen, M., Jr. (1982). *The child with multiple birth defects.* New York: Raven Press.

Dion, K. (1972). Physical attractiveness and evaluation of children's transgressions. *Journal of Personality and Social Psychology, 24,* 207–213.

Dion, K. (1973). Young children's stereotyping of facial attractiveness. *Developmental Psychology, 9,* 183–188.

Dion, K., & Berscheid, E. (1974). Physical attractiveness and peer perception among children. *Sociometry, 37,* 1–12.

Eliason, M., & Richman, L. (1987). *Behavioral characteristics of cleft children related to age, sex, and cleft type.* Paper presented at the American Cleft Palate Association, San Antonio.

Estes, R., & Morris, H. (1970). Relationship among intelligence, speech proficiency, and hearing sensitivity in children with cleft palates. *Cleft Palate Journal, 7,* 763–773.

Goodstein, L. (1961). Intellectual impairment in children with cleft palate. *Journal of Speech and Hearing Research, 4,* 287–294.

Harper, D., & Richman, L. (1978). Personality profiles of physically impaired adolescents. *Journal of Clinical Psychology, 34,* 636–642.

Harper, D., Richman, L., & Snider, B. (1980). School adjustment and degree of physical impairment. *Journal of Pediatric Psychology, 5,* 377–383.

Kapp, K. (1979). Self-concept of the cleft lip and/or palate child. *Cleft Palate Journal, 16,* 171–176.

Kommers, M., & Sullivan, M. (1979). Written language skills of children with cleft palate. *Cleft Palate Journal, 16,* 18–85.

Lamb, M., Wilson, F., & Leeper, H. (1972). A comparison of selected cleft palate children and their siblings on the variables of intelligence, hearing loss, and visual–perceptual–motor skills. *Cleft Palate Journal, 9,* 218–228.

Lamb, M., Wilson, F., & Leeper, H. (1973). The intellectual function of cleft palate children compared on the basis of cleft type and sex. *Cleft Palate Journal, 10,* 367–377.

Langlois, J., & Downs, A. (1979). Peer relations as a function of physical attractiveness: The eye of the beholder or behavioral reality? *Child Development, 50,* 409–418.

Langlois, J., & Stephan, C. (1977). Effects of physical attractiveness and ethnicity on children's behavioral attributions and peer preferences. *Child Development, 48,* 1694–1698.

Lencione, R. (1980). Psychosocial aspects of cleft lip and palate. In M. Edwards & A. Watson (Eds.), *Advances in the management of cleft palate.* New York: Churchill Livingstone.

Lerner, R., & Lerner, J. (1977). Effects of age, sex, and physical attractiveness on child–peer relations, academic performance, and elementary school adjustment. *Developmental Psychology, 13,* 585–590.

Lewis, R. (1961). A survey of the intelligence of cleft palate children in Ontario. *Cleft Palate Bulletin, 11,* 83–85.

Lis, E., Pruzansky, S., Koepp-Baker, H., & Kobes, H. (1956). Cleft lip and cleft palate perspectives in management. *Pediatric Clinics of North America, 3,* 995–1025.

Livneh, H. (1982). On the origins of negative attitudes toward people with disabilities. *Rehabilitation Literature, 43,* 338–345.

Lochman, J., Haynes, S., & Dobson, E. (1981). Psychosocial effects of an intense summer communication program for cleft palate children. *Child Psychiatry and Human Development, 12,* 54–62.

MacDonald, S. (1979). Parental needs and professional responses: A parental perspective. *Cleft Palate Journal, 16,* 188–192.

McWilliams, B., & Matthews, M. (1979). A comparison of intelligence and social maturity in children with unilateral complete clefts and those with isolated cleft palates. *Cleft Palate Journal, 16,* 363–372.

McWilliams, B., & Paradise, L. (1973). Educational, occupational, and marital status of cleft palate adults. *Cleft Palate Journal, 10,* 223–229.

Means, B., & Irwin, J. (1954). An analysis of certain measures of intelligence and hearing in a sample of the Wisconsin cleft palate population. *Cleft Palate Newsletter, 4,* 2–4.

Munson, S., & May, A. (1955). Are cleft palate persons of subnormal intelligence? *Education Research Journal, 48,* 617–622.

Musgrave, R., McWilliams, B., & Matthews, M. (1975). A review of the results of two different surgical procedures for the repair of clefts of the soft palate only. *Cleft Palate Journal, 12,* 281–290.

Peter, J., & Chinsky, R. (1974a). Sociological aspects of cleft palate adults: I. Marriage. *Cleft Palate Journal, 11,* 295–309.

Peter, J., & Chinsky, R. (1974b). Sociological aspects of cleft palate adults: II. Education. *Cleft Palate Journal, 11,* 443–449.

Peter, J., Chinsky, R., & Fisher, M. (1975a). Sociological aspects of cleft palate adults: III. Vocational and economic aspects. *Cleft Palate Journal, 12,* 193–199.

Peter, J., Chinsky, R., & Fisher, M. (1975b). Sociological aspects of cleft palate adults: IV. Social integration. *Cleft Palate Journal, 12,* 304–310.

Podol, J., & Salvia, J. (1976). Effects of visibility of a prepalatal cleft on the evaluation of speech. *Cleft Palate Journal, 13,* 361–366.

Richardson, S. (1970). Age and sex differences in values towards physical handicaps. *Journal of Health and Social Behavior, 11,* 207–214.

Richardson, S. (1971a). Children's values and friendships: A study of physical disability. *Journal of Health and Social Behavior, 12,* 253–258.

Richardson, S. (1971b). Handicap, appearance, and stigma. *Social Science and Medicine, 5,* 621–628.

Richman, L. (1976). Behavior and achievement of cleft palate children. *Cleft Palate Journal, 13,* 4–10.

Richman, L. (1978a). The effects of facial disfigurement on teachers' perception of ability in cleft palate children. *Cleft Palate Journal, 15,* 155–160.

Richman, L. (1978b). Parents and teachers: Differing views of behavior of cleft palate children. *Cleft Palate Journal, 15,* 360–364.

Richman, L. (1980). Cognitive patterns and learning disabilities in cleft palate children with verbal deficits. *Journal of Speech and Hearing Research, 23,* 447–456.

Richman, L. (1983). Self-reported social, speech, and facial concerns and personality adjustment of adolescents with cleft lip and palate. *Cleft Palate Journal, 20,* 108–112.

Richman, L., & Eliason, M. (1984). Type of reading disability related to cleft type and neuropsychological patterns. *Cleft Palate Journal, 21,* 1–6.

Richman, L., & Eliason, M. (1985). *Incidence of reading disability in a cleft palate population.* Unpublished manuscript, Department of Pediatrics, University of Iowa, Iowa City.

Richman, L., & Eliason, M. (1986a). Development in children with cleft lip and/or palate. *Seminars in Speech and Language, 7,* 225–239.

Richman, L., & Eliason, M. (1986b). Psychological characteristics of cleft lip and palate children. *Cleft Palate Journal, 19,* 249–258.

Richman, L., & Harper, D. (1978a). Observable stigmata and perceived maternal behavior. *Cleft Palate Journal, 15,* 215–219.

Richman, L., & Harper, D. (1978b). School adjustment of children with observable disabilities. *Journal of Abnormal Child Psychology, 6,* 11–18.

Richman, L., & Harper, D. (1979). Self-identified personality patterns of children with facial or orthopedic disfigurement. *Cleft Palate Journal, 16,* 257–261.

Richman, L., & Harper, D. (1980). Personality profiles of physically impaired young adults. *Journal of Clinical Psychology, 36,* 668–671.

Richman, L. C., Holmes, C. S., & Eliason, M. J. (1985). Adolescents with cleft lip and palate: Self-perceptions of appearance and behavior related to personality adjustment. *Cleft Palate Journal, 22,* 93–96.

Richman, L., Michele, J., & Lindgren, S. (1988). Reading disability in children with clefts. *Cleft Palate Journal, 25,* 21–25.

Rist, R. (1970). Student social class and teacher expectations: The self-fulfilling prophesy in ghetto education. *Harvard Educational Review, 40,* 411–451.

Robson, K., & Moss, H. (1970). Patterns and determinants of maternal attachments. *Journal of Pediatrics, 76,* 976–985.

Rubin, R. (1963). Maternal touch. *Nursing Outlook, 11,* 828–831.

Ruess, A. (1965). A comparative study of cleft palate children and their siblings. *Journal of Clinical Psychology, 21,* 354–360.

Shontz, F. (1975). *Psychological aspects of physical illness and disability*. New York: Macmillan.

Slutsky, H. (1969). Maternal reaction and adjustment to the birth and care of the cleft palate child. *Cleft Palate Journal, 6*, 425–427.

Smith, R., & McWilliams, B. (1968). Psycholinguistic abilities of children with clefts. *Cleft Palate Journal, 5*, 238–249.

Snyder, M., Tanke, E., & Berscheid, E. (1977). Social perception and interpersonal behavior: On the self-fulfilling nature of social stereotypes. *Journal of Personality and Social Psychology, 35*, 656–666.

Spriestersbach, D. C. (1973). *Psychosocial aspects of the "Cleft Palate Problems"* (Vols. 1 and 2). Iowa City: University of Iowa Press.

Tisza, V., & Gumpertz, E. (1962). The parents' reaction to the birth and early care of children with cleft palate. *Pediatrics, 30*, 86–90.

Weachter, E. (1959). Concerns of parents related to the birth of a child with a cleft of the lip and palate with implications for nurses. Unpublished master's thesis, University of Chicago.

Author Index

Abbe, R., 73, 76
Abdelmalek, L., 260, 298
Abyholm, F. E., 26, 46
Adams, L. E., 161, 186
Adisman, I. K., 181
Aduss, H., 122, 131, 142
Ahlgren, J., 89, 90, 117
Albery, E., 276, 297
Allison, D. L., 160, 181
Altemus, L. A., 26, 46
Amato, J., 42, 48
Angle, E. H., 122, 142
Aram, A., 174, 181
Aramany, M. A., 168, 186
Araujo, A., 106, 115
Arndt, W. B., 172, 187, 303, 350, 356
Aronson, A. E., 179, 183
Artz, J. S., 29, 47
Ashley, M., 279, 297
Aten, J. L., 175, 179, 181

Backdahl, M., 90, 115
Baer, T., 26
Baken, R., 290, 291, 292, 298
Bandt, C. L., 90, 92, 116
Banks, P., 99, 115
Bankson, N. W., 331, 333
Bardach, J., 65, 76
Barker, L. F., 6, 15, 22
Barnes, M., 253, 304, 316, 335
Barney, H., 253, 303
Barocas, R., 365, 376
Bartlett, D. M., 166, 183
Bauer, B. S., 63, 76
Bear, J. C., 46, 268, 270, 298
Beaumont, K., 345, 356
Becker, M., 224, 245
Beder, O., 371, 376
Beery, Q., 301
Beiter, A. L., 309, 334
Bell, W. H., 106, 115
Bell-Berti, F., 279, 281, 298, 300
Bennett, J., 276, 297
Bennett, M. E., 106, 115

Bensen, J., 255, 298
Berkowitz, S., 89, 115, 122, 131, 142
Berlin, C., 210, 216
Bernhardt, B., 316, 333
Bernstein, L., 212, 215
Bernthal, J. E., 157, 181, 231, 245, 331, 333
Berry, Q. C., 197, 199, 215
Berscheid, E., 365, 367, 376, 377, 380
Bess, F. H., 201, 215
Beukelman, D. R., 157, 181, 231, 245
Beumer, J., 171, 182
Bevis, R. R., 90, 92, 116, 121
Billig, A., 368, 376
Bishara, S. E., 93, 115
Bixler, D., 38, 40, 46, 47, 48
Bjork, L., 285, 298
Black, H., 365, 376
Blake, G. B., 38, 46
Blakeley, R. W., 168, 172, 181
Blank, J. L., 164, 187
Bleiberg, A. H., 4, 22
Bless, D., 164, 181, 295, 300
Bloem, T., 252, 301
Blomain, E., 299
Bloomer, H. A., 163, 175, 181, 183, 284, 298
Bluestone, C. D., 157, 185, 195, 197, 199, 214, 215, 216
Bonaiti, C., 40, 46
Bonaiti-Pellie, C., 40, 46
Bond, E. K., 163, 184
Boo-Chai, K., 52, 76
Boone, D. R., 156, 182
Boothroyd, A., 287, 304
Borden, G. J., 166, 181
Bosma, J. F., 174, 183
Bouhuys, A., 156, 185
Boyce, S., 268, 298
Boyne, P. J., 88, 89, 90, 115
Brackett, I., 279, 297
Bradford, L., 284, 298
Bradley, D. P., 159, 185, 264, 291, 301, 302

Bralley, R., 299
Branemark, P. I., 154, 186
Brantley, H., 364, 371, 376
Brauer, R. D., 61, 76
Braun, T. W., 107, 115
Brazelton, T., 363, 376
Brennan, D., 369, 377
Briard, M. L., 40, 46
Brodie, A., 86, 115
Broen, P. A., 69, 219, 224, 232, 236, 240, 245, 246, 247, 325, 326, 330, 333
Brooks, A. R., 261, 265, 284, 298, 303, 313, 333
Brooks, R., 265, 303
Brookshire, B. L., 225, 247
Broomhead, M., 90, 117
Broude, D. J., 89, 115
Brown, A. S., 20, 22
Brown, C., 305
Brown, J. B., 52, 76
Brown, K. S., 30, 47
Brown, W., 294, 302
Buckingham, R. A., 212, 215
Bull, G., 299
Bundgaard, M., 90, 116
Burrell, K., 343, 344, 354
Burston, W. R., 122, 131, 142
Byrne, M. C., 229, 245
Bzoch, K. R., 170, 171, 182, 186, 188, 222, 261, 298, 229, 230, 245, 314, 319, 333, 347, 355

Campbell, W. E., 19, 22
Cantekin, E. I., 197, 199, 215
Carlstrom, J. E., 189
Carollo, D., 86, 115
Carrell, J., 264, 298
Cervenka, J., 29, 42, 46, 47
Charles, D. H., 145
Chase, R., 305, 340, 349, 350, 356
Chaudhry, A. P., 126, 143
Chierici, G., 149, 182
Chin, L., 253, 304
Ching, G. H., 40, 46, 253, 304
Chinsky, R., 373, 374, 378
Chir, J., 90, 117
Chisholm, T., 90, 117
Chisum, L., 172, 187, 303, 350, 356
Chomsky, N., 245
Chosack, A., 28, 46
Christiansen, R., 280, 281, 302, 347, 355

Christie, F. B., 88, 117
Christoplos, F., 5, 9, 11, 15, 16, 23
Chung, C. S., 40, 46
Churchill, J. D., 309, 333
Cichoke, A., 264, 305
Clemis, J., 198, 199, 216
Clifford, E., 360, 361, 364, 365, 367, 369, 371, 373, 376
Clodius, L., 61, 76
Cohen, A. B., 64, 78
Cohen, M. A., 20, 22
Cohen, M. M., Jr., 36, 43, 46, 47, 360, 377
Cohn, E., 159, 187, 260, 298
Cole, R., 338, 355
Coleman, R. F., 156, 182
Colton, J., 253, 304
Compton, A. J., 223, 246
Compton, M., 299
Conneally, P. M., 40, 47
Cook, D., 103, 115
Cooper, H. K., 4, 5, 6, 7, 8, 22
Cooper, J., 236, 248
Counihan, D. T., 170, 182, 284, 298, 229, 246, 351, 355
Crabb, J. J., 131, 143
Crocker, E., 360, 361, 373, 377
Croft, C., 253
Croft, C. B., 316, 333, 335
Croft, C. V., 159, 182, 275, 298
Cronin, T. D., 59, 76
Crutchfield, E., 302
Cullinan, W. L., 170, 182, 284, 298, 351, 355, 369, 377
Curran, J., 79
Curtin, J. W., 15, 21, 22, 66, 76, 236, 246, 310, 333
Curtis, A., 198, 199, 216
Curtis, J. F., 157, 171, 182, 284, 298
Curtis, T. A., 182, 171
Cutting, C., 279, 301

D'Antonio, L. L., 160, 177, 182, 185, 276, 299
Dalston, E., 161, 182, 213, 217, 287, 298,
Dalston, R. M., 156, 160, 161, 182, 184, 186, 188, 276, 277, 278, 279, 284, 286, 287, 291, 292, 294, 297, 298, 300, 301, 302, 305, 341, 355
Daly, D., 188
Daniel, B., 155, 186

Daniller, A., 159, 182, 275, 298
Daniloff, R., 253, 299
Darley, F. L., 161, 158, 188, 222, 248, 282, 302, 319, 335
Davis, J. M., 210, 216
Davis, W. B., 90, 116
Dawson, W., 284, 304
DeBlanc, G. B., 29, 46
Dellon, A. L., 200, 216
Desai, S. N., 66, 76
Dibbell, O., 164, 181
Dickson, D. R., 252, 284, 285, 299
Diedrich, W., 229, 245, 265, 303,
Dieffenbach, J. F., 64
Dinnsen, D. A., 223, 225, 246
Dion, K., 365, 367, 377
Dixon-Wood, V. L., 4, 23
Dobie, R., 210, 216
Dobson, E., 372, 378
Dolan, E. A., 177, 186
Dolan, K., 262, 301
Dooley, P., 345, 356
Dorf, D. S., 66, 76, 164, 186, 236, 246, 310, 333
Downs, A., 365, 378
Downs, M. P., 206, 216
Drachter, R., 89, 90, 116
DuBois, A. B., 160, 188, 292, 305
Ducanis, A. J., 5, 6, 11, 12, 15, 16, 20, 21, 22
Dunn, C., 308, 318, 326, 335
Dunn, V., 268, 269, 299

Eckel, F., 156, 182
Edgerton, M., 287, 289, 299
Edwards, M. L., 316, 318, 320, 333
Egyedi, P., 103, 116
Ehrhardt, J., 268, 269, 299
Eidelman, E., 28, 46
Eilers, R. E., 231, 247
Eisenbach, C., 258, 261, 265, 299, 305
El Deeb, M., 79, 84, 89, 90, 91, 92, 93, 94, 99, 107, 116
El Deeb, M. E., 116
Elbert, M., 303, 325, 331, 333, 350, 356
Elbert, M. A., 172, 187
Eliason, M. J., 357, 367, 368, 369, 370, 372, 377, 379
Ellwood, P., 21, 22
Elster, B., 314, 334
Emanuel, F. W., 156, 183
Emanuel, I., 26, 42, 46

Enemark, H., 90, 116
Epker, B. N., 100, 103, 105, 106, 110, 115, 116, 118, 119
Epstein, L. J., 90, 116
Estes, R., 368, 377
Estrem, T., 232, 246, 325, 330, 333
Ewanowski, S., 164, 181

Falter, J. W., 172, 182
Farrange, J., 175, 186
Farwell, C. B., 226, 234, 246
Feingold, J., 40, 46
Felden, H., 199, 216
Felsenfeld, S., 236, 245
Ferguson, C. A., 226, 234, 246
Feth, L., 253, 299
Fey, M., 246
Fiala, K. H., 160, 187
Figueroa, A., 131, 142
Finch, D., 13, 23
Firtell, D. N., 171, 182
Fish, L. C., 110, 116
Fisher, H. A., 158, 182
Fisher, M., 374, 378
Fishman, L. S., 84, 86, 116
Fitch, H., 166, 181
Fletcher, S. G., 174, 183, 188, 229, 246, 285, 286, 299, 342, 343, 344, 355
Flint, M., 116
Fogh-Andersen, 38, 40, 46, 47, 48
Folkins, J. W., 155, 183, 252, 264, 279, 297, 299, 300, 301, 303, 305
Fox D. R., 225, 247
Fox, A., 149, 168, 187
Franco, P., 52, 76
Fraser, F. C., 40, 47
Freihofer, H. P. M., 101, 103, 116
Friede, H., 89, 90, 117
Fristoe, M., 158, 183
Fritzell, B., 279, 299
Fujika, Y., 264, 305
Fujimura, O., 166, 183, 284, 299
Furnas, D. W., 54, 76
Furr, M., 345, 356

Gallia, L., 106, 119
Gandour, J., 226, 246
Garber, S. R., 166, 183
Gay, W. D., 177, 185
Geoffrey, V. C., 166, 183
Georgiade, N. G., 53, 61, 76
Gibbons, P., 175, 183

Gierut, J., 325, 331, 333
Gilbert, S., 272, 299
Girdany, B., 264, 301
Glaser, E., 291, 299, 301
Gnoinski, W. M., 93, 117, 131, 142
Gold, D. P., 40, 48
Gold, H. O., 164, 186
Goldberg, R. B., 42, 48
Goldin, H., 22, 90, 117
Golding-Kushner, K. J., 160, 183, 275,
    299, 322, 333
Goldman, M., 156, 183, 184
Goldman, R., 158, 183
Golin, A. K., 5, 6, 11, 12, 15, 16, 20, 21
Gonzalez, J. B., 179, 183
Gooch, V., 19, 22
Goodstein, L., 368, 377
Gore, J., 268, 298
Gorlin, R. J., 25, 29, 36, 38, 41, 42, 47,
    48
Grabb, W. C., 65, 77
Graber, T. M., 122, 142
Gradfield, S., 345, 356
Graham, J., 284, 304
Graham, W. P., 54, 78
Graves, D. K., 157, 184
Griffith, B. H., 89, 118
Grossman, W., 90, 117
Gruber, H., 131, 142
Grunewell, P., 126, 139, 143, 326, 333
Gumpertz, E., 367, 380
Gutierrez, R., 175, 179, 181
Gutman, L. T., 26, 42, 46
Guyette, T. W., 160, 187

Hagedorn, M., 52, 58, 77
Hagerty, R. F., 53, 77
Hairfield, W. M., 174, 185, 213, 217
Hall, H. D., 90, 116
Hall, P., 316, 333
Halle, M., 245
Hallock, G. G., 53, 77
Hamlet, S. L., 157, 166, 183
Hanson, W., 156, 183
Hardy, J. C., 174, 175, 179, 183, 184
Harper, D., 364, 370, 371, 372, 374,
    377, 379
Harrington, D., 20, 23
Harrington, J., 264, 299
Harris, F., 28, 47, 166
Harris, K. S., 166, 181, 184, 345, 356
Haskins, R. C., 174, 183

Hassell, J. R., 30, 47
Hattori, S., 284, 299
Hawkins, C., 270, 271, 299, 303
Haynes, S., 372, 378
Hayward, J. R., 92, 116
Hebda, T. W., 84, 89, 90, 91, 93, 99,
    116
Heckler, F. R., 29, 47
Hedrick, D. L., 236, 248, 326, 335
Heiner, H., 29, 47
Henderson, D., 106, 116, 148, 149, 152,
    179, 183
Henningson, G. E., 322, 333
Hess, D. A., 53, 77, 300, 350, 351, 355
Hinrichs, J. E., 90, 92, 116
Hinrichsen, G., 103, 115
Hinson, J. K., 156, 182
Hirschberg, J., 258, 300
Hixon, E., 259, 300
Hixon, T. J., 156, 157, 183, 184, 187,
    255, 271, 295, 300, 301, 305
Hoch, L. M., 322, 330, 331, 333
Hodgson, W. R., 216
Hodson, B. W., 225, 246, 324, 326, 331,
    333, 334
Hoffman, R., 86, 115
Hofmann, F., 264, 305
Hogan, V. M., 69, 77
Hogeman, K. E., 89, 117
Hoke, J. A., 90, 119, 177, 186
Holder, M., 156, 188
Hollien, H., 156, 158, 184
Holmes, C. S., 367, 379
Honjo, I., 267, 300
Honjow, I., 225, 246
Hoppe, W., 47
Hopper, J. E., 200, 216
Horiguchi, S., 281, 300
Horii, Y., 156, 184, 287, 289, 300, 344,
    355
Hotz, M. M., 93, 117, 131, 142
Huang, S. W., 26, 42, 46
Hubbard, T., 314, 334
Huddart, A. G., 131, 143
Huebner, D. V., 131, 143
Hultzen, L., 287, 300
Humes, L. E., 215
Huston, K., 223, 246
Hyman, L., 222, 246

Ibuki, K., 160, 184, 275, 300, 346, 356
Iglesias, A., 253, 263, 300

Ikeoka, N., 264, 305
Ingram, D., 223, 225, 226, 246, 324, 334
Irwin, J., 368, 378
Isaacson, R. J., 126, 143
Isberg, A. M., 322, 333
Isshiki, M. D., 225, 231, 246
Isshiki, N., 156, 184

Jabaley, M. E., 29, 47
Jackson, I. T., 65, 69, 77, 88, 90, 106, 116, 117
Jacobson, B. N., 89, 118
Jacobson, R., 122, 143
Jacobsson, S., 89, 117
Jaffe, B. F., 29, 47
Jakobi, P., 20, 23
Jakobson, R., 223, 246
James, D., 126,143
Janson, T., 154, 186
Jobe, R., 349, 356
Johanson, B., 63, 78, 89, 90, 117
Johnston, M. C., 4, 23, 30, 36, 47
Jolleys, A., 63, 77, 89, 90, 117, 118
Jones, B. W., 309, 333
Jones, D., 278, 300
Jones, J. E., 64, 78
Jones, J. W., 28, 47
Jones, R. N., 175, 184
Jons, S. M., 224, 245
Jordan, R., 82, 117
Jordan, W., 13, 23

Kahn, S., 61, 77
Kalikow, D., 287, 304
Kaplan, J., 40, 46
Kapp, K., 371, 377
Karnell, M. P., 160, 184, 264, 272, 273, 275, 279, 282, 300
Kastner, C., 291, 301
Kawai, T., 28, 47
Kawano, M., 267, 300
Kelsey, C., 271, 301
Kelso, J. A. S., 166, 184
Kemp-Fincham, S. I., 310, 334
Kent, K., 86, 117
Kent, R. D., 16, 23, 284, 303, 320, 335
Kern, C. A., 236, 248, 326, 335
Kernahan, D. A., 118, 143
Kersten, R. B., 6, 90, 119
Khan, L. M., 324, 334
Kimberling, W. J., 43, 47

Kipfmueller, L. J., 175, 184
Kistler, E., 93, 117
Kittelson-Bacon, C., 245
Knox, A. W., 172, 187, 303
Koberg, W. R., 89, 117, 118
Kobes, H., 3, 23, 360, 378
Koch, H., 89, 118
Koch, L., 93, 117
Koepp-Baker, H., 3, 4, 10, 11, 14, 16, 19, 23, 229, 248, 261, 304, 360, 378
Koguchi, H., 40, 46
Kommers, M., 369, 370, 377
Krakow, R., 281, 298
Kraus, B., 82, 117
Krogman, W., 4, 23
Kuehn, D. P., 156, 159, 184, 188, 252, 253, 260, 262, 264, 279, 280, 282, 284, 285, 300, 301, 305, 310, 334, 341, 355
Kufner, J., 103, 117
Kuhl, P., 228, 246
Kwiatkowski, J., 223, 225, 248, 308, 318, 324, 335
Kwon, H. J., 90, 117

Lagu, R., 276, 302
Laine, T., 160, 184, 291, 294, 301
Lamabadusuriya, S., 126, 143
Lamb, M., 368, 369, 377
Lang, B. R., 175, 184
Lang, J., 344, 355
Lange, K., 40, 48
Langlois, J., 365, 378
LaRossa, D., 64, 78
Laskin, R., 316, 334
Lass, N., 302
Latham, R. A., 53, 61, 76, 126, 143
LaVelle, W. E., 174, 175, 179, 184
Lavorato, A. S., 157, 185, 214, 216, 301
Lawrence, C., 301, 313, 314, 334
Lawson, W. A., 163, 184
Leck, I., 26, 47
Leeper, H. A., 145, 157, 160, 161, 168, 175, 176, 177, 178, 181, 184, 186, 187, 368, 369, 377
Lehman, J. A., 29, 47
Lehnert, M. W., 84, 89, 90, 91, 93, 99, 116
Lehr, R., 279, 297
LeMesurier, A. B., 52, 77
Lencione, R., 159, 187, 360, 378
Leopold, W. F., 223, 226, 227, 246, 247

Lerner, J., 365, 378
Lerner, R., 365, 378
Letcher, L., 240, 247
Leubling, H. E., 4, 22
Leutert, G., 29, 47
Levin, L. S., 36, 47
Levinson, C., 339, 355
Lewin, J. L., 159, 182, 298
Lewin, M., 275
Lewis, N. P., 324, 334
Lewis, R., 368, 378
Lexer, E., 52, 77, 89, 117
Lin, C. C., 26, 42, 46
Lindblom, B., 284, 285, 301
Lindemann, G., 28, 47
Lindgren, S., 370, 379
Lindquist, A. F., 172, 187
Linville, R. N., 157, 188, 305
Lippmann, R., 287, 301
Lis, E., 360, 378
Lis, E. F., 3, 23
Livneh, H., 365, 378
Lloyd, R. S., 174, 184, 187
Lochman, J., 372, 378
Locke, J. L., 232, 247, 308, 315, 326,
   334
Logemann, J. A., 158, 182, 236, 247,
   310, 334
Loney, R., 252, 301
Louis, H., 172, 188
Lowry, R. B., 26, 47
Lubit, E., 339, 354
Lubker, J., 252, 256, 261, 264, 284,
   294, 301
Lynch, H. T., 43, 47, 247
Lynch, J. I., 225

Mabis, J. H., 156, 182
MacDonald, S., 364, 378
MacIntosh, R. B., 103, 117
MacKenzie-Stepner, K., 316, 334
Maier, N. F., 51, 77
Makepeace, A., 272, 276, 303
Malgaine, J. F., 52, 77
Mann, M., 160, 170, 186
Margolis, R. H., 204, 216
Mars, M., 126, 139, 143
Marsh, J. L., 131, 143, 160, 177, 182,
   185, 276, 299
Marshall, R. C., 175, 184
Martin, R., 280, 281, 302
Mason, R., 105, 117, 156, 185, 261, 301

Massengill, R., Jr., 89, 90, 118, 339,
   355
Matkin, N. D., 210, 216
Matsuya, T., 159, 160, 172, 185, 346,
   355, 356
Matthews, D., 90, 117
Matthews, M., 368, 369, 378
Maue-Dickson, W., 216
May, A., 368, 378
Mazaheri, E. H., 172, 174, 185
Mazaheri, M., 168, 172, 174, 185
McCall, G. N., 159, 187, 253, 304, 316,
   335, 347, 356
McCarty, T., 166, 183
McClelland, K., 345, 356
McCormack, R., 264, 305
McDonald, A., 175, 179, 181
McDonald, W., 299
McDowell, F., 52, 76
McGrath, C. O., 334
McGregor, J. C., 88, 117
McKinney, P., 89, 118
McLennan, C., 65, 71
McLennan, J. G., 88, 90, 117
McNeil, C. K., 131, 143
McParland, F., 90, 117
McReynolds, L. V., 223, 247
McWilliams, B. J., 4, 23, 157, 159, 168,
   185, 186, 188, 214, 216, 229, 230,
   247, 252, 255, 258, 260, 266, 282,
   283, 286, 291, 294, 295, 297, 301,
   302, 313, 314, 334, 338, 350, 355,
   368, 369, 373, 378, 380
McWilliams-Neely, B., 264, 302
Mead, J., 156, 183, 184, 185
Means, B., 368, 378
Melnick, M., 40, 47
Meltzoff, A. N., 228, 246
Menn, L., 221, 227, 247
Menyuk, P., 223, 247
Messer, L. B., 84, 89, 90, 91, 93, 99,
   116
Meyer, M. W., 106, 107, 116, 117
Michele, J., 370, 379
Middleton, G., 302
Migne-Tufferand, G., 40, 46
Millard, D. R., 52, 55, 62, 73, 77
Millard, R. T., 174, 185
Mills, A., 228, 247
Minifie, F., 271, 301
Minsley, G. E., 174, 185
Mirault, G., 52, 77

Mitoma, T., 267, 300
Miyazaki, T., 159, 160, 172, 185, 346,
    348, 355, 356
Moll, K. L., 159, 170, 184, 229, 247,
    248, 256, 264, 284, 301, 302
Moller, K. T., 1, 69, 158, 185, 219, 240,
    247, 280, 281, 302, 304, 326, 347,
    355
Molt, L. F., 161, 185
Monroe, C. W., 89, 118
Moon, J. B., 159, 185, 251, 267, 268,
    276, 278, 290, 293, 294, 297, 299,
    302, 304
Moore, J., 351, 355
Morgan, R. F., 200, 216
Moriarity, J., 90, 119
Morimoto, M., 225, 246
Morley, M. E., 230, 247
Morr, K. E., 160, 182, 184, 185, 291,
    292, 301, 302
Morris, H. L., 4, 5, 8, 20, 23,65, 76,
    160, 170, 175, 183, 184, 188, 222,
    229, 247, 248, 252, 253, 261, 264,
    272, 275, 282, 291, 300, 301, 302,
    334, 338, 355, 368, 377
Morton, N. E., 40, 48
Moser, H., 282, 287, 302
Moskowitz, A., 223, 247
Moss, H., 363, 379
Mourino, A., 253, 302
Moyce, A., 195, 216
Muller, E., 294, 302
Munro, I., 105, 119
Munson, S., 368, 378
Muntz, H. R., 160, 177, 182, 185, 276,
    299
Musgrave, R., 369, 378
Mylin, W. K., 53, 77

Nackashi, J. A., 4, 23
Natsume, N., 28, 47
Neiman, G., 253, 302
Nelson, C. L., 64, 78
Nelson, R. L., 106, 117
Neptune, C., 82, 117
Netsell, R., 155, 156, 175, 183, 186,
    295, 300
Nickerson, R., 287, 304
Nishio, J., 346, 355, 356
Nissen, G., 103, 117
Noll, J. D., 222, 248
Nordin, K. D., 89, 90, 118

Nordin, K. E., 63, 78, 115
Northern, J. L., 206, 216
Novak, M. A., 309, 334
Novak, R. E., 309, 333
Noyes, F. B., 122, 143
Nussbaumer, H., 93, 117
Nye, P., 268, 298
Nylen, B., 88, 90, 115, 118, 285, 298

O'Gara, M. M., 236, 247, 310, 334
Obwegeser, H., 103, 118
Oeschlaeger, M., 100, 105, 118
Oesterle, L. G., 29, 47
Ogle, R., 106, 117
Ohala, J., 276, 278, 302
Ohlson, A., 89, 90, 117
Olin, W. H., 65, 76, 93, 115, 122, 143
Oller, D. K., 231, 232, 247, 310, 334
Olson, D. A., 229, 248
Oral, K., 168, 186
Osberg, P. E., 172, 186
Ostry, D., 270, 302
Owen, E., 52, 78
Owens, J. R., 28, 47

Paden, E. P., 225, 246, 309, 326, 331,
    334
Paesani, A., 345, 356
Palmer, J., 163, 186
Pannbacker, M., 188, 262, 267, 282,
    295, 302
Paradise, J. L., 199, 212, 215, 216, 314,
    334
Paradise, L., 373, 378
Pare, A., 52, 78
Parel, S. M., 154, 186
Parush, A., 270, 302
Path, M., 106, 117, 302, 347, 355
Pauli, S., 284, 301
Paulus, G. W., 103, 110, 116, 118
Paulus, P. J., 110, 116
Pavy, B., 40, 46
Paynter, E., 13, 23
Peagler, F. D., 29, 48
Peet, E., 64, 78
Perry, C. C., 149, 168, 187
Perkom M., 131, 142
Peter, J., 373, 374, 378
Peters, A. M., 226, 248
Peterson, G., 253, 284, 298, 303
Peterson, S. J., 170, 186, 316, 334, 340,
    349, 355, 356

Petrovic, S., 90, 118
Philips, B. J., 283, 284, 303, 313, 314, 334
Phillips, C., 160, 182, 276, 299, 301
Pickrell, K., 88, 89, 90, 118, 339, 355
Pigott, R. W., 159, 186, 258, 272, 276, 297, 299, 303
Podol, J., 366, 378
Polpelka, G. R., 204, 216
Pope, B., 373, 377
Posnick, J. C., 90, 116
Poswillo, D., 30, 47
Powers, G. N., 313, 335
Powers, G. R., 229, 248, 339, 356
Prather, E. M., 236, 248, 326, 335
Priestly, T. M. S., 226, 235, 248
Primosch, R. E., 83, 118
Proctor, D. F., 156, 185
Province, M., 160, 182, 276, 299
Pruzansky, S., 3, 42, 23, 47, 122, 131, 143, 174, 184, 360, 378
Psaume, J., 40, 46
Putnam, A. H. B., 156, 184, 291, 301

Quinn, G., 88, 89, 90, 118, 339, 355

Rakoff, S. J., 253, 298, 316, 333, 335
Randall, P., 54, 56, 58, 60, 64, 65, 78
Ranta, R., 86, 118
Redenbaugh, M., 289, 290, 303, 344, 356
Rehrmann, A. H., 89, 118
Reich, A., 289, 290, 303, 344, 356
Reich, T., 40, 48
Reichenbach, E., 103, 118
Reisberg, D. J., 164, 186
Richardson, S., 366, 379
Richman, L. C., 357, 364, 367, 368, 369, 370, 371, 372, 374, 377, 379
Riis, B., 29, 47
Riski, J. E., 177, 186
Rist, R., 365, 379
Robertson, N. R. E., 63, 77, 89, 90, 117, 118
Robson, K., 363, 379
Rollins, A., 287, 304
Rood, S. R., 195, 198, 216, 260
Rose, W., 52, 55, 78
Rosen, M. S., 171, 186
Rosenbek, J. C., 155, 186
Rosenstein, S., 122, 131, 132, 143
Rosenstein, S. W., 89, 118

Ross, M., 211, 216
Ross, R. B., 4, 23, 122, 131, 143
Rouse, V., 222, 248
Rowe, N. C., 115, 118
Rubin, R., 379
Ruess, A., 368, 379
Ruscello, D. M., 156, 187, 338, 356
Rutherford, D., 229, 249
Ryan, W., 270, 303

Sadove, A. M., 64, 78, 299
Sakuda, M., 171, 172, 187
Salvia, J., 366, 378
Salyer, K., 322, 346, 356, 336
Sands, N. R., 88, 89, 90, 115
Sarnas, K. V., 89, 117
Sato, M., 176, 186
Sato, Y., 176, 186
Schaaf, N. S., 86, 117
Schaumann, B. F., 29, 48
Scheker, L. R., 90, 117, 65, 77
Schendel, S. A., 100, 103, 105, 106, 115, 118, 119
Scherbick, K., 302
Schmid, E., 89, 119, 63, 78
Schmidseder, R., 103, 117
Schneider, E., 158, 186, 257, 262, 266, 282, 287, 291, 295, 303
Schneiderman, C. R., 160, 170, 186
Schuckers, G., 253, 299
Schwartz, M., 256, 284, 303
Schwartz, R. H., 217
Schweckendiek, W., 38, 48, 64, 78
Schweiger, J., 175, 183
Scott, J. H., 126, 143
Seaver, E. J., 160, 186, 264, 278, 279, 298, 300, 303, 305
Sell, D., 126, 139, 143
Senturia, B., 199, 217
Sewerin, I., 29, 47
Shanks, J. E., 204, 216
Shapiro, B., 29, 46
Sharry, J. J., 176, 186
Shaughnessy, A. L., 175, 186
Shaw, R., 264, 303
Shelton, R. L., 4, 159, 164, 172, 174, 182, 187, 252, 261, 265, 284, 285, 291, 298, 301, 302, 303, 23, 229, 245, 247, 313, 333, 338, 345, 350, 355, 356
Sher, A., 316, 335
Sherman, D., 4, 23, 222, 248

Shields, E. D., 38, 40, 47, 48
Shiere, F. R., 149, 168, 187
Sholes, G., 345, 356
Shons, A. R., 49
Shontz, F., 371, 380
Shprintzen, R. J., 20,23, 42, 48, 158,
    159, 186, 187, 253, 257, 262, 266,
    282, 287, 291, 292, 295, 298, 299,
    303, 304, 316, 322, 345, 347, 348,
    356, 333, 335
Shriberg, L. D., 223, 225, 231, 308,
    309, 318, 320, 324, 335, 248
Siegel, G. M., 16, 23, 166, 183
Siegel-Sadewitz, V. L., 42, 48, 322, 345,
    356, 333, 335
Sills, P. S., 145, 168, 175, 176, 177,
    178, 184, 187
Silverton, J. S., 69, 77
Simmons, R., 276, 297
Simon, C., 156, 185
Simpson, M., 175, 179, 181
Simpson, R., 253, 302, 304
Sindet-Pedersen, S., 90, 116
Skaar, S., 284, 304
Skolnick, E. M., 65, 78
Skolnick, M. L., 159, 187, 253, 260,
    265, 298, 301, 304, 347, 356, 335
Skoog, T., 89, 119, 48, 52, 58, 78
Slutsky, H., 360, 363, 367, 380
Smit, A. B., 326, 335
Smith, A. J., 231, 248, 309, 335
Smith, B., 294, 304
Smith, C., 40, 46
Smith, B. E., 160, 187
Smith, L., 292, 302
Smith, L. R., 160, 182
Smith, N. V., 223, 226, 248
Smith, R., 369, 380
Smith, W., 267, 268, 302
Smith, W. L., 159, 185
Smitheran, J., 157, 187
Snider, B., 372, 377
Snyder, M., 365, 380
Solomon, M., 64, 78
Sonderman, J., 253, 306
Sotereanos, G. C., 107, 115
Speidel, T. M., 166, 183
Spence, M. A., 40, 48
Spriestersbach, D. C., 4, 18, 23, 222,
    229, 248, 282, 302, 304, 350, 351,
    356, 362, 364, 371, 380
St. Louis, K. O., 156, 187

Stampe, D., 223, 225, 248
Stark, R. B., 125, 143
Starr, C. D., 158, 163, 185, 187, 284,
    302, 304, 229, 248, 337, 339, 356
Stathopoulos, E., 255, 304
Stea, G., 103, 119
Steffel, V. L., 148, 149, 152, 179, 183
Steinhauser, E., 103, 118
Stenberg, D. J., 103, 119
Stenstrom, S. J., 89, 90, 119
Stephan, C., 365, 378
Stevens, K., 287, 304
Stick, S. L., 172, 187
Stickel, F. R., 90, 117
Stoel-Gammon, C., 236, 248, 308, 315,
    318, 326, 335
Stoelinga, P., 106, 119
Stone, M., 166, 183
Stool, S. E., 195, 198, 216
Stringer, D., 316, 334
Stringer, D. A., 159, 187, 265, 304
Strombeck, J., 90, 115
Studdert-Kennedy, M., 227, 248
Stutz, M., 272, 305
Subtelny, J. D., 122, 131, 143, 171,
    172, 174, 187, 229, 248, 261, 264,
    304, 305
Subtelny, Jo. D., 171, 172, 174, 181,
    184, 187, 261, 264, 304, 305, 229,
    248
Sulik, K. K., 30, 36, 47
Sullivan, M., 369, 370, 377
Swisher, W., 270, 271, 299

Tanke, E., 365, 380
Taub, S., 159, 187, 272, 305
Taylor, F., 314, 334
Templin, M. C., 158, 161, 188, 222, 248
Tennison, C. W., 52, 58, 78
Tharp, R. F., 159, 188, 260, 305
Thilander, B. L., 89, 90, 119
Thompson, A., 255, 305
Thompson, J. F., 52, 55, 78
Thompson, L. W., 90, 116
Tideman, H., 106, 119
Tisza, V., 367, 380
Tobe, J., 322, 346, 356, 336
Tolarova, M., 40, 48
Tomblin, J., 316, 333
Tondury, G., 125, 143
Topic, M., 13, 23
Trapp, D., 302

Trefler, M., 267, 305
Trier, W., 65, 78, 156, 159, 187, 188, 265, 303, 345, 356
Trimble, B. K., 26, 47
Trost, J. E., 222, 230, 248, 314, 315, 316, 331, 335
Trost-Cardamone, J. E., 307, 310, 313, 314, 316, 319, 323, 324, 327, 334, 335, 336
Tsuru, H., 176, 186
Tuller, B., 166, 184
Turvey, T. A., 90, 105, 117, 119, 122 144

Ulvestad, R. F., 189
Ushiro, K., 267

Valletutti, P. J., 5, 9, 11, 15, 16, 23
Van Demark, A. H., 229, 249
Van Demark, D. R., 159, 160, 161, 162, 170, 184, 188, 260, 275, 282, 300, 305, 229, 249
Van Hattum, R., 350, 356
Vandehaar, C., 170, 188
Vanderas, A. P., 26, 48
Vandervord, J. G., 88, 90, 117
Vannier, M., 268, 305
Vargervik, K., 122, 144
Veau, V., 52, 78, 125, 144
Velten, H. V., 223, 249
Vig, K. W., 90, 119, 122, 144
Vihman, M. M., 325, 336
Von Eiselberg, F. W., 89, 119
Von Graefe, C. F., 52, 64, 78
Von Langenbeck, B. R. K., 64, 78

Wada, T., 264, 305
Waite, D. E., 79, 84, 89, 90, 91, 92, 93, 99, 106, 107, 115, 116, 117, 119
Walster, E., 365, 367, 376, 377
Ward, P., 253, 306
Warren, D. W., 105, 117, 156, 160, 161, 170, 172, 174, 182, 184, 185, 188, 213, 217, 255, 261, 264, 284, 286, 287, 291, 292, 293, 294, 297, 298, 301, 302, 305, 342, 347, 355, 356
Watanabe, T., 40, 46
Weachter, E., 361, 367, 380

Weber, J., 349, 356
Weinberg, B., 188, 253, 293, 294, 302, 304
Weiner, F. F., 225, 249, 324, 331, 336
Weinstein, P., 371, 376
Weismer, G., 255, 304
Weiss, A., 285, 305
Weiss, C. E., 168, 172, 188
Wells, C., 4, 7, 23, 229, 249,
Werth, L., 302, 347, 355
Westlake, H., 229, 249
Westlake, J., 40, 48
Westra, S. E., 13, 24
Whitehouse, F. A., 6, 15, 17, 18, 19, 24
Willemain, T., 287, 304
Williams, J. Ll., 115, 118
Williams, W. N., 158, 188, 258, 261, 265, 299, 305
Willis, C., 272, 305
Willmar, K., 103, 119
Wilson, F., 368, 369, 377
Winsten, J., 61, 77
Witzel, M. A., 105, 119, 159, 172, 186, 187, 265, 304, 316, 322, 346, 356, 334, 336
Wolford, L. M., 100, 103, 105, 106, 110, 115, 116, 118, 119
Wong, L. P., 168, 172, 188
Wood, M. T., 160, 188
Woolf, C. M., 40, 48
Wreakes, G., 38, 46
Wright, V. L., 172, 187

Yamamoto, K., 284, 299
Yamaoka, M., 159, 160, 172, 185, 346, 348, 355, 356
Yasumoto, M., 264, 305
Yoshida, K., 176, 186
Yoshinaga, R., 264, 305
Yoshioka, H., 166, 181
Youngstrom, K. A., 172, 187, 261, 265, 303, 313, 350, 356, 333
Yu, F-C., 26, 42, 46
Yules, R., 305, 340, 349, 350, 356

Zajac, D. J., 157, 188
Zimmerman, G., 279, 305
Zwitman, D., 253, 306

Subject Index

Abbe flap, 51,73, 74
Accelerometer, 285, 286, 287, 288, 289, 341, 344
Adenoid hypertrophy, 197
Alveolar cleft defects
  associated dental problems, 82, 83, 84, 85, 86
  definition, 82
  incidence, 82
  management, 87, 88, 89, 90, 91, 92, 93, 94, 95, 96
Alveolar cleft surgery
  associated orthodontic treatment, 91, 93
  definition, 88
  history, 87, 88, 89
  postsurgical considerations, 98
  presurgical considerations, 93, 94
  procedures-techniques, 94, 95, 96, 97, 98
  rationale and indications, 63, 64, 89, 90
  timing considerations, 88, 89, 90, 91
American Cleft Palate-Craniofacial Association
  beginnings, 7
  history, 7
  mission, 2
Anterior palatal appliance
  adaptation, 165
  fistulae obturation, 164
  kinesthetic feedback, 166
  speech production, 163
  speech test protocol, 164
  tactile feedback, 166
Appliances
  orthodontic expansion, 124, 131, 133, 135, 136, 137
  presurgical orthopedic, 131, 132, 133
  See also Anterior palatal appliance; Prosthetic speech appliance; Prosthetic appliance, 161
Articulatory backing, 313, 314, 324

Articulation/Phonology
  evaluation, 161, 228, 310, 324, 325
  tests, 39, 158, 161, 169, 317, 318, 319
  treatment, 326, 327, 328, 329, 330, 331, 332
  See also Assessment of sound systems
Assessment of sound systems
  analyzing speech samples, 321
  developmental norms comparison, 322
  intelligibility, 321, 322
  nasendoscopy (nasopharyngoscopy), 316, 328
  oronasal fistulae, 316
  phonetic inventory, 323
  phonological assessment protocol, 317, 318
  phonological pattern analysis, 323
  speech sample, 318
  speech sound inventories, 319
  stimulability testing, 319, 320
  tonsils, 316, 317
  transcription scoring, 320, 321
  velopharyngeal sphincter, 316
  videofluoroscopy, 317
  videonasendoscopy, 316
Audiological evaluation
  acoustic immittance, 203
  acoustic reflex testing, 204
  auditory behavior index for infants, 207
  auditory brainstem response (ABR), 204, 206
  behavioral hearing tests, 206
  behavioral observation audiometry, 206
  conditioned orienting response audiometry (COR), 206, 207, 208, 209
  conditioned play audiometry, 209
  eustachian tube function, 204
  infants at risk, 201
  sensorineural hearing loss, 209
  speech awareness thresholds, 209
  speech reception thresholds, 209
  speech recognition tests, 209
  tympanogram, 203, 204, 205

tympanometry, 203
visual reinforcement audiometry
    (VRA), 206
Audiological follow-up and monitoring
    indications for amplification, 210, 211
Audiologist
    role on interdisciplinary team, 8
    See also Audiological evaluation
Auditory (eustachian) tube
    changes in inclination with age, 192,
        193, 194
    cleft palate effects, 195, 196, 197, 198
    dilation, 192, 194
    fluid & by-products outlet, 191, 192,
        193
    pressure equalization in middle ear,
        191, 192
    role in swallowing, 192, 194
    structure and function, 191
    ventilation of middle ear, 191
Autogenous bone, in alveolar cleft
    repair, 95

Babbling, 310, 311, 312
Barium, in fluoroscopic assessment,
    260
Behavior, and clefting
    anxiety, 372
    independence, 371
    inhibition, 371, 372
    psychopathology, 371
    self-perception and appearance, 371
    treatment, 372
Bone grafting
    alveolar clefts, 88, 89, 90, 91, 92, 93,
        94, 95, 96, 97, 98, 99
    associated orthodontic treatment, 91,
        93, 94
    evaluation studies, 91, 92, 93, 99
    history, 87, 88, 89
    indications, 90
    maxillary advancement, 106
    periodontal status-postsurgery, 92
    postsurgical considerations, 98
    presurgical considerations, 92, 93, 94
    procedures-techniques, 94, 95, 96, 97,
        98
    terminology, 88
    timing considerations, 88, 89, 90, 91
    See also Alveolar cleft surgery
Buccopharyngeal membrane, in
    prenatal development, 32

Bzoch Error Patterns Diagnostic, 319
    See also Articulation/Phonology, tests

Cephalometrics, 122, 127, 128, 129,
    131, 158, 259
    See also Radiography
Cineradiography, 158, 264
    See also Radiography
Cleft lip surgery
    bilateral cleft lip repair, 59, 60, 61,
        62, 63
        Millard technique, 62, 63
        principles (Cronin), 59, 60
        straight line muscle repair-forked
            flaps, 62, 63
        straight line repair, 61, 62
        timing, 60, 61
        Veau III technique, 61, 62
    combined upper and lower flap
        repair, 58, 59, 60
        Skoog technique, 58, 59, 60
    history, 52
    lower ⅓ flap repair, 57, 58, 59
        Tennison-Randall technique, 57, 58 59
    objectives, 51
    preoperative care, 53
    preoperative maxillary positioning, 53
        feeding, 53
        maxillary orthopedics, 53
    timing of repair, 53
    unilateral cleft lip repair, 54, 55, 56,
        57, 58, 59
        lip adhesion, 54
        Randall technique, 54
        Rose-Thompson technique, 55
        straight line lip repair, 55, 56
        upper one-third lip repair, 55, 56, 57
        Millard rotation advancement
            technique, 55, 56, 57
        Randall muscle flap technique, 56, 57
Cleft palate hearing problems
    See Hearing problems and clefting
Cleft palate speech characteristics
    See Speech characteristics and cleft
        palate
Cleft palate surgery
    effects of early surgery on speech , 65
    effects on speech, 65
    goals, 65, 66
    history, 64, 65
    primary, 66, 67
    secondary, 74, 75

timing, 65
V-Y pushback technique, 66, 67
Cleft(s)
  associated anomalies, 41, 43
  causes, 35, 36, 40
  coarticulation, 314
  columella lengthening, 71, 72, 73
  genetics, 38, 39, 40, 41
  incidence, 2, 26, 40
  mechanisms involved, 35, 36
  nature, 2
  types, 2, 26, 27, 28, 29, 30
  variability in formation , 26
Compensatory articulation, 221, 230,
  310, 313, 314, 315, 316, 324, 327,
  328, 329, 330, 331, 332, 333
  See also Speech, characteristics in
    children with clefts
Compliance with treatment
  recommendations, 13
Computerized tomography, 129, 130,
  131, 267, 268
  See also Radiography
Concordance of clefting, in twin
  studies, 38, 39

Dental conditions, effects on speech, 162
Dental hygienist, on interdisciplinary
  team, 8
Dental implants, 154
Dentition
  alveolar clefts, 83, 84
  early mixed , 133, 134, 135, 136
  later mixed, 136
  orthodontic intervention, 133, 134,
    135, 136, 137, 138, 139, 140
  permanent, 137, 138, 139, 140
Dentoalveolar problems in clefting
  bone support, 83
  fistulae, 81, 87
  malformed teeth, 82
  malposed teeth, 83, 84
  missing teeth, 83, 84
  panoramic radiographs, 86
  periapical radiographs, 85
  speech problems, 86
  supernumerary teeth, 83, 84
  tooth eruption, 84
Dentures, 148
Distinctive features model, of
  phonological development
  normal vs. non-normal speech, 223, 224

phonemic contrasts, 223
problems, 223, 224

Ear, medical evaluation, 200, 201, 202
  binocular microscope, 200, 201
  otoscopy, 200
  See also Middle ear disease,
    treatment
Early secondary osteoplasty
  definition, 88
  See also Bone grafting
Edwards/Falconer approximation, in
  multifactorial disorders, 37
Effects of cleft palate on auditory tube
  function
  lymphatic system obstruction, 198
  morphology of tube and clefting, 195
  mucous lining of tube, 195, 196, 198
  tube collapse, 195
  tube surface fluids, 195
  See also Auditory tube
Embryology of clefting
  neural crest, 31
  primary palate, 30, 31, 32
  secondary palate, 32, 33, 34, 35
  timing and development of clefts, 32, 33
Endoscopy
  evaluation of velopharyngeal
    function, 271, 272, 273, 274, 275,
    276
  flexible fiberoscope, 161, 344
  flexible laryngoscope, 214, 215
  rigid scope, 272
Eustachian tube
  See Auditory tube
Expansion appliances, in orthodontic
  treatment, 131, 133

Feeding problems, 361, 362
Fiberoptic laryngoscope
  See Endoscopy
Fisher-Logemann Test of Articulation
  Competence, 158
  See also Articulation/Phonology, tests
Fistulae
  alveolar clefts, 82
  effects, 164, 258, 316, 323
  indications for repair, 90
  prosthetic treatment, 74, 164, 165,
    166, 167, 168
  surgical repair with alveolar cleft
    repair, 90
  surgical treatment, 74, 75

Frankfort horizontal plane, in presurgical oral and maxillofacial analysis, 100

Genetic counseling, in cleft palate
approaches, 44
caveats, 45
definition, 43
role on team, 43
the law, 46
training, 43
Geneticist
parent counseling, 43, 46
role on interdisciplinary team, 8, 43
Glottal stops
See Speech characteristics and clefting
Glottal valving, 314
Goldman-Fristoe Test of Articulation, 158
See also Articulation/Phonology, tests
Growth and development, of facial structures
effects of surgical repair, 126
prenatal, 30, 31, 32, 33, 34, 35, 125, 136
postnatal, 126, 127
nasal septum, 126
posterior maxillary segments, 126
premaxilla, 126

Hearing aids, 210, 211
Hearing loss
nature and implications, 210, 211
conductive loss audiogram, 210
fluctuating conductive hearing loss, 210
Hearing problems and clefting
conductive loss, 230
middle ear effusion, 230
recurrence of problems, 230
relation to speech, 230, 231
HONC (Horii Oral Nasal Coupling), 287, 289, 290, 344
Hypernasality
See Speech characteristics and clefting
Hypernasality, relation to articulation, 313
Hyponasality, 354

Intellectual ability and clefting, 368, 369, 370
association with type of cleft, 368
verbal versus nonverbal, 368

Interdisciplinary care
benefits, 4, 15, 81, 94, 122, 123
definition , 4, 5
future, 19, 22
goals, 21
outcomes, 14, 21
problems, 18, 19
therapy concepts, 151
See also, Teams
Intermaxillary segment, in prenatal facial development, 32
Intrauterine-healed clefts, 26
Iowa Pressure Articulation Test, 319
See also Articulation/Phonology, tests

Jaw discrepancies in clefting, 99, 100, 101, 102, 103, 104. 105, 106, 107, 108, 109, 110, 111, 112, 113, 114

Language learning and clefting, 369
Laryngeal evaluation, 156
Laryngeal problems, in clefting, 214
Late secondary osteoplasty
definition, 88
See also Bone grafting
Le Fort I, II, III, defined, 115
Levator palatini, 196, 200

Magnetic resonance imaging, 131
Magnetometrics, 156
Mandibular osteotomy, in jaw discrepancy management
associated with orthodontic treatment, 139, 140, 141
goals, 100
relapse, 103, 111
timing, 99, 101, 102, 103, 104, 105, 106, 107
Maxillary osteotomy, in jaw discrepancy management
associated with orthodontic treatment, 139, 140, 141
diagrams depicting, 106, 107, 108, 109, 110
goals, 100
indications, 99, 100
postsurgical considerations, 111, 112, 113, 114
presurgical considerations, 104, 105
procedures-techniques, 105, 106, 107, 108, 109, 110

speech effects, 105
timing, 99, 100, 101, 102, 103, 104
Maximum phonation time (MPT), 157
Meckel's cartilage, in prenatal
    development, 34
Microforms of clefts, 29, 30
Middle ear disease, treatment
    antibiotics, 211
    antihistamine, 211
    corticosteroids, 211
    decongestants, 211
    mastoidectomy, 213
    myringotomy, 211
    PE tubes, 212
    prevention, 211
    tympanoplasty tube insertion, 211,
        212, 213
Mid-dorsum palatal
    See Speech characteristics and clefting
Middle ear muscles, 197
Middle ear pathology
    effusion, 199, 200
    exudate, 199
    hemorrhage, 199
    mucosal change, 199
    mucosal edema, 198
    negative pressure, 199
    otitis media, 194, 199, 210
    transudate, 199
Mother infant attachment (bond), 363
Multifactorial inheritance
    definition, 36, 37
    Edwards/Falconer approximations, 37
    quasicontinuous variation, 37
    recurrence risks, 37
    role in clefting, 36, 37, 38, 39
    versus single gene inheritance, 38

Nasal emission
    See Speech characteristics and clefting
Nasal fricatives
    See Speech characteristics and clefting
Nasal olfactory pits, in prenatal
    development, 32
Nasal placodes, in prenatal
    development, 32
Nasal problems
    alar collapse, 213
    nasal septum deviation, 213
    orthodontic treatment, 213
    pharyngeal flap, 213

Nasal snorts
    See Speech characteristics and
        clefting
Nasal surgery, timing, 68
Nasality
    behavioral management approaches,
        338
    client selection recommendations,
        352, 353, 354
    muscle change therapy, 338
    acoustic feedback techniques, 341
    airflow and pressure feedback
        techniques, 347
    effects of airflow and pressure
        feedback therapy, 347, 348
    effects of electrical stimulation
        therapy, 349, 350
    effects of visual feedback therapy,
        345, 346, 347
    electrical stimulation techniques, 348
    muscle change exercise effects, 339,
        340
    muscle change exercises, 339
    muscle control change therapy, 340
    visual feedback techniques, 344,
        345, 346, 347
    perceptual change therapy, 350, 351,
        352
    articulation modification, 350
    loudness change, 351
    oral resonance change, 352
    pitch change, 350, 351
Nasometer, 161, 285, 286, 287, 342,
    343, 344
NAVI (Nasal Accerleromic Vibrational
    Index), 344
Neural crest cells, in clefting, 31
Neurosurgeon, on interdisciplinary
    team, 8
Nodules, vocal, 214
Nose, and cleft lip, 68
NRI (Nasal Resonance Index), 289
Nurse, on interdisciplinary team, 8

Obturator
    See Anterior palatal appliance,
        Prosthetic appliance
OME-otitis media with effusion, 194,
    199, 210, 309
    See also Middle ear pathology
Ophthalmologist, on interdisciplinary
    team, 8

Oral and maxillofacial surgeon
    definition, 80
    education and training, 80
    role on team, 81, 82
Oral defects, treatment, 167
Oral manometer, 291
Orthodontic treatment and clefting
    principles, 123, 124
    records, 127, 128, 129, 130, 131
        cephalometric, 127, 128, 129
        models of teeth, 127
        panoramic, 129
        photographs, 127
        tomograms, 129
    treatment phases, 131, 132, 133, 134,
        135, 136, 137, 138, 139, 140, 141
        early mixed, 133, 134, 135, 136
        later mixed, 136
        permanent, 137, 138, 139
        presurgical, 131, 132, 133
        premaxillary repositioning, in
            bilateral cleft of primary palate,
            60, 133
        presurgical orthopedics, 131, 132, 133
        appliances, 124, 131, 133, 135,
            136, 137
        bone grafting, 131, 132, 133, 134,
            135, 136, 137
        cuspid guidance, 139
        speech effects, 124
        psychosocial issues, 139, 142
Orthodontist
    concerns for clefting, 125
    definition, 122
    education/training, 122
    relationship with other team
        members, 124, 125
    role on team, 8, 122, 124, 125
Otolaryngologist
    certification, 190
    education/training, 190
    role on cleft palate team, 8, 190

Palatal lift, treatment, 147, 170, 173, 176
Parents(family), and alveolar cleft
    repair, 94
Parent-child interactions, 363, 364
Parents (families)
    communication, 3, 13, 18
    compliance with treatment, 13
    cooperation, 2, 13
    understanding of team
        recommendations, 18

Parents reactions and concerns, early,
    360, 361, 362, 363
Pediatric/family dentist, on
    interdisciplinary team, 8
Pediatrician, on interdisciplinary team, 8
PERCI (Palatal Efficiency Ratio
    Computed Instantaneously), 292
Personality, and clefting
    See Behavior, and clefting
Pharyngeal affricatives
    See Speech characteristics and
        clefting
Pharyngeal flap
    effect on speech, 238, 239, 240, 241,
        242, 243, 244
    surgical procedure, 67, 70, 71
Pharyngeal fricatives
    See Speech characteristics and
        clefting
Pharyngeal stops
    See Speech characteristics and
        clefting
Pharyngeal valving, 314
Phonetic
    control development, 311, 312
    distortions, 313
    substitutions, 313
Phonology/Articulation
    See Articulation/Phonology
Phonological acquisition
    autonomic/taxonomic model, 222
    distinctive feature model, 223, 224
    early development, 310
    effect of surgery on, 310
    phonological learning, 227, 228, 229
    phonological processes, 225, 226, 227,
        309, 310, 316
    phonological rules, 224, 225
Phonological analysis procedures, 324,
    325
Phonological assessment of toddlers,
    325
    See also Assessment of sound
        systems, phonological assessment
        protocol
Phonological disorders, 308, 309, 316
Phonological learning models
    applied to cleft palate speech, 227,
        228, 229
    multiple level analysis, 228
    normal vs. non-normal speech, 227,
        228, 229

Phonological patterns
in young children, 325
treatment, 326
See also Articulation/Phonology,
evaluation, treatment
Physical attractiveness
children with physical disabilities,
365
normal children, 365
persons with clefts, 366, 367
Plastic and reconstructive surgeon
education/training, 50
role at child's birth, 51
role on interdisciplinary team, 9, 50
Plastic surgery
analysis of results, 50
effects on growth, 50
goals of treatment, 51, 52
prosthetic (speech appliance)
management, 67
timetable of care, 51
See also Cleft lip surgery; cleft palate
surgery
Plethysmography, 156
Pneumotachograph, 291
Premaxilla, in prenatal development, 32
Premaxillary management in alveolar
clefts, 92, 93
Premaxillary repositioning, in bilateral
primary palate clefts, 133
Presurgical orthopedic treatment, 131,
132, 133
disadvantages, 131, 132
procedures, 132, 133
rationale, 131, 132
Primary osteoplasty
definition, 88
See also Bone grafting
Primary palate
Prosthesis
See Prosthodontic appliance;
Prosthetic speech appliance
Prosthodontic appliance, 179
dental, 179
speech, 67, 179
Prosthetic clinical procedures, 152
Prosthetic management, for soft palate
defects
complete soft palate clefts, 170
considerations, 168
partial soft palate clefts, 171
speech considerations, 169

Prosthetic speech appliance, 147
assessment modifications, 178
definition, 147
design considerations, 174
optimizing speech, procedures, 171
reduction, 173
soft palate defects, 168, 169
Prosthetic therapy
influence of oral factors, 149
influence of patient factors, 150
Prosthetic-speech team, 177
Prosthodontic assessment, 151
Prosthodontics, definition, 147
Prosthodonist, on interdisciplinary
team, 8
Psychological adjustment, in adults
with clefts
aspirations, 373
education, 373
family status (marriage, children),
373, 374
self-satisfaction, 373
socioeconomic status, 374
Psychological aspects of clefting, 359
effects of clefting on family, 51
intervention at birth, 361
Psychologist, role on interdisciplinary
team, 8, 359
Psychosocial issues and orthodontic
treatment, 139, 142
Pterygoid plate, 195

Radiography
cephalometric, 122, 127, 128, 129,
131, 158, 259
cineradiography, 158, 264
computerized tomography, 129, 130,
131, 267, 268
panoramic, 86, 129
periapical, 85
tomographic, 129, 262, 263
videofluoroscopic, 158, 264, 265, 266
Radiologist, on interdisciplinary team, 8
Respiratory evaluation, 155
Rigid endoscopy
See Endoscopy; Velopharyngeal
closure, evaluation

School achievement and clefting, 368,
369, 370
reading, 370
remedial intervention, 370

Secondary lip surgery, 73, 74
Secondary osteoplasty
    definition, 88
    See also Bone grafting
Secondary palate, 2
Secondary procedures for
    velopharyngeal incompetence
    diagnosis of velopharyngeal
        incompetence, 69, 70
    pharyngeal flap, 67, 70, 71
    speech prosthesis (speech appliances),
        70
    sphincter pharyngoplasty, 70, 71, 72
    See also Cleft palate surgery,
        secondary
See-Scape, 290, 347, 348
Skeletal growth patterns in clefting
    arch discrepancies, 126
    documentation, 126, 127
Social worker, on interdisciplinary
    team, 8
Soft palate defects and prosthodontics,
    168
Sound systems
    See Assessment of sound systems
Speech
    assessment principles, 154
    characteristics in children with clefts,
        229, 230
    back patterns, 221
    compensatory patterns, 230
    maladaptive patterns, 221, 230
    posterior patterns, 230
    dentoalveolar problems, 86
    maxillary advancement, 105
    models of learning speech, 222, 223,
        224, 225, 226, 227, 228, 229
    autonomic model, 222
    distinctive features model, 223, 224
    phonological learning, 227, 228, 229
    phonological processes, 225, 226, 227
    phonological rules, 224, 225
    sound acquisition process, 221, 222,
        223, 224, 225, 226, 227, 228, 229
Speech bulb
    See Prosthetic speech appliance
Speech characteristics and clefting
    delayed development, 230
    error patterns, 230
    glottal stops, 11, 230, 313, 314, 315
    hypernasality, 309, 313, 317
    individual variability, 230

mid-dorsal palatal, 315
nasal emission, 309, 313, 317, 323,
    324, 328
nasal fricatives, 230, 314, 315, 316
nasal snorts, 316
oral structures, 230
    dental hazards, 231
    fistulae, 231
    jaw discrepancies, 231
pharyngeal affricatives, 314, 315
pharyngeal fricatives, 230, 314, 315
pharyngeal stops, 314, 315
rate of sound acquisition, 230
velar fricatives, 315
velopharyngeal closure, 231, 232
vocabulary acquisition, 232, 233
vowel distortions, 324
weak consonants, 313
Speech studies of young children, 232,
    233, 234, 235, 236, 237, 238, 239,
    240, 241, 242, 243, 244
Speech treatment decisions
    deciding how to treat speech errors, 327
    establishing baselines, 327
    modifying compensatory articulations,
        330, 331, 332
    velopharyngeal closure and error
        patterns, 327, 328, 329, 330
Speech-language pathologist, on
    interdisciplinary team, 8
Sphincter pharyngoplasty, 70, 71, 72
Spirometer, 156
Stomodeum, in prenatal facial
    development, 32
Submucous cleft palate, 29, 67, 68, 258
Surgery
    adenoids; *See* Adenoid hypertrophy
    alveolar process; *See* Alveolar cleft
        surgery
    cleft lip; *See* Cleft lip surgery
    cleft palate; *See* Cleft palate surgery
    fistulae; *See* Palatal fistulae
    jaw; *See* Mandibular osteotomy,
        maxillary osteotomy
    nasal; *See* Nose and cleft lip
    tonsils; *See* Tonsils
Syndromes associated with clefting, 41,
    42, 43

Teams, 8
    cleft palate versus craniofacial, 8
    composition, 8, 9, 17

core versus "desirable," 8
function, 10, 14
future, 19, 20
history, 6
leadership, 9
problems, 4, 18, 19
procedures, 9, 10
quality, 16, 22
research, 15,16
structure, 7, 10
value, 15, 16
Templin-Darley Test of Articulation,
    158, 161, 169, 319
    See also Articulation/Phonology, tests
Temperomandibular joint (TMJ), 129
Tensor palatini, 192, 194, 195, 196
Tensor tympani, 197
Tonar II, 285, 286, 342
Tonsils, 197
Tympanic membrane, 191

Velar biomechanics, 179
Velar fricative
    See Speech characteristics and clefting
Velopharyngeal function-evaluation
    direct primary measures, 256, 257
    computed tomography (CT scan),
        267, 268
    endoscopy, 159, 271, 272, 273, 274,
        275, 276
        data interpretation, 275, 276
        flexible fiber endoscopes, 272, 273
        nasal endoscopy, 272
        oral endoscopy, 272
        panendoscope, 272
        rigid endoscopes, 272
    frontal still radiography
        (tomography), 262, 263
    lateral still radiography
        (cephalometrics), 158, 259
        interpretation, 260
    magnetic resonance imaging (MRI),
        268, 269, 270
    motion picture radiography
        (cineradiography), 158, 264
    ultrasound, 270, 271
    videofluoroscopy, 158, 264, 265
        base view, 265, 266
        frontal plane, 265, 266
        lateral view, 265
        multiview, 265, 266
    visual examination, 257

indirect primary measures, 256, 257,
    276
    electromyography (EMG), 279, 280
    movement transduction, 280, 281
    strain gauge transducer, 280
    velotrace, 281
    phototransduction, 276, 277, 278,
        279
secondary measures, 281, 282, 283, 284
    acoustic measures, 282
    accelerometry (HONC-NAVI-NRI),
        287, 288, 289, 290, 344
    Nasometer (nasalance), 161, 285,
        286, 287
    Oral Nasal Acoustic Ratio
        (TONAR), 285, 286
    perceptual judgments, 158, 282,
        283, 284
    sound pressure, 285, 286, 287,
        288, 289, 290
    spectography, 284, 285
    aerodynamic measures, 160, 290
    airflow detection, 290, 291
    air pressure detection, 291, 292
    orifice area estimation, 292, 293,
        294, 295, 296
Velopharyngeal closure acoustics, 253
Velopharyngeal closure aerodynamics,
    160, 255
Velopharyngeal closure judgments,
    325, 326
Velopharyngeal closure kinematics,
    253, 254
Velopharyngeal inadequacy, 230
Velopharyngeal inadequacy (VPI) &
    laryngeal function, 157
Velopharyngeal incompetence (VPI)
    without clefts, 174
    treatment considerations, 175
Velopharyngeal incompetence,
    inadequacy, insufficiency; defined, 252
Videofluoroscopy
    See Velopharyngeal function evaluation,
        direct primary measures
Vocabulary acquisition in children
    with cleft palate, 232, 233
Vowel distortions
    See Speech characteristics and clefting

Weak consonants
    See Speech characteristics and
        clefting